George D. LeMaitre

M.D., F.A.C.S., DIPLOMATE AM. BD. OF SURGERY

*Senior Surgeon, Lawrence General Hospital; Senior Surgeon,
Bon Secours Hospital; formerly Chief Surgical Resident,
Carney Hospital, Boston, Massachusetts*

Janet A. Finnegan

R.N., M.S.

*Associate Professor, Northeastern University College of Nursing;
Boston, Massachusetts*

THE PATIENT IN SURGERY:
a guide for nurses

THIRD EDITION

Illustrated by Robert Fredrickson

W. B. SAUNDERS COMPANY

Philadelphia, London, Toronto

W. B. Saunders Company: West Washington Square
Philadelphia, PA 19105

1 St. Anne's Road
Eastbourne, East Sussex BN21 3UN, England

1 Goldthorne Avenue
Toronto, Ontario M8Z 5T9, Canada

Library of Congress Cataloging in Publication Data

LeMaitre, George D.

  The patient in surgery.

  Includes index.

  1. Surgical nursing.   I. Finnegan, Janet A., joint author.
    II. Title.   [DNLM: 1. Surgical nursing. WY161 L547p]

RD99.L35 1975   610.73'677   74-31838
ISBN   0-7216-5717-6

The Patient in Surgery: A Guide for Nurses   ISBN 0-7216-5717-6

Last digit is the print number: 9   8   7   6   5

This book is dedicated to the memory of Leon Vincent, of the Department of Biology of Boston College: a great teacher, a dedicated biologist, and a true humanist

Preface to the Third Edition

The third edition of *The Patient in Surgery* remains a comprehensive guide for the surgical nurse.

The section divisions in Part II have been reorganized in accordance with the present classification of surgical specialties. Each description of operative procedures has been updated to meet the changes in concepts that have occurred as surgery continues to evolve, but the format remains the same.

For this edition, a chapter on anesthesia has been added to Part I (an earlier version of this chapter appeared in the first edition). A new chapter, "Surgical Drains, Tubes, and Catheters," has been added to Part I in an effort to delineate the general principles of drainage, a factor of great importance in all phases of surgery.

Many new chapters have been added to Part II, and each chapter retained from the second edition has been carefully revised.

Because of the enormous difficulties in keeping up with the literature and the increasing number of excellent reference guides in modern medical libraries, the bibliographic references found at the end of each chapter in previous editions have been deleted. The student nurse should become familiar with the reference indices available in the medical library and become aware of the enormous help a medical librarian can provide. (A guide to these indices and to texts of special value is provided at the end of this book.)

The Patient in Surgery remains a guide to surgical principles, and it is expected to lead to more comprehensive investigation by the student. The study questions at the end of each chapter have been revised and expanded to stimulate this investigation.

The continued popularity of *The Patient in Surgery* is due in part, we believe, to its concise structure as an outline for surgical and operating room nurses, and every effort has been made to preserve this original concept. The temptation to expand the book into an encyclopedic text covering every field of surgery has been resisted, as has been the twin temptation to deal in depth with the complete preoperative and postoperative care of the surgical patient. Our goal remains an introductory but comprehensive guide, geared to the student nurse, that will emphasize the preoperative evaluation and preparation for surgery, the operative procedure itself, and the early postoperative recovery phase.

George D. LeMaitre, M.D., F.A.C.S.
Janet A. Finnegan, R.N., M.S.

Acknowledgments

One of the most difficult tasks an author has is to compile a list of people who have contributed, in one way or another, toward the completion of a book. In this case the authors have a doubly difficult job in that so many people were kind enough to give of their time in encouragement, reading of manuscripts, criticisms, et cetera.

The book would never have gotten beyond infancy had it not been for the encouragement and persistence of Miss Mary Sullivan, R.N., of Carney Hospital in Boston. The senior author spent many a day seeking reassurance on certain aspects of the manuscript, and Miss Sullivan's experience and excellence as a surgical nurse were often called upon for crucial decisions.

We received a great deal of help from several members of the nursing staff at the Peter Bent Brigham Hospital in Boston. We are grateful for the advice and encouragement we received from:

Marion Metcalf, R.N., M.S.
Director of Nursing Service and Associate Director
Peter Bent Brigham Hospital
Boston, Massachusetts

Eleanor Toohey, R.N., M.S.
Assistant Director for Special Services
Peter Bent Brigham Hospital
Boston, Massachusetts

Barbara Lacey Arbene, R.N.
Assistant Supervisor of the Operating Room
Peter Bent Brigham Hospital
Boston, Massachusetts

Elizabeth Nagel, R.N.
Head Nurse, Recovery Room
Peter Bent Brigham Hospital
Boston, Massachusetts

Libby Battit, R.N., M.S.
Thoracic Nurse Clinician
Peter Bent Brigham Hospital
Boston, Massachusetts

Special thanks are due Jane Aroian, Assistant Professor, Northeastern University College of Nursing, for her comments and suggestions. Carolyn Tamer, R.N., enterostomal therapist at Massachusetts General Hospital, gave generous help, advice, and guidance regarding the care of the patient with a stoma.

Dolores Allicon, Operating Room Supervisor, and Agatha Lane, Operating Room Coordinator, both of Lawrence General Hospital, Lawrence, Massachusetts, proofread a considerable portion of the sections dealing with the operating room and offered many important suggestions and revisions.

William Lane, Administrator of Bon Secours Hospital, and Ashton Smith, Administrator of Lawrence General Hospital, were extremely helpful in obtaining the full cooperation of every department in their respective institutions, and the senior author wishes to extend his personal thanks for all that they have done over the years to be of service to our patients and, thereby, to the full development of this book.

The members of the medical staffs of Peter Bent Brigham Hospital, Lawrence General Hospital, and Bon Secours Hospital contributed in a variety of ways, often providing informal suggestions and, occasionally, thorough evaluations. A special note of thanks is due Dr. Lowell Rosman, Department of Neurosurgery, for his comprehensive and most detailed contribution to the chapter on rupture of cerebral aneurysms. Dr. Neville Rosen, Department of Anesthesiology, and Dr. Santos Cataudella, Department of Oral Surgery, were also very helpful in those sections dealing with their fields of expertise.

The philosophy of nursing education and the characteristics of the conscientious nurse, so well exemplified in Jo Cavallerro, Head Nurse of the Intensive Care Unit at Bon Secours Hospital, Lawrence, Massachusetts, permeate this book and must be acknowledged.

We are extremely pleased with the quality of the illustrations and, particularly, with the patience of our illustrator, Mr. Robert Fredrickson, who spent many a long night completing these illustrations for us.

The senior author wishes to thank his secretary, Mrs. Diane Anderson, for the many manuscript revisions which she so gladly typed. Lastly, both the authors wish to thank their spouses for their encouragement and proofreading.

George D. LeMaitre, M.D., F.A.C.S.
Janet A. Finnegan, R.N., M.S.

Preface to the First Edition

The surgical patient passes through three distinct phases during his hospitalization: preoperative evaluation and preparation for surgery, the operative procedure itself, and the postoperative recovery phase. While theoretically distinct, these phases must be integrated into one continuous psychological and physiological experience for the patient.

Nursing education must therefore follow this pattern of continuity and, consequently, the student nurse learns *total patient care and follow-through* while on the surgical service.

The senior author has long felt the need for a concise surgical nursing manual which would bring these three phases together under one cover. Such a manual would integrate the many facets of surgical preparation, operative technique, and postoperative management, and would create a sense of continuity and chronological progression for the student. The authors believe that such a manual must incorporate the viewpoints of the medical as well as the nursing profession; hence the need for a co-authored text seemed appropriate.

The Patient in Surgery has been structured with these needs in mind. Part I introduces the student to the surgical milieu or environment within which the surgical experience occurs. A sense of *chronology* is attempted. The student is first oriented to the general philosophy of surgery. The physical structure of an operating room suite and the nature of surgical sepsis and its control are then alluded to. Chapter 5 describes the physiological and psychological preparation for surgery in general terms. This *first phase* logically blends into the operative experience or second phase as the student is taken, gradually, through progressively more complicated nursing experiences. Throughout this chapter, the authors have attempted, as specifically as possible, to portray the student's experiences chronologically and realistically. Finally, the third or postoperative phase is presented.

Part II of the manual is devoted to specific operative procedures, covering a wide variety of cases to be seen by the student. Here, again, the emphasis is on continuity and chronological progression throughout the surgical experience. A brief history and physical examination of each patient is described, along with pertinent diagnostic studies. When necessary, a description of the rationale and methodology of the diagnostic test is given.

The probable hospital course and preparation for surgery constitute an important aspect of the preoperative course. The manual attempts to deal with this area as concretely as possible, allowing for minor variations as necessary. Every effort has been made to consider the whole patient, his anxieties, his family, and the like. The physiological and psychological preparations for surgery are described, along with the timing of these events.

The rationale and details of the operative procedure itself are then alluded to and correlated with the nurse's responsibilities in the operating room. In addition, the surgical hazards of each procedure are examined, as they will have an important bearing on the postoperative phase.

The immediate postoperative management of the patient constitutes the third phase of the surgical experience. In this section, reference is made to specific postoperative problems and their management.

The study questions at the end of each chapter constitute a vital part of the manual. These questions have been carefully structured to stimulate maximum initiative for research and discussion on the student's part. Many of these questions will require guidance by the *nursing instructor,* and the student should be encouraged to seek her experienced judgment.

The student should note any dissimilarities between her experiences on the surgical service and those as described in the manual. While every effort has been made to minimize "local customs," these inevitably creep into every textbook.

The Patient in Surgery should be used as a guide and should be carried by the student while on the surgical pavilions as well as while in the operating room. It should afford the student a concise summary or digest of the surgical experience and a stimulus for further collateral reading.

The authors firmly believe that this new approach to surgical nursing education will help bridge the gap between available study hours and the knowledge explosion in nursing.

George D. LeMaitre, M.D., F.A.C.S.
Janet A. Finnegan, R.N., M.S.

Contents

PART II _____

SPECIFIC OPERATIVE PROCEDURES

Section I   ABDOMINAL AND PELVIC SURGERY

Part I

GENERAL CONSIDERATIONS IN THE CARE OF THE SURGICAL PATIENT

THE MEANING OF SURGERY

DEFINITION AND TYPES

DEFINITION

Surgery may be defined as a "planned anatomic alteration of the human organism designed to arrest, alleviate, or eradicate some pathologic process." While no one could seriously quarrel with the accuracy of this definition, its comprehensiveness leaves much to be desired. The profound psychological and physiological ramifications of surgery are not even suggested by this concept.

It might be better to consider some of the implications of surgery as they are viewed by the patient, the surgeon, and the nurse.

The Patient's Viewpoint

Surgery Is an Act of Faith.   Regardless of his station in life or his intellectual gifts, the patient cannot really know that he must have surgery or what type of surgery must be done. He can only trust to his surgeon's knowledge and judgment. He cannot adequately appreciate the complexities and necessities of certain acts of nursing care, but must believe in the expertness and professional knowledge of his nurses. Lastly, the patient cannot comprehend the workings of a hospital, its operating rooms, and its facilities. He must only resign himself to accepting this vast organization as something created for his safety and benefit.

Consider, then, how total this act of faith must be to a patient! His very life and happiness are suddenly entrusted to a group of people he hardly knows and to a highly complex institution he cannot begin to understand. The obvious corollary may be stated thus: let no one, through ignorance, negligence, or malice, fail his patient's faith. Adequate training, conscientiousness, and a completely selfless dedication to patient care are the primary obligations and responses to the patient's act of faith.

Surgery Is an Act of Submission.   This is closely akin to the act of faith, as it represents the first external effect of the internal act of faith. The patient is saying: "Since I believe completely in my doctor and nurses (internal act of faith), I will now submit myself (external act of submission) to all the actions and procedures necessitated by my illness as determined by my doctor and nurses." The vast majority of patients will submit completely because they have complete faith. When submission seems only partial, or when the patient rejects the doctor or nurse, the act of faith has been weakened somewhere along the line. The doctor and nurse must thoroughly examine their abilities, motivations, and actions to determine whether the inadequacy is on their part before branding the patient as "uncooperative" or "foolish." It will often be found that misunderstandings due to faulty communication have breached the chain of faith and resulted in an "uncooperative" patient or family.

Lack of submission is not to be confused with hesitancy or reluctance. These are perfectly normal and healthy mental attitudes, considering the stakes to be lost if all does not go well. The patient who hesitates in agreeing to an amputation of his leg is far from uncooperative or foolish. His reaction is normal and healthy, and must be appreciated as such. The act of faith is still intact, but the patient is desperately trying to understand his act of faith. While no amount of medical discussion will completely satisfy the patient, frank and thorough explanations will boost the patient's faith, and submission will follow.

Surgery Is a Radical Invasion of Privacy. Since the total mental, physical, and, at times, moral structure of a patient must be evaluated prior to major surgery, the intimate life of a human being is invaded and the knowledge derived therefrom is inscribed on a chart. The patient's body becomes a drawing board, as it were, for the surgeon, and is exposed to a complete perusal by medical and nursing personnel. Grave moral and legal consequences are attached to negligence and thoughtlessness in this area. The hospital chart, for example, is the property of authorized personnel only. Its contents are not to be discussed with or displayed to anyone not directly concerned with the medical, nursing, or administrative care of the patient.

All attempts must be made to preserve the patient's modesty within the limits imposed by sound medical and nursing care. For example, physical examination of the female is necessary, but a nurse ought to be in attendance during this examination. Pelvic or rectal examinations should be done with adequate draping of the patient. The same considerations must be given in the operating room even after the patient has been anesthetized.

Surgery Induces Fear. It is an obvious but easily forgotten fact that surgery is frightening to a patient. The root of this fear may be ignorance, false knowledge, or even true knowledge:

Fear Rooted in Ignorance. This is the most common cause of preoperative fear, and may take several forms. Often the patient expresses his fear through a disguised question. The disguise must be recognized and answered accordingly. Some typical questions are:

> *Disguised Question:* "Will the operation take very long?"
>
> *Real Question:* "Doesn't a long operation mean a serious illness?" or, "Isn't a long operation dangerous?"
>
> *Answer:* "It is a very difficult thing to estimate the length of an operation. This depends on so many factors which may or may not occur in your case. At any rate, it doesn't make much difference, as the length of an operation has no definite relationship to the nature of the illness. Moreover, with anesthesia being what it is today, the operation will be as safe as can be expected regardless of the length of the procedure."
>
> *Disguised Question:* "Do you (the nurse) think I have cancer?"
>
> *Real Question:* "Is my doctor telling me the truth when he says he is not certain what is wrong with me?" or, "Wouldn't they be able to treat my condition with drugs if there was no thought of cancer?"
>
> *Answer:* "I'm really in no position to say. Your doctor is doing this exploration in order to make that decision. He'll be able to tell you more only after the operation."
>
> *Disguised Question:* "Is the anesthesia comfortable?"
>
> *Real Question:* "Will I awaken from the anesthesia?"

Answer: "Anesthesia is much more comfortable and pleasant than it used to be. You will go to sleep almost naturally and with no irritating gases to bother you before or after the operation. These agents are quite safe and you will be in competent hands throughout your period of unconsciousness."

Fear Rooted in False Knowledge. The patient often tends to compare his problem with some remotely similar problem a friend or relative had and, if the latter suffered a misfortune, the patient is liable to expect the same. In many cases, the comparison lacks validity, but the patient is naturally unaware of the dissimilarities.

Disguised Question: "My uncle underwent serious intestinal surgery. Do you think I have something wrong with my intestines?"

Real Question: "My uncle has a colostomy. Do you think I will have one?"

Answer: "Although both you and your uncle apparently had something in common, your intestinal operation may be completely different from that of your uncle. It is not wise to anticipate the same problem since there are so many possible situations. Just try to trust in your doctor and believe that he will do all that is possible to restore you to a completely normal state of health."

Disguised Question: "I was told that my sister talked while under anesthesia. Do you think I will?"

Real Question: "What if I say terribly embarrassing things or reveal a well-guarded secret while asleep?"

Answer: "It is extremely rare for people to speak under anesthesia. Those who do speak are usually speaking in mumbled phrases that are barely understandable. Besides, the operating team is much more concerned with your well-being than with what you may say, and spoken words are not even noticed. Keep in mind also that any words overheard are strictly confidential."

Fear Rooted in True Knowledge. Some patients are preoccupied with fears based on known facts. The worst way of handling these fears is to deny their validity. This breaks the patient's faith in your honesty. These fears are best handled by placing them in their true proportion:

Disguised Question: "Will this operation be painful?"

Real Question: "How can I possibly tolerate the terrible pain of an operation?"

Answer: "Naturally there is some discomfort for a few days following an operation. But we have many strong drugs at our disposal and these will be used as necessary to minimize your discomfort. We shall be available at all times to assist you in your convalescence and make you as comfortable as possible."

Disguised Question: "Do I really need a colostomy?"

Real Question: "Won't a colostomy be an unholy mess and make me a social outcast?"

Answer: "Your doctor feels a colostomy is absolutely necessary. You're going to be surprised at how rapidly and completely you will learn to adapt to a colostomy, and how clean and odorless it will be."

In *summary,* then, from a patient's viewpoint, surgery has four characteristics:
1. It is an act of faith.
2. It is an act of submission.
3. It is a radical invasion of privacy.
4. It induces fear.

Considerable thought should be given to this four fold view of surgery as interpreted by the patient. It will help to explain the profound psychological changes which can affect the patient about to undergo a surgical procedure.

The Surgeon's Viewpoint

Surgery Is a Necessary Evil. No one can rightfully deny the misfortune of surgical illness and the fundamental crudity of the surgical act. Were it possible to eradicate illness without forcibly entering the human body, any alternative would be superior and fundamentally more in keeping with the sanctity of the person's body. In this respect, then, surgery may almost be looked upon as a basic inadequacy or failure to achieve health by less radical and more rational means. It is only when all other means fail and surgery becomes necessary that one can justify it. The surgeon must therefore be conservative in his approach to illness, using his surgical skills only when and to the extent that they become absolutely necessary.

Surgery Is Both Art and Science. Surgical skill is a neat fusion of many faculties. It must include some very real but often difficult-to-define considerations, as well as some calculation of statistics and objective facts. Thus, the woman about to undergo a radical mastectomy must be looked upon as an unfortunate person whose breast must be removed in order to restore her to good health. The grave psychological and social ramifications must be appreciated and managed accordingly. One may hesitate to recommend this cosmetically deranging procedure, but the scientific side of surgery insists that there is no other alternative consistent with life and good health.

Surgery Is a Risk of Human Life. However minor the procedure may be, there are definite and, at times, considerable risks attending every surgical procedure. The surgeon must be confident of his training, conservative in his approach, and extremely cautious in his every surgical act. The physiological and biochemical alterations of every procedure undertaken must be anticipated and treated accordingly. This can be done only in the context of adequate facilities and with the help of efficient and well-trained personnel. From a surgeon's point of view, then, surgery has three characteristics:
1. It is a necessary evil.
2. It is both art and science.
3. It is a risk of human life.

If a nurse would understand the compulsiveness of the surgeon, his anger when things seem to be going wrong, and his tendency, at times, to blame others when the procedure is mentally and physically frustrating, she would do well to reflect on these characteristics of surgery as seen by the surgeon.

The Nurse's Viewpoint

Surgery Is a Psychological Act. From all we know of the patient's viewpoint, it is manifest that the anticipation of surgery creates great psychological "storms" within every patient, however stable or mature he may be. We have already considered fear. Equally important is the creation of resentment in the surgical patient. This resentment is, paradoxically, a by-product of the act of submission, which we have previously considered. The patient may subconsciously resent the fact that he must submit himself to the care of the physician and nurses. This may seem destructive of his self-esteem, dignity, and independence. It is best managed by considering those factors which will emphasize to the patient your belief in his dignity and independence. Treating him as an equal; showing sincere interest in his work and family; maintaining a nonclinical conversational level with the patient—all these factors restore dignity and create a wholesome rapport between nurse and patient. The nurse who talks on a level with the patient, neither too simply—for this will insult his intelligence, nor too clinically—for this will frustrate him, is most apt to minimize any resentment the patient may be harboring.

Surgery Is a Physiological Act. The nurse must be more than a psychotherapeutist or a confidante. She is also a professional clinician with well-trained faculties for observing any signs or symptoms of physiological stress in her patient. She integrates and applies her knowledge of physiology, pharmacology, bacteriology, and nutrition toward the well-being of her patient. It is axiomatic that the safest surgery is performed on the patient who physiologically approaches normal health. The nurse must aid the surgeon in accomplishing this end for her patient.

Surgery Is a Social Act. The patient is not a social appendage, suddenly cut off from family and friends. He is a father, a brother, or a son. His family has every right to be informed of his state of health at any time. Failure to communicate is just as productive of fear and resentment on the part of the patient's family as it is with the patient. When, for example, emergency surgery is suddenly decided upon by the surgeon, someone must be certain that the family is notified. This responsibility generally falls to the surgeon, but the nurse ought also to prevent oversights by either reminding the surgeon or notifying the family directly.

The family may direct a barrage of questions toward the nurse. She must distinguish between those questions best left for the surgeon to cope with and those which she ought to answer immediately. There are no definite rules to follow, and only experience can lead the way. Those questions pertaining to diagnosis, surgical technique, and prognosis are certainly best left for the surgeon to answer, though here again, one may give general and indirect answers pending the arrival of the surgeon.

Relatives can become extremely anxious over intravenous set-ups that are not working or other mechanical devices that appear not to be operating well. A little patience and reassurance will often calm the situation. Again, the key words are tact and discretion in dealing with these situations, however irritating they may be during a busy work day.

Surgery Is a Legal Act. Medical liability grows more common every day. There was a time when almost no lawsuits were brought against the medical or nursing profession. However one may argue as to their advantages or disadvantages in the general scheme of things, one thing is certain: lawsuits are here to stay and are likely to increase in frequency and scope.

The general and local laws are far too complex to be covered in this manual, nor would it be safe to depend on any interpretation made other than by competent counsel. Nevertheless, the nurse must be aware of possible areas of liability in her profession. Certainly a good number of difficulties will be assignable to negligence, engaging in the practice of medicine without a license, and so forth. The most important rule of thumb is to be extremely circumspect about any proposed procedure which appears to be out of the ordinary for a nurse to be doing. When in doubt about the legality of a procedure (e.g., starting an intravenous infusion, or giving a blood transfusion) the nurse should check with her floor supervisor before acting.

If surgery involves invasion of privacy, then most assuredly much liability can be attached to the surgeon and his team for the act performed. This often takes the form of assault and battery charges. A permit for inducing anesthesia and performing surgery must be signed by the patient prior to surgery. This permit must be witnessed by a duly authorized person, usually appointed by the hospital. The surgical ward nurse and, later, the circulating operating room nurse should be certain that this permit has been signed prior to surgery.

Acts of omission or commission may involve liability, depending on the situation. The nurse should thoroughly chart everything she does to a patient as well as every drug she administers, and should make adequate daily nurse's notes describing her patient's progress. Failure to keep adequate records is frequently the cause of a lost lawsuit.

Surgery Has Religious Connotations.   Almost without exception and without regard to creed, most people undergoing surgery will harbor some religious thoughts. Some may formalize these thoughts according to their church affiliations. Others merely think out their own spiritual concepts. Whatever the form of it, there are religious connotations to anticipated surgery, and the nurse must recognize these and work with them as best she can. Many hospitals have chaplains of the major denominations, and cooperation between chaplain and nurse is all to the patient's benefit. An understanding of the general nature of the patient's creed may help immensely in meeting the patient's preoperative and postoperative spiritual needs.

As the nurse looks at surgery, then, it takes on five characteristics:
1. It is a psychological act.
2. It is a physiological act.
3. It is a social act.
4. It is a legal act.
5. It bears religious connotations.

The nurse would do well to reevaluate periodically her viewpoint of surgery. A good deal of implication exists in these five characteristics, and the good nurse appreciates and applies them daily in her work.

Summing up this entire section, then, we can define or characterize surgery according to many points of view, realizing that these viewpoints all overlap and interdigitate into one complex, comprehensive view:

From the patient's viewpoint, surgery has four characteristics:
1. It is an act of faith in a surgeon, a nurse, and a hospital.
2. It is an act of submission to doctors and nurses.
3. It is a radical invasion of mental, physical, and moral privacy.
4. It induces fear and resentment.

From the surgeon's viewpoint, surgery has three characteristics:
1. It is a necessary evil called into play when all else fails.
2. It is both art and science; the surgeon must be artist and scientist.
3. It is a risk of human life to be taken most seriously.

From the nurse's viewpoint, surgery has five characteristics:
1. It is a psychological act, and she must be a psychologist.
2. It is a physiological act, and she must be a professional clinician.
3. It is a social act, and she must consider the patient's family and friends.
4. It is a legal act, and she must be aware of her legal rights and responsibilities.
5. It bears religious connotations which she must consider most seriously.

TYPES OF SURGERY

Surgery may be arbitrarily divided into several types for convenience of discussion. While there are many overlaps and arbitrary distinctions in the divisions to follow, the various types do serve to illustrate certain basic implications found in them. Accordingly, surgery may be classified into four categories.

1. According to whether it is evident or not evident to the patient, surgery may be designated as:

a. External Surgery. E.g., a radical mastectomy.

b. Internal Surgery. E.g., a gastrectomy.

Implication. As a general rule, external procedures carry with them a greater degree of psychic stress for the simple reason that the patient is able to appreciate the result by direct observation. In the case of external reconstructive surgery, the psychic stress may be one of elation or depression, depending, of course, on whether the anticipated results were fulfilled. For the surgical nurse, the most important aspect of this division into external and internal types is the anticipation and recognition of the psychological problems that may arise. In the example of a radical mastectomy, one can fully expect a great deal of preoperative anxiety over the possibility of breast removal, and this must be handled with sympathy and discretion. The patient must, of course, be forewarned of the possibility of mastectomy by the surgeon, but the nurse must attempt to focus the patient's attention on the more probable course of events (that is, assuming the surgeon feels that the breast lesion is benign).

Internal procedures affecting reproductive organs may or may not have serious psychic overtones, depending primarily on the functional or supposed functional importance ascribed to these organs at the time of surgery. A hysterectomy in a childless woman would certainly be expected to have greater significance than one in a 50-year-old mother of four children. This factor of functional importance of an organ to be removed must be evaluated by the nurse as she estimates the psychological effects of a given procedure on her patient. No less important is the supposed functional importance of an organ in the mind of the patient. Thus, for example, a woman—although several times a mother—might infer that hysterectomy will in some mysterious way affect her womanhood, making her physically or sexually unattractive. This false inference may be at the root of her anxieties over the anticipated procedure. A few explanatory words concerning the function of the uterus would go far toward dispelling her fears.

2. According to its degree of hazard or physiological effects, surgery may be designated as:

a. Minor Surgery. E.g., excision of a sebaceous cyst of the scalp.

b. Major Surgery. E.g., an abdominal-perineal resection.

Implication. The intensity of preoperative and postoperative management of the surgical patient necessarily varies directly with the extent of the procedure and the general health of the patient. With experience, the surgical nurse will develop a sense of what to expect for each given surgical procedure. The early postoperative abdominal-perineal patient who is pale and has a pulse of 110 per minute will come to be regarded as "normal" or as "doing well," as this is a very shocking procedure to the average patient. The same clinical picture in a lesser procedure would alert the nurse to a possible impending complication, such as shock.

Likewise, in the preparation for surgery, a more extensive evaluation and psychological preparation will attend the patient undergoing major surgery. This is not to say that minor surgical patients can be neglected, but that a realistic sense of proportion should be encouraged.

3. According to its effect on the pathologic process, surgery may be designated as:

a. Curative surgery, in which the basic disease is arrested or eradicated: e.g., an appendectomy.

b. Palliative surgery, in which the symptoms are alleviated but the disease is unaffected: e.g., a by-pass intestinal operation to relieve the obstructing symptoms of an unresectable carcinoma of the bowel.

Implication. It is often difficult to make the distinction preoperatively. One usually operates with the hope of cure, although occasionally the lesion is known to be incurable preoperatively. Often the operative finding of advanced unresectable disease creates the need for palliative surgery. The great difficulty in palliative surgery is that the patient, relieved of his pain or uncomfortable symptoms, becomes temporarily elated and optimistic about his future. The decision as to how much truth this patient can tolerate is an extremely difficult one, as no two cases are alike. Considerations are given to age, employment, family, psychic structure, anticipated survival time, and so forth. The decision must be made by the surgeon in conjunction with the patient's family. The nurse should be extremely cautious regardless of her personal convictions. She should discuss the matter with the surgeon, ascertaining what he plans to tell the family and the patient. At any rate, her conversations with the patient must be sympathetic, tactful, and discreet.

    4. According to its mode of operation, surgery may be designated as:

    a. Reconstructive surgery, in which a damaged organ is partially or fully restored to its previous anatomic and functional status: e.g., the badly damaged hand is reconstructed.

    b. Constructive surgery, in which a congenitally defective organ is improved in function or apperance: e.g., a congenitally small ear is improved.

    c. Ablative surgery, in which a diseased tissue or organ is removed: e.g., nephrectomy for chronic pyelonephritis.

Implication. Reconstructive and constructive surgical procedures are particularly apt to be disrupted by postoperative sepsis. The highest degrees of aseptic technique must be practiced in these surgical fields. Very frequently they are staged procedures, and it is not uncommon for a patient to undergo several separate procedures for constructive or reconstructive purposes. The fact that the patient has safely undergone several procedures of a similar nature in the past is no excuse for a casual approach toward his impending surgery. A thorough evaluation must attend the preoperative state for each procedure.

    The degree of risk incurred by ablative surgery depends, naturally, on the organ being removed and the surgical ease or difficulty encountered in its removal. Whenever a major organ is removed there is, of course, a double risk involved — that of the procedure itself, and that related to the physiologic state resulting from the removal of the organ in question. These risk factors must be compounded in assessing the true risk for a given procedure, and the degree or intensity of preoperative preparation must be in direct proportion to the estimated risk.

GENERAL EFFECTS OF SURGERY ON THE PATIENT

    From what has already been said, one realizes that certain procedures carry with them greater risks than others. The nurse must ask herself how this procedure will affect her patient psychologically as well as physiologically. Her entire preoperative and postoperative management is dependent on her ability to understand and anticipate the sequelae of various surgical procedures. While differing with each procedure, certain basic bacteriological, physiological, and psychological events underlie all surgery. These events are first to be understood if one would gain a comprehensive knowledge of surgery and the surgical patient. These events may be considered under five broad headings.

    Penetration of the Bacterial Barrier. The skin represents the patient's first line of defense against the invasion of bacteria and the establishment of a clinical infection. Intact, this organ is impervious in its texture and practically infallible in its protective abilities. Surgery, however minor it may seem, immediately and necessarily destroys the continuity of this barrier and sets the stage for surgical sepsis. A wound infection in certain procedures, while inconvenient and undesirable, is tolerable. For example, a minor wound infection occurring after an otherwise successful gastrectomy may be accepted with calm resignation. To the contrary, reconstructive surgery, however successful it may at first appear, can be ruined by the occurrence of wound sepsis.

    Regardless of the nature of the procedure, all precautions must be taken to maintain sepsis at a minimum. Thus it becomes important for the surgical nurse to be thoroughly familiar with the nature of surgical sepsis, the principles of aseptic technique, and the means of achieving sterilization in the operating room. These matters will be considered in subsequent chapters.

Penetration of the Vascular Tree. As long as the vascular tree remains intact, blood volume is maintained and organ nourishment is achieved. Surgery interrupts this system by its severance of arteries and veins. Left unchecked, these severed vessels would result in excessive blood loss, shock, and, ultimately, death. Controlling this blood loss — *hemostasis* — is therefore an essential act of surgery. A thorough understanding of hemostasis can be achieved only through surgical experience. It is one of the prerequisites of a good surgical nurse.

Removal of Tissues and Organs. During an operation, the surgeon will dissect and identify a tissue or organ in order to examine and work on the local pathology. Certain tissues or organs must be sacrificed as a necessary part of many surgical procedures. The potential physiological defect resulting from the removal of a specific tissue or organ must be thoroughly understood by the surgical nurse in order to make her postoperative management of the patient adequate and logical. In the case of nephrectomy, to cite one example, knowledge that temporary malfunction of the remaining kidney may lead to anuria and severe electrolyte disturbances will place the nurse on careful guard for such a sequence of events. If she is further aware that the elevated serum potassium accompanying anuria may forebode or precipitate a cardiac arrest, all the more efficient and vigilant will her observation of vital signs and general well-being become.

The potential physiological defects resulting from specific organ removal will be covered in Section II of this manual.

In addition, the removal of a given organ or tissue often requires the use of specialized instruments. In the example of nephrectomy, a renal pedicle clamp must be used on the renal vessels. Efficient assistance from the surgical nurse requires that she know the names of all instruments needed in a given case, their construction, and their function.

Initiation of the Stress Response. Largely because of the work of endocrinologists and other physiologists, clinicians have come to understand a complex, diffuse physiological response to stress which is probably mediated through the pituitary and adrenal glands. Any one of a number of stressful situations can elicit the "stress response" from the organism. This response appears to be a defense mechanism against a threatened change in *homeostasis.* The response is extremely widespread, and almost every organ in the body is affected. The blood pressure and pulse may rise; the pupils dilate; the blood sugar is increased; the basal metabolic rate is quickened; the tonus of the muscles is increased; the mental faculties become more acute; the gastrointestinal activity is decreased; urinary excretion is decreased; and a host of other changes may occur.

This stress reaction may become very obvious following major surgery and must be recognized for what it is. The surgical factors resulting in this reaction are poorly understood, and may be a combination of the psychic stimuli set in motion by the fear of surgery, the premedications and anesthetic medications used, and the responses to the surgery itself.

At times the stress response seems to serve a useful purpose as it maximally prepares the patient to accommodate himself to the otherwise threatening problems of surgery. At other times, the mechanism seems to run amiss, and various complications may threaten the patient as a direct result of the stress response. It therefore behooves the nurse to acquaint herself fully with the meaning and nature of this stress response as well as its manifestations. In this way she will be better able to anticipate complications and deal with them adequately. A complete description of the stress response is largely outside the scope of this manual. Standard surgical and nursing texts should be consulted.

Precipitation of Anxieties and Depressions. Surgery may have profound psychological effects on the patient both pre- and postoperatively. At times the problems are clear-cut and simple to handle. At other times they are subtle, and may have far-reaching effects on the ego. A great deal of experience, common sense, and training is required to properly manage and prevent these difficulties, and this must form an important phase of the nurse's education. The very outcome of the surgical procedure may be dependent on how well the patient deals with his anxieties. The psychological preparation of the patient for surgery will be examined in Chapter 5.

SUMMARY AND CONCLUSIONS

Surgery represents a profound challenge to surgeon, nurse, and patient. The three objectives of surgical patient care are:

1. The delivery of a psychologically and physiologically prepared patient for surgery.

2. The safe, efficient, and sound alleviation of the patient's disease.

3. The careful guidance of the patient's postoperative period until he is safely recovered from his anesthesia and the immediate shocking effects of surgery.

Upon these three principles rests the success or failure of any surgical procedure. As simple and obvious as they may appear, a failure to appreciate these principles or the adoption of an all-too-casual attitude toward them is directly related to most surgical tragedies. Careful reflection will reveal that these objectives can be attained only through the concerted efforts of a well-functioning team, each member of which fully appreciates his or her individual responsibilities.

The surgical nurse must participate in all phases of the surgical experience, and her professional training and experience must be correspondingly complete. No part of this training can be lacking if she is to have a total picture of surgery, so necessary for the proper management of her patient. The psychological, physiological, social, and moral facets of surgery form an integrated whole which permeates the preoperative, operative, and postoperative course of the surgical patient. The remainder of this manual will attempt to focus on this total surgical experience of the surgical nurse and her patient.

STUDY QUESTIONS

1. A 32-year-old housewife is about to undergo excision of a breast mass which has been present for three months. In the course of your admitting her and taking her vital signs, she asks whether *you think* her breast will be removed. Discuss *your* reactions to her question and how you would answer her.

2. This same patient's mother died one year after a radical mastectomy. How would you respond to the patient if she pointed out this family history to you?

3. A 43-year-old male is admitted to your surgical ward following an auto accident in which he is seriously injured. You receive a telephone call from the city desk of the local newspaper requesting information concerning your patient's condition. How would you handle this situation?

4. A 50-year-old carpenter suffered traumatic amputation of his right thumb while at work. He is very resentful of the fact that you are changing the dressings frequently throughout the day. Discuss the factors that may have led to his resentment and how you would handle them.

5. A palliative by-pass intestinal procedure has been done on a 50-year-old woman for inoperable carcinoma of the cecum. She now asks whether you think she is going to be well. What are some of the factors you must consider before giving her an answer?

6. Surgical sepsis is always to be avoided. Nevertheless, sepsis is much more catastrophic in some operations than in others. Rearrange the following procedures in proper order according to *increasing hazard* from sepsis:
   a. Open reduction of fractured femur.
   b. Appendectomy.
   c. By-pass arterial graft for femoral artery obstruction.
   d. Rhinoplasty.
   e. Abdominal-perineal resection.
What important lessons can be learned from this exercise?

7. Discuss how socioeconomic factors affect the surgical patient and how a knowledge of them will aid in your nursing of the surgical patient.

8. A surgeon calls in and asks you to remove the sutures from his patient prior to discharge. You have never done this before, but feel quite competent from repeated observations. What factor or factors will govern your response to his request?

9. How would you compare the psychological implications of a gastrectomy versus an oophorectomy in a given patient? What factors must you consider in making your comparison? How does this knowledge affect your relationship with the patient undergoing these procedures?

10. Review the nature of the "stress response" in any standard textbook of physiology or surgery. List as many physiological alterations in the organism brought about by the stress reaction as you can. How does this list affect your nursing care of the surgical patient?

11. It is in vogue to talk of a patient's "bill of rights." What are some of these rights? What part does *trust* play in dealing with these rights?

THE SURGICAL ENVIRONMENT

2

FUNDAMENTAL PURPOSES OF AN OPERATING ROOM SUITE

The novice often conceives of the operating room suite as some mysterious aggregation of rooms located in a far-off corner of the hospital and usually set off by a sign such as: "Danger — only authorized personnel allowed beyond this point." Surgery was not always conducted under such isolated conditions. Indeed, the era of "kitchen table surgery" still lingers in the senior surgeon's memory.

The modern operating room suite serves *four fundamental purposes,* and an understanding of these will go far toward removing the cumbersome mystery surrounding surgery. These purposes are:

To Obtain Geographical Isolation. By placing the operating room in an isolated section of the hospital, one acquires a private, relatively quiet, and clean place to perform surgery. The operating room suite is best located in a blind wing, on the top floor or in the basement of the hospital, and is sealed off from unauthorized personnel with appropriate signs. The patient's privacy is thereby guaranteed, confusion and sepsis are minimized, and the entire environment becomes more conducive to safe and effective surgery.

To Obtain Bacteriological Isolation. Ideally, the operating room suite uses a separate water supply, as well as a separate laundry and disposal system. In addition, special clothing and footwear must be used by all operating room personnel within certain distances of the operating rooms, as designated by appropriate signs. These measures insure that serious hospital infection will not affect sterility in the operating rooms.

To Centralize Equipment. The operating room suite, in essence, represents a series of carefully integrated, fully equipped, and well-lit rooms whose sole function is to help facilitate safe and effective surgery. By setting off this area from the remainder of the hospital, one is able to store and maintain all necessary equipment in maximum operating condition. The supervisor is responsible for keeping a careful inventory of equipment and for seeing that all instruments are functioning properly.

While not differing in essentials, the operating room suite of each hospital is unique, and the staff nurse must acquaint herself with all its features. It is particularly important that she know the following:

1. The location of certain emergency items:
   Electrocardiogram and cardiac monitors.
   Pacemakers and defibrillators.
   Oxygen tanks.
   Laryngoscopes and endotracheal tubes.
   Emergency drug trays.
   Suctioning equipment.
   Tracheostomy and thoracotomy sets.
   Transfusion and infusion equipment.
2. The equipment, instruments, and linens found in the supply room.
3. The facilities found in the recovery room.
4. The location and operation of various sterilizers.

To Centralize Trained Personnel. Modern surgery requires the combined talents of many groups of trained specialists who, by working together frequently in a special setting, acquire a great deal of efficiency, cooperation, and skill in their common labor. This can be accomplished only in the context of an isolated, restricted environment.

BASIC DESIGN AND EQUIPMENT OF AN OPERATING ROOM SUITE

The Floor Plan

Most hospitals have diagrams illustrating the plan of each floor. These plans are found in convenient locations on the wards and are used to show escape routes for patients and personnel in the event of a fire. The floor plan of the operating room suite should be studied carefully. This will show the relative locations of the supervisor's office, the surgeons' and nurses' lounges, the corridors and entrance ways for patients, the instrument and work rooms, the recovery room, the anesthesia suite, the substerilizing rooms, the major and minor operating rooms, the pathology laboratory for studying frozen sections, the instrument preparation and packing rooms, and the scrub areas.

Familiarity with this floor plan will eliminate the confusion which often attends the student's first days in the operating room.

The Supervisor's Office

The supervisor's office is usually centrally located in the operating room suite, thus affording more efficient control of traffic and personnel in all directions. The surgeon schedules his cases with the secretary. She records these cases in a master schedule book, which also contains the time of surgery, the room assignment, the type of anesthesia to be administered, and the assistants for the surgeon. Assignments for nursing duties in the operating room are also made at this desk. The student will receive her assignments here from the instructor.

The Surgeons' and Nurses' Lounges

The lounges are conveniently located at the perimeter of the suite and away from the operating rooms. They are equipped with individual clothing lockers. In addition, they usually have wash facilities, scrub suits, protective footwear, and shower facilities. In most hospitals, fire laws permitting, smoking is allowed in these lounges only. Under no conditions should smoking be tolerated in open rooms or corridors. The lounges should be kept uncluttered, as they can easily become a source of dust-borne bacteria.

Corridors and Entrance Ways for Patients

The main corridor should be wide enough to comfortably accommodate two patients' litters standing side by side. It must be kept scrupulously clean and dust-free, as the traffic load is necessarily heavy in this area and can lead to serious problems with dust-borne bacteria. The corridor should be kept as free as possible from equipment which tends to clutter and obstruct the free flow of traffic. Entrances and exits should be conveniently located near patients' elevators. *Emergency exits* are clearly labeled, and their locations should be known by all personnel. Fire alarm boxes and extinguishers are placed for easy access, as required by law. All personnel should be familiar with their location.

The Patient Receiving Area

The premedicated patient is brought on a litter to a special waiting area outside the operating room proper. Here the nurse makes the final checks before the patient is delivered to the operating room, making certain that everything is ready for the anticipated surgery. The nurse should check the ID bracelet, the skin preparation, and the vital signs; she should determine what medications have been given and whether the patient has voided prior to surgery. All prostheses not heretofore removed are checked and removed at this point. These include dentures, removable bridgework, contact lenses, eye prostheses, and so forth. The patient's hair is checked for pins. All valuables are removed and labeled.

A thorough review of the medical record will establish whether everything is in order. The patient's history and the results of the physical examination should be on the chart, along with the anesthesiologist's preoperative notes. If preoperative tests such as chest x-ray or electrocardiogram were ordered, the results should be available. Any apparent abnormality is reported to the operating room supervisor or the responsible anesthesiologist. All laboratory work ordered by the attending surgeon should be recorded on the patient's chart. The availability of typed and cross-matched blood should be double-checked.

The patient will need psychological support while he is in the receiving area. Premedications notwithstanding, very few patients are without anxieties about safety, pain, death, cancer, and other concerns. A few moments spent in honest conversation with the patient here are often worth many hours at less critical times. Specific questions cannot always be answered in detail, but often just general supportive care and reassurance are all that is necessary and can be extremely important to the patient.

A Typical Major Operating Room and Its Basic Equipment

The size of a major operating room will vary, depending on the available space in each hospital (Fig. 2-1). The walls, the floor, and the ceiling are constructed as soundproof as possible and of a material that is easily cleaned. In addition, the floor is constructed in such a fashion as to conduct static electricity efficiently. The conductive qualities of this floor must be checked periodically by the engineering department of the hospital. Wear and tear, dirt and debris, and various waxes and polishes can all decrease the conductivity of the operating room floor and create a serious explosion hazard.

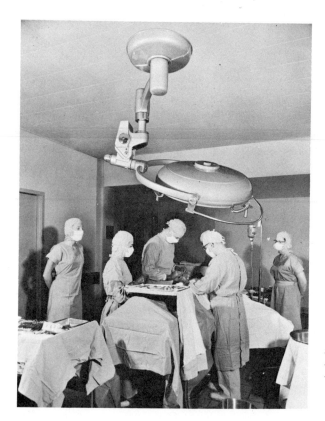

FIGURE 2-1 Scene in a modern operating room. Note the position of the surgeon, the assistant, and the scrub nurse. Also note the student nurses observing the procedure. (Courtesy Wilmot-Castle Company.)

Most operating rooms have three doors: a main door to admit the patient on his litter, a door connecting the operating room with the adjacent scrub room or scrub area, and a door leading to the adjacent substerilizing room. These doors must be kept closed at all times, and are to be used only by personnel directly involved in the management of the case.

Each operating room possesses a flexible and versatile operating table. Efficient functioning of this table demands a thorough understanding of its working parts. This will form part of the instruction in the operating room (Fig. 2-2).

Proper lighting is indispensable for safe surgery. Each room is equipped with one main overhead lamp and one or more portable spotlights. A good overhead lamp supplies approximately 1800 foot candles of light. The lamp is adjustable in all directions and is suspended from a sliding rotating track which, in turn, is attached to the ceiling (Fig. 2-3). The light head should be controllable from outside the sterile field by a handle attached to the reflector.

Portable spotlights are also available to supplement the overhead lamp. These are usually necessary when the operative site is within a body cavity which the overhead light cannot reach. These spotlights will require adjusting from time to time at the request of the surgeon (Fig. 2-4). They are equipped with explosion-proof interlocking electrical outlet switches.

All operating rooms are equipped with emergency accessory lighting signals. Should the normal electrical power fail, an accessory power source immediately takes over, and lighting is resumed.

Oxygen and suction apparatus may be from a wall source or dispensed from a separate portable unit. If separate suction apparatus is used, it must be explosion-proof.

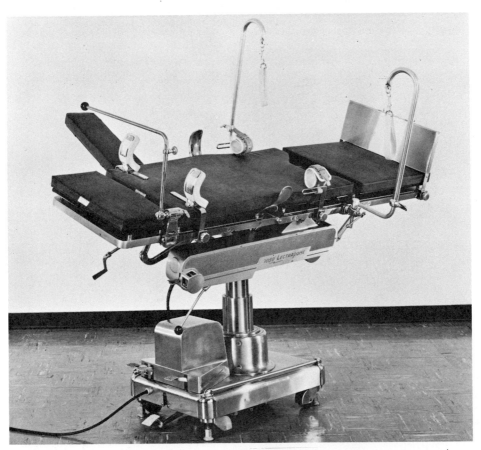

FIGURE 2-2 A modern electric operating table. (Courtesy American Sterilizer Company.)

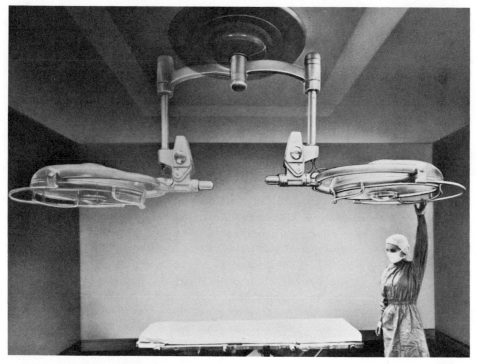

FIGURE 2–3 Overhead main light, adjustable to all positions. (Courtesy Wilmot-Castle Company.)

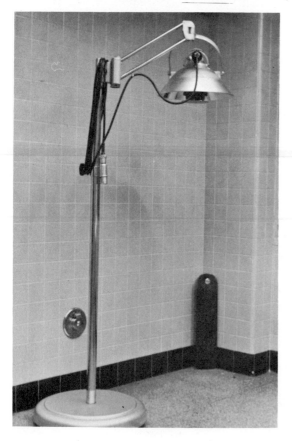

FIGURE 2–4 A portable spotlight for supplementary lighting in the operating room.

Temperature and humidity control switches are usually found adjacent to the main entrance door in each operating room. Comfortable and safe operating temperatures range from 60 to 75°F. Proper air hygiene is insured by adequate and clean ventilating devices which are also checked periodically by the engineering department. Faulty or nonfunctioning ventilators have been incriminated in the epidemiology of surgical sepsis. Some operating rooms are additionally supplied with air conditioning for patient and personnel comfort.

Other standard equipment of a major operating room includes:

1. *Equipment Shelves.* These hold various types of sutures, sterilizing solutions, and lubricants.

2. *Linen Cabinets.* These hold clean sheets, pillow cases, towels, gloves, sterile linen, and paper supplies.

3. *Anesthesia Cabinets.* These hold spinal trays, intravenous set-ups, and various types of intravenous infusion fluids.

4. Explosion-proof x-ray viewing box.

5. Two or three revolving adjustable stools.

6. One large and one small foot stand.

7. Two or three kick buckets with swivel casters.

8. Two utility tables, one medium-size and one large, with shelves for gowns, gloves, and skin prep equipment.

9. Two Mayo stands.

10. Two instrument tables

11. One anesthesia table

12. One sponge basin on swivel casters.

All equipment making contact with the floor must be furnished with explosion-proof casters to prevent the discharge of static electricity in the vicinity of explosive gases.

A substerilizing room is found adjacent to each major operating room, and can be reached through an adjoining door. This room contains a steam flash sterilizer for rapid sterilization and decontamination of instruments.

A Typical Minor Operating Room

The minor operating room is similar to the major operating room but is on a smaller scale. All lighting is usually from one or more portable spotlights. The precise equipment in the room will depend on whether it is used for fracture work, cystoscopy, tonsillectomy and adenoidectomy, or minor plastic and excisional surgery. However, a properly equipped minor operating room will contain oxygen and suction apparatus, cardiac arrest and tracheostomy sets, an emergency drug table or tray, and a linen supply cabinet. In addition, each room will have its own adjacent substerilizing unit similar to that found with the major operating rooms. These minor operating room units should be in a wing away from the main line of traffic through the major operating rooms. In this way outpatient surgery can be done without fear of contaminating the main operating room suite.

Scrub Areas

Adjacent to each operating room is a scrub area, and access to the operating room is through a separate door. The scrub area may be closed off from the main corridor, but often is not. Usually one scrub area serves two nearby operating rooms.

Each scrub area consists of several separate sinks and faucets. Hot and cold water should be from separate sources, and their control must be through foot or elbow valves so as to leave the hands free. The trough or sink basin must be deep enough to prevent dirty water and soap from splashing on the cleansed hands. Appropriate soap or detergent dispensing units are found with each sink, and these are usually controlled by foot pedals.

Automatic brush dispensers or individually packaged nail files and disposable brushes impregnated with scrub solution are attached at convenient levels on nearby walls.

The Recovery Room

Most modern operating room suites are equipped with a recovery room. This is fully equipped and staffed for the immediate postoperative recovery period.

The basic equipment of a recovery room is as follows:

1. Oxygen and suctioning units, appropriately placed adjacent to each recovery room litter.
2. A medication cabinet, containing all emergency drugs, intravenous set-ups, and infusion fluids.
3. Emergency equipment, including cardiac arrest trays, tracheostomy sets, cardiac pacemakers, and defibrillators.
4. Suctioning devices.
5. A central charting desk.
6. A wash basin or sink.
7. A linen cabinet, with gowns, draw sheets, pillows, and so forth.

The recovery room is staffed by a supervisor, a head nurse, and one or more graduate nurses, depending on the size and patient load of the operating and recovery rooms. These nurses have specialized preparation in this phase of surgical nursing. In addition, the anesthesiologist is immediately available for emergency consultations.

The Instrument Room

After any operation, all surgical instruments not disposed of undergo some sterilization and are sent to the instrument room. Here they are cleansed in an ultrasonic unit and then sorted for repacking. Individual set-ups are made consisting of a designated assortment of instruments which are wrapped in muslin, taped, and labeled: e.g., "laparotomy set," "thoracotomy set." The packs *have still not been rendered fully sterile* at this point, and care must be taken to avoid mixing them with sterile packs.

Some institutions send instruments to a central supply room for sorting and repackaging immediately after decontamination.

Instrument and Sterile Supply Room

Following sterilization, the set-ups are stored in a clean, well lit, and conveniently located supply room adjacent to the main operating rooms. The staff nurse should familiarize herself with the location of the various instruments and packs in this room.

Frozen Section Room

From time to time the surgeon will require a rapid microscopic analysis of a surgical specimen. This specimen will be analyzed by the pathologist, who performs a frozen-section study. This consists of freezing the specimen with carbon dioxide under pressure, then cutting it into thin slices with a microtome. The specimen is then stained with appropriate tissue stains and examined under the microscope. The pathologist usually performs this study in a small room located in the operating room suite (Fig. 2–5).

SUMMARY

The student nurse will usually be given a guided tour through the operating rooms by her instructor. She should observe all the points that have been mentioned and try to see the operating room suite as an integrated and fully equipped series of rooms. Particular note should be made of the sterilizing areas, the cleanliness of all the rooms, the safety devices on all equipment to prevent explosions, and the specialized functions of each member of the operating room staff.

STUDY QUESTIONS

1. Obtain a floor plan of your hospital's operating room suite. How does it compare with the general outline described in this chapter?

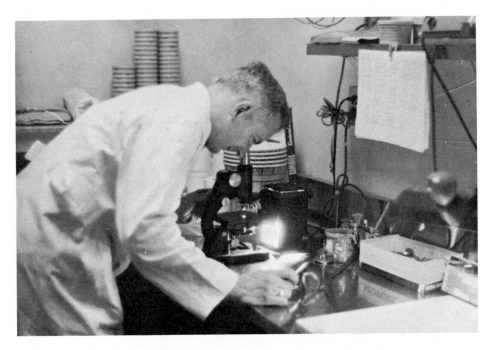

FIGURE 2–5 Pathologist examining frozen section.

2. List the personal *safety precautions* which you, as a member of the operating room team, must take against the hazards of explosive gases. Which anesthetic gases are explosive?

3. What is meant ·by "conductive" and "nonconductive," with respect to operating room equipment?

4. How is the operating room floor made conductive? Can it lose its conductivity and, if so, how?

5. What equipment is likely to be sterilized in a substerilizing room, and under what circumstances?

6. Can you list five *situations* in which the surgeon is apt to call for a frozen section analysis of a surgical specimen?

7. What are the *advantages* and *disadvantages* of a frozen section as compared with a permanent section on a surgical specimen?

3   SURGICAL SEPSIS

HISTORICAL CONSIDERATIONS

The modern surgeon takes aseptic technique and antisepsis for granted, and fully expects his incisions to heal cleanly and *per primam intentionem* (by first intention). This healthy situation was not always so, and it is instructive to review the historical development of the concepts of surgical sepsis and aseptic technique.

In the early years of the nineteenth century, a bleak picture could have been painted of surgical wounds and the complications of sepsis. Wound infection was so common an event as to be considered "normal." Indeed, when pus broke through the incision, thereby evacuating the under-lying abscess, it was referred to as "laudable pus" for it usually signaled the beginning of clinical improvement. The wound became septic, threatening the patient's life, frequently ruining the surgical procedure, always lengthening the hospital stay, and usually marring the surgical site cosmetically. In some clinics, fully 80 per cent of all clean wounds developed sepsis, and the mortality from limb amputation, for example, was formidable. High on the list of problems of sepsis was that of puerperal fever. The mortality and morbidity rates from postpartum uterine sepsis reached truly epidemic proportions throughout European hospitals in the 1820's and 1830's.

Several clinicians were responsible for the elimination of this dreaded obstetrical complication, and their contributions taught us much concerning the etiology, epidemiology, and prophylaxis of other surgical infections. The first breakthrough must be credited to the Manchester surgeon Charles White (1728–1813), who conceived of puerperal fever as arising from putrefying lochia within the uterus. Even though he had no knowledge of the bacterial world as we know it, he advocated cleanliness and isolation of the postpartum patient based on his empirical observation of a higher incidence of puerperal fever among women in overpopulated dirty hospitals.

Other clinicians added to White's concepts of the disease, and common to all these early investigators was an emphasis on cleanliness, the use of disinfectants, and "aseptic conduct" in the management of the infected patient. However, it is to Ignaz Semmelweis that the credit must go for precisely defining the epidemiology of puerperal fever. By 1847 he had established that puerperal fever was conveyed from one woman to another by the examining finger of the doctor. By advocating the disinfection of the hands between examinations, the isolation of infected patients, and the nontraumatic examination of the patient's uterus, Semmelweis reduced the incidence of puerperal fever in his clinic from 18 per cent in 1847 to 1 per cent in 1848!

In 1857 Louis Pasteur offered abundant evidence that fermentation of alcohol was due to airborne bacteria. In England the surgeon Joseph Lister took note of Pasteur's theories and first used the antiseptic carbolic acid for sterilizing instruments and surgical wounds. He also introduced the surgical wound dressing as a prevention against the airborne bacteria theorized by Pasteur.

Other concepts of aseptic technique developed rapidly. Ernst von Bergmann (1880) advocated sterilization of surgical instruments, dry goods, and the surgeon's hands with bichloride of mercury; Gustav Neuber (1881) first used the cap and gown in the operating room; Curt Schimmelbusch first used the steam sterilizer for cleansing instruments, linen, and scrub brushes. In 1894 Joseph Bloodgood donned sterile gloves, as did all the members of his scrub team. Among William Halsted's innumerable contributions to surgical technique was his observation on the proper management and closure of the wound. He advocated perfect hemostasis, evacuation of all debris, prevention of "dead spaces," and the avoidance of strangulation ligatures. The surgical mask was first used by Johann von Mikulicz in 1896.

To Louis Pasteur and Robert Koch must go some of the highest laurels for their contributions concerning heat sterilization and sterilizers. Pasteur had demonstrated clearly that heat destroyed microorganisms. In 1878 Robert Koch demonstrated that the organisms described by Pasteur actually were present in infectious lesions. He helped develop and improve the hot air sterilizer. Soon it was realized that the original steam sterilizers were ineffective against certain spores, and it was soon shown that the temperature of steam in a sterilizer could be raised by increasing its pressure and that this was effective against spores.

The modern era of asepsis and antisepsis is characterized by a refinement of previously developed techniques and is reinforced by the development and proliferation of chemotherapeutic agents and antibiotics. There is danger of relying too heavily on antibiotics while relaxing aseptic surgical technique. No drug is a substitute for meticulous attention to aseptic technique and thorough sterilization of all items contacting the surgical wound.

Infection developing in clean wounds is becoming increasingly rare. The use of disposable materials, better sterilizing procedures, and a vigilant nursing staff, combined with cleaner and better ventilated operating rooms, undoubtedly spells success.

FACTORS PREDISPOSING TO WOUND INFECTION

On a well-run surgical service, approximately 1 per cent of initially clean wounds will become infected. This theoretical minimum is the ideal toward which all operating room teams must strive. One often underestimates the incidence of sepsis, and such "clinical impressions" are notoriously unreliable. Only a carefully documented study, repeated at frequent intervals, is liable to give one an idea of how efficiently the operating room team is maintaining an acceptably low infection rate.

Several factors, taken singly or together, predispose to wound infection. If one clearly and thoroughly understood the operation of all these factors, wound sepsis could be eliminated from the surgeon's vocabulary. Such a situation, though theoretically possible, cannot be realized in the present state of our knowledge. Nevertheless, each "infection survey" should attempt to define the most likely factor or factors responsible for any given infection. Only in this way can light be shed on the weak links in the aseptic chain and appropriate corrective measures undertaken.

Some of the more common factors predisposing to surgical infection are described.

Factors Intrinsic to the Patient

Debilitation. Any pathological condition that causes debilitation may predispose the patient to the development of a surgical infection. The exact reasons for this relationship are poorly understood. General immunity to infection appears to reside in the globulin fraction of the body's proteins and in the cells of the reticuloendothelial system. It may be that these immune mechanisms are somehow less effective because of the loss of proteins which occurs in the debilitated patient. Defects in phagocytosis due either to a deficiency of serum opsonins or to an abnormality of the phagocyte itself have also been suggested. Such conditions as malignancy, chronic intestinal disease with malabsorption, ulcerative colitis, or chronic infection are particularly apt to debilitate the patient and lower his resistance to infection. All attempts must be made to restore the patient's general health to normal prior to surgery. This may require a high protein diet, blood transfusions, albumin, high caloric infusates, vitamins, and antibiotics.

Anemia. Regardless of the cause of the anemic state, the patient with a low red cell volume is prone to infection. This may be indirectly due to the debilitating state attending the anemic condition or may be related to the anemia itself. Again, the mechanism of low resistance is not clearly understood but, empirically, red cell volume should be returned to normal, when feasible, prior to surgery.

Obesity. Some studies have associated obesity with a doubling of infection rate. Fat is notoriously avascular and for this reason probably has a low resistance to infection.

Leukopenia. Resistance to infection is intimately bound to the quantitative and qualitative status of the white corpuscles of the body. The phagocytic activity of the leukocyte, which engulfs and destroys invading bacteria, partially accounts for this resistance. Leukopenic states, accompanying blood loss, debilitation, or bone marrow depression, as well as faulty leukocyte development, as found in leukemia, are accompanied by a high incidence of wound sepsis following surgery.

Certain Metabolic Conditions. Two common conditions should be mentioned here.

Diabetes Mellitus. This is a very common metabolic disorder characterized by an insufficient supply of insulin which causes defective utilization of glucose and results in high levels of blood sugar. How this state results in a higher surgical sepsis rate is not clear. It may be related to the higher growth rate of bacteria in the presence of abnormally high glucose levels in the tissues. Moreover, the diabetic is prone to atherosclerosis which, of itself, predisposes to sepsis.

Vascular Insufficiency. Any condition resulting in poor blood supply to a part or organ of the body predisposes that part or organ to infection. In the aged patient, atherosclerosis is the most common cause of vascular insufficiency, and hence this disease becomes a frequent factor predisposing a patient to sepsis. The vascular insufficiency results in poor tissue nourishment and a decrease in all those general factors which bring about resistance to infection. In effect, the poorly vascularized organ or part is comparable to a debilitated, anemic patient.

Concurrent Infections. In spite of an otherwise clean surgical site, a patient with concurrent infections becomes a candidate for wound sepsis postoperatively. The most common such infection is a chronic pulmonary condition, such as bronchitis or a low-grade bronchopneumonia.

With each cough, such patients spread pathogenic bacteria on their clothing, bed linens, and surgical dressings, and frequently contaminate and infect their own wounds.

Local Tissue Factors. Tissues of high vascularity (e.g., the head and the face) are much more resistant to infection than those with a lower blood supply (e.g., the feet). As a general rule, tissue resistance is highest in the head and the neck, and becomes progressively lower as one approaches the feet. Location of a tissue near a contaminated area of the body (e.g., the groin, the axilla, the perineum) is also more apt to lead to infection than relatively cleaner areas.

Miscellaneous Factors. Other conditions which can result in a higher incidence of infection include prematurity, agranulocytosis, hypogammaglobulinemia, cutaneous anergy, deficiency in the cellular community, and lupus erythematosus.

Factors Relating to the Patient's Preparation for Surgery

Medical Preparation. From what has already been said, it is obvious that the detailed attention given to the patient's general state of health is related to his chances of resisting a wound infection. Such factors as general hygiene and nutrition, state of blood volume, presence or absence of infection, regulation of diabetes, etc., must be evaluated and controlled whenever feasible prior to surgery. For example, the patient with chronic lung disease who is about to undergo gastric resection should have a careful evaluation of his chest to determine the presence or absence of chronic bronchitis or low-grade bronchopneumonia. Sputum cultures should be taken preoperatively. If a serious pathogen (e.g., *Staphylococcus aureus,* coagulase positive) is isolated from the sputum, surgery should be deferred and chemotherapy instituted in an attempt to eradicate or minimize the pulmonary infection. Elderly males with chronic prostatic obstruction frequently harbor dangerous pathogens in their bladders. If there is the slightest suspicion of infection, a urine culture should be obtained preoperatively.

Preparation of Skin. Hair follicles harbor a high concentration of resident bacteria, and can be a source of wound infection. Failure to thoroughly shave all hair follicles may well make the difference between a clean wound and a secondarily infected one. If the skin is shaven more than 6 hours prior to surgery, extreme care must be used to prevent nicking or abrading the skin, as minor wounds permit rapid proliferation of resident bacteria from the skin and often become subclinically infected by the time the surgical incision is made.

Factors Relating to the Surgical Procedure

Breaks in Aseptic Technique. The innumerable potential breaks in aseptic technique constitute, as a whole, a most important predisposing cause of wound infection. These factors will be considered in later chapters. Suffice it to say here that the chain of aseptic technique is no stronger than its weakest link, and perpetual vigilance must be maintained in all areas of the technique.

Poor Surgical Technique. Local tissue resistance is directly related to the health of the local tissue. Any poorly conceived surgical technique which results in mishandling of tissues predisposes to surgical infection. This includes:

1. Rough handling of tissues.
2. Excess foreign body left in the wound which results from mass ligature of small bleeders, use of heavier suture than necessary, and failure to irrigate wounds.
3. Inadequate hemostasis, resulting in wound hematomas.
4. Failure to eradicate all dead spaces.
5. Inappropriate use of drains.

Factors Relating to the Causative Microorganism

Virulence. A given species or strain of pathogenic microorganisms will have a certain virulence or potency to infect. The incidence of wound sepsis following contamination is proportional to the relative virulence of the contaminating organisms.

Size of Inoculum. The body's resistance may be able to overcome a given number of bacteria or bacterial colonies. When this number is exceeded, resistance is destroyed and sepsis is established. Hence the size of the inoculum bears some direct relationship to the incidence of wound sepsis. From a practical point of view, this implies: (1) that surgery should be conducted as rapidly as is safely possible to minimize the number of contaminating organisms falling into the wound; and (2) that wounds should be thoroughly and frequently irrigated to reduce the size of the inoculum.

MICROORGANISMS OF SURGICAL IMPORTANCE

The student should have a general idea of the most important types of microorganisms capable of harming the surgical patient. Surgical sepsis, as here defined, will be limited to *those infections arising in a previously clean surgical site and related causally to the act of surgery.*

Although any pathogenic microorganism is capable — at least theoretically — of causing surgical sepsis, certain bacteria are frequent offenders (see Fig. 3-1), and this discussion will be limited to these bacteria. Each microorganism or group of microorganisms will be considered under four headings:

1. *Morphology and Types.* A brief description of the growth characteristics and major types found within a given class.

2. *Sources.* Knowledge of the major sources of these microorganisms serves to make the student more keenly aware of the rationale behind various aspects of aseptic technique.

3. *Pathogenicity.* This will include a description of the types, locations, and clinical manifestations of infections arising from each microorganism.

4. *Resistance.* The relative resistance of each microorganism to various methods of sterilization or disinfection will be mentioned.

THE STAPHYLOCOCCI

The staphylococci are ubiquitous microorganisms and represent the commonest cause of localized suppurative infections.

Morphology and Types

Staphylococci are gram positive cocci which occur in groups and resemble grape clusters under the microscope. They do not form spores and are almost always nonmotile. They fall into the class of organisms referred to as pyogenic (pus-forming), which also includes the streptococci, the pneumococci, the gonococci, and the meningococci.

One system of classifying the various types of staphylococci depends on the fact that different species form different types of pigmentation which are visible on agar media. Basically, there are three pigment types:

Staphylococcus aureus — golden pigmented forms.

No. of Isolates	Species	PENICILLIN P	BACITRACIN B	ERYTHROMYCIN E	TETRACYCLINE TE	CHLORAMPHENICOL C	STREPTOMYCIN S	NEOMYCIN N	LINCOMYCIN L	METHICILLIN DP	POLYMIXIN-B PB	COLISTIN CL	GENTAMYCIN GM	NITROFURANTOIN F/M	KANAMYCIN K	CEPHALOTHIN CR	AMPICILLIN AM	SULFATHIA ZOLE ST	CARBENICILLIN CB	CEPHALOGLYCIN CG
233	E-Coli	3			73	99	75				99	99	99	95	92	87	84	70	86	83
184	Staph Aureus	34	92	90	81	98	94	100	95	95						98	37			
92	Klebsiella				94	97	93				96	99	100	78	97	94	16	83	26	81
88	Enterobacter				80	98	91				91	97	100	80	98	38	29	85	65	48
83	Prot. Mirab.	73			3	94	93						100		98	92	94	89	94	85
78	S Epidermidis	51	93	92	55	94	93	91	92	95						97	57			
72	Pseud. Aerug.				18	25	44				100	99	100		13	4	3	90	91	
66	Strep Faecalis	83	65	69	31	90	3	6	6	1				83		66	93		19	67
10	Herellea				91	14	83				100	100	100		91	14	29	75	91	50
10	Escherichia				76	87	89				83	100	100	100	89	89	69	73	76	78
8	Serratia				20	100	100						100		100				80	
3	Mima				100	100	100				75	75	100		50	25	25		25	

SENSITIVITY
(PERCENT)

FIGURE 3-1 Microorganisms of surgical importance. This is a typical monthly report on organisms cultured throughout a community hospital. It indicates the frequency of the types of bacteria that are cultured and their sensitivity (in per cent) to commonly used antibiotics. This chart includes a profile of useful antibiotics for the staphylococcus organism.

Staphylococcus citreus — lemon-yellow pigmented forms.

Staphylococcus albus — white forms.

This classification is of clinical importance in that, for practical purposes, the only pathogenic form is *Staphylococcus aureus.*

When cultured on blood agar, some staphylococci will cause hemolysis of the red cells, while other types do not. This hemolytic characteristic of some types also divides staphylococci into *hemolytic* and *nonhemolytic* types. Most hemolytic forms are also of the golden variety, and we may speak of *hemolytic Staphylococcus aureus* organisms.

Finally, some staphylococci are able to coagulate plasma, and this *coagulase-positive* characteristic is found associated with pathogenic forms of the organism. Thus the *hemolytic Staph. aureus coagulase positive* type is the most important pathogenic form.

Sources

Staphylococci are truly ubiquitous microorganisms, being found on walls, floors, ceilings, bed linens, and the patient's skin. They are also present as normal inhabitants of the upper respiratory tract. While most of these staphylococci are of the benign varieties (*Staph. albus* and *Staph. citreus*), nasal carriers are probably the most important single reservoir of pathogenic strains and hence the most important single source of staphylococcal infection in man. Nasal carrier rates within a hospital may reach 50 to 60 per cent. The nasal carrier transmits the organisms in the form of finely dispersed moisture droplets as he breathes, talks, or coughs.

Within the modern hospital, in which staphylococcal infections are often very prevalent, pathogenic strains are frequently found on wards, bed linens, and on the skin and clothing of carriers. These strains can be transmitted through the air clinging to dust particles, and rapidly make their way from one source, sometimes contaminating the entire hospital.

Pathogenicity

Wound Infections. These microorganisms can enter the body through the intact skin at the bases of hair follicles or sweat ducts. Localized pustules, furuncles, and carbuncles may result. The surgical incision also affords the staphylococci opportunity to invade the subepidermal tissues where localized necrotic abscesses may become established. The typical staphylococcal wound infection is odorless, erythematous, tender, and fluctuant, and creamy-yellow pus is produced in great abundance. This abscess may drain spontaneously, in which instance there may be very little in the way of fever, rapid pulse, or other signs of systemic toxicity.

Septicemia. More virulent strains of staphylococcus may break down local tissue barriers and invade the circulating blood. Marked systemic toxicity may result, with high fever, rapid pulse, and leukocytosis. Metastatic abscesses to various organs may occur, leading to the death of the patient. Sometimes these abscesses may be localized (e.g., perirenal abscess or subdiaphragmatic abscess), and treatment consists of appropriate surgical drainage.

Pneumonia. Staphylococcal pneumonia secondary to surgery is uncommon. It may result from a debilitating postoperative course or may be secondary to thoracic surgery. It is frequently characterized by multiple pulmonary abscesses and empyema.

Enteritis. Following a mechanical and chemical sterilization of the bowel for intestinal surgery, a fulminating overgrowth of highly resistant staphylococcal organisms may occur within the bowel. This leads to a widespread enterocolitis which is characterized by voluminous diarrheal stools, generalized sloughing of the intestinal mucosa, and a severe fluid and electrolyte imbalance. This condition is most apt to occur in the debilitated patient who has been maintained on a prolonged antibiotics sterilization regimen of the bowel prior to surgery.

Resistance

The staphylococci are more resistant to heat and chemical disinfectants than the vegetative forms of many other bacteria. Temperatures as high as 80°C. for 1 hour are often required to destroy all staphylococci. Nevertheless they do not form spores, and steam under pressure, at proper levels of temperature and time, is most effective.

THE STREPTOCOCCI

Streptococci may cause a variety of surgical infections, depending on the type of streptococcus, its virulence, and its location in the body.

Morphology and Types

These organisms are also gram positive cocci which appear in long chains resembling a necklace. They do not form spores and are almost always nonmotile. They are considered under the pyogenic class of microorganisms.

Classification of streptococci is very complex. On the basis of hemolysis, there are three types of streptococci:

1. *Beta hemolytic streptococci,* which produce a clear zone of hemolysis around each colony on the blood agar plate.

2. *Alpha hemolytic streptococci,* or *Strep. viridans,* which produce a zone of greenish discoloration around each colony.

3. The *anhemolytic* or *nonhemolytic type.*

The highly virulent pathogenic streptococci are usually of the *beta hemolytic* type.

Streptococci may also be classified, according to their optimum growth medium, into aerobic and anaerobic types (and a small group of microaerophilic ones). By far the majority of infections are due to the aerobic varieties, although very severe infections may result from anaerobic streptococci.

Sources

The primary source of pathogenic streptococci is the human upper respiratory tract. Direct hand-to-hand contact, moisture droplets, and dust-borne bacteria represent the three modes of contamination from one person to another. Measures to suppress dust formation and dust circulation are very important in the prevention of these infections in surgery. *Streptococcus faecalis* (Group D enterococci) is a normal inhabitant of the gastrointestinal tract and often causes infection when there is perforation of the intestinal tract.

Pathogenicity

Wound Infections. Pure cultures of streptococci are rarely found in surgical wound infections. Nevertheless the organism is frequently found in association with other infecting organisms. The streptococcus is less of a pus-former than the staphylococcus. The infection tends also to be less localized, and a diffuse erythema and cellulitis frequently surround the wound.

Several rarer and more virulent forms of streptococcal wound infections should be mentioned.

1. *Surgical Scarlet Fever.* This lesion is characterized by a spreading cellulitis with erythema, swelling, and bullous formation around the wound margins.

2. *Necrotizing Fasciitis.* This is an infection involving the epifascial areas of the surgical incision. Undermining of the skin by a spreading cellulitis occurs, and the skin margins become gangrenous. The final result may show multiple draining sinuses connected with necrotic underlying fascia.

3. Other lesions due to microaerophilic streptococci include chronic burrowing ulcer and chronic progressive cutaneous gangrene (Meleney's gangrene). This latter is due to the synergistic activity of the microaerophilic streptococci and an aerobic hemolytic staphylococcus.

Septicemia. Signs of systemic involvement, with lymphangitis, lymphadenitis, and frank septicemia are more frequent with streptococcal than with staphylococcal infections.

Puerperal Fever. This is due to infection of the postpartum uterus with streptococcus.

Resistance

Streptococci are quite fastidious with respect to nutritive requirements and growth characteristics. They are easily destroyed with steam under pressure at proper levels of time and temperature. They are nonspore-formers, existing only in the vegetative forms.

THE ENTERIC BACILLI

The enteric bacilli are a large family of gram negative, nonspore-forming bacilli whose major source of origin is the gastrointestinal tract of man and animals. Often these gram negative bacilli are fairly innocuous, but in the presence of necrotic tissue and debilitation or when they migrate outside the gastrointestinal tract, serious wound infections, peritonitis, or cystitis may occur. It is not possible to describe the entire group of enteric bacilli in this manual. Four common pathogenic bacilli will be described. For more detailed discussion of these and other enteric bacilli, the student is referred to any standard textbook of bacteriology.

Morphology and Types

Four groups of organisms are common causes of surgical infections. These are: *Escherichia coli, Proteus vulgaris, Alcaligenes faecalis,* and *Aerobacter aerogenes.* They are all gram negative, nonspore-forming bacilli. Individual morphological differences will not be described.

Sources

The major source of these four organisms, as stated, is the gastrointestinal tract of man and animals. Patients undergoing any type of lower intestinal surgery may autoinfect their wounds. The organisms may also be transmitted to the wound from the hands of the scrub team. Other hospital sources include the linens and instruments used in the management of a patient with established gram negative bacilli infection.

Pathogenicity

Wound Infections. These are often necrotic purulent infections with a distinctly fecal odor. Such wound infections frequently follow intestinal surgery of a nonsterilized bowel, drainage of a ruptured appendix, or diverticulitis. They may sometimes arise without any apparent contamination from the gastrointestinal tract.

Urinary Tract Infections. Such infections often occur in the debilitated patient following catheterization of the urinary bladder. They may be relatively mild and asymptomatic infections or, at times, virulent and invasive, leading to gram negative septicemia and shock.

Peritonitis. Following perforation of the appendix or bowel, a severe form of generalized or localized peritonitis may occur. This is usually due to a mixed bacterial flora, with gram negative bacilli being frequent offenders.

Septicemia. The gram negative bacilli may become extremely virulent when in the presence of necrotic tissue. Frequently, following a urinary tract infection or an infected burn or wound, a gram negative septicemia occurs, with shaking chills, tachycardia, prostration, and profound circulatory collapse and shock.

Resistance

As with other nonspore-forming organisms, the enteric bacilli are highly susceptible to appropriate measures of sterilization and disinfection.

PSEUDOMONAS AERUGINOSA

The genus pseudomonas includes about 30 species found in water, soil, and decomposing organic matter. The only species pathological to man is *Pseudomonas aeruginosa.*

Morphology

The bacilli are usually small slender rods frequently united in pairs and short chains. They are gram negative bacilli, and are nonspore-formers. They form a blue-green pigment which diffuses throughout the growth medium.

Sources

Water, soil, and decomposing organic matter are the major sources. A large necrotic burn may contaminate an entire surgical ward and be the source of later infections in clean incisions. Likewise, the terminal patient with secondarily infected bed sores and urinary tract infection may be the offending source. Pseudemonas contamination of respirator and ventilator equipment is often a hazard to the comatose patient who not infrequently succumbs to a pseudomonas pneumonia.

Pathogenicity

Wound Infections. These organisms are frequently found as secondary invaders in an already infected, necrotic wound. Their presence is signaled by the development of a blue-green discoloration of the wound associated with an acrid musty odor.

Septicemia. Following a wound or burn infection with secondary overgrowth of virulent pseudomonas organisms, a generalized septicemia may develop, with metastatic abscesses occurring throughout the body and subcutaneous spaces. These abscesses cause local necrosis and vascular thrombosis which result in characteristic tender purple spots on the skin. This type of septicemia is extremely intractable to therapy and is usually a preterminal event.

Pneumonia. As has been mentioned, pneumonia caused by pseudomonas contamination can be fatal to the comatose patient. Respirator and ventilator equipment must be kept free of the pseudomonas pathogen.

Resistance

The vegetative bacteria are very susceptible to standard sterilizing measures.

CLOSTRIDIA

The spore-forming anaerobes are by far the most dangerous group of organisms in that they are highly resistant to all but the most intensive sterilization measures. This family of microorganisms includes the causative agents of tetanus and gas gangrene.

Morphology and Types

Clostridia are gram positive bacilli and are all spore-formers. The most common types are *C. welchii, C. novyi, C. septicum, C. sordelli,* and *C. tetani.*

Sources

The bacteria occur in the soil, particularly in manured soils, and in the intestinal tracts of men and animals. The spore forms may remain viable for years. Consequently, any patient infected with these clostridial organisms could conceivably act as a hospital focus for months or years after his discharge.

Pathogenicity

Tetanus. This is a disease characterized by marked spasms of the voluntary muscles of the body, particularly those associated with movements of the jaw (hence the synonym "lockjaw"). It is due to the clostridial organism *Clostridium tetani.* The clinical manifestations are due to a neurotoxin released by the tetanus organisms (exotoxin). The mortality rate following established infection may approach 50 per cent.

Gas Gangrene. This is a clinical syndrome which may follow dirty infected wounds. However, the organism may be a secondary invader of surgical incisions if contamination has occurred. The most frequently found clostridial organism is *Clostridium welchii,* but *C. novyi* and *C. septicum* may also be found in established cases. The clinical picture of gas gangrene is variable, usually consisting of a widespread necrotic, gangrenous, and crepitant wound, destroyed muscle and subcutaneous tissue; extreme prostration, profound shock, and death follow. The mortality rate is extremely high.

Resistance

The spore forms are highly resistant to sterilization and disinfection measures. A number of strains of *C. tetani,* for example, can resist steam at 100°C. for 40 to 60 minutes.

OTHER ORGANISMS OF SURGICAL IMPORTANCE

The discussion presented by no means exhausts the number of microorganisms capable of complicating surgical procedures. Other organisms occasionally causing postoperative surgical complications include the pneumococcus, the spirochetal organisms, the tubercle bacillus, the bacillus anthrax, and the virus of serum hepatitis.

MODES OF CONTAMINATION

The previous discussion of organisms responsible for surgical sepsis should give the student a healthy respect for these organisms and the disastrous results that follow any carelessness in aseptic techniques.

In spite of constant threat of surgical sepsis, it is axiomatic that infection *cannot occur* unless contamination exists. There are several modes of contamination which should be understood by the entire operating room team.

Direct Contact between a Nonsterile and a Sterile Surface

1. The surgeon's nonsterile back contacting sterile wash basin.
2. Bacterial seepage through moist linen.
3. A puncture in a sterile glove.
4. Possible contact by the circulating nurse with any sterile item passed to the scrub nurse.
5. The anesthetist contacting the top of the anesthesia screen.
6. Infected fluids from the patient contacting sterile gloves or instruments.
7. The surgeon's glove contacting the exposed skin of the patient.

Note. The student would do well to make a list of the countless other examples of this and other modes of contamination. (See Figs. 3–2 to 3–4).

Nonsterile Moisture Droplets Falling on a Sterile Surface

1. Droplets passing through the surgeon's or scrub nurse's mask.
2. Beads of perspiration falling into the wound from a member of the scrub team.
3. Respirations from the patient's unmasked mouth.
4. Perspiration occurring through a sterile gown.

Nonsterile Air Circulating over a Sterile Surface

Hematogenous.   From the patient's circulating blood.

SOURCES OF CONTAMINATION

The modes of contamination describe the way by which infecting organisms reach a sterile surface. The *sources* of contamination represent the reservoir from which these organisms arise. A

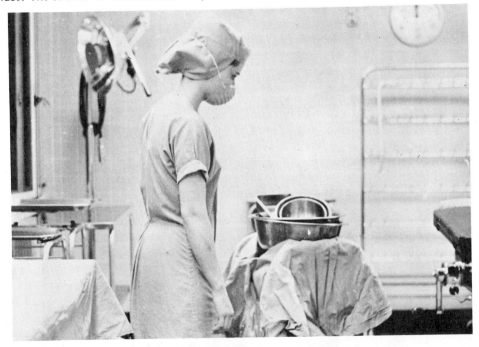

FIGURE 3–2 Mode of contamination: the nurse is passing too close to the sterile basin and the instrument table. The back of her non-sterile dress has contacted the sterile edge of the instrument table cover and contaminated it.

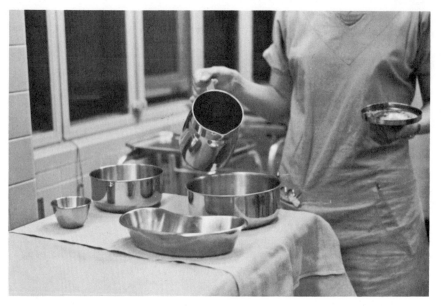

FIGURE 3–3 Mode of contamination: the nurse is standing too close to the sterile table. In addition, the non-sterile container she is holding is too close to the basin.

thorough understanding of the modes and sources of contamination will go far toward minimizing surgical sepsis. In Chapter 4, sterilization procedures will be discussed. Actually, the essence of aseptic technique consists of eliminating all the modes and sources of contamination to the extent that this is possible in the operating room. Therefore, the beginning of a knowledge of aseptic technique consists in a full knowledge of these sources of pathogenic bacteria.

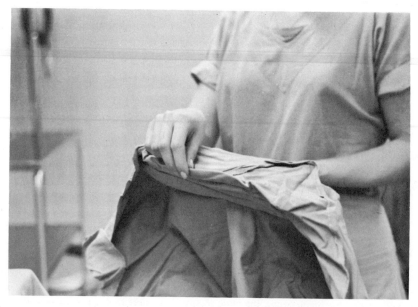

FIGURE 3–4 Mode of contamination: the nurse's index finger is contacting the sterile undersurface of the drape wrap.

There are fundamentally *ten sources* of contamination. These will be listed here along with a brief allusion to the method used to eliminate the source.

The Patient's Skin. All skin surfaces are contaminated with an abundance of pathogenic organisms, particularly the staphylococcus. The surgical incision will carry these organisms into the subcutaneous tissues of the body, thereby contaminating the deep surfaces of the incision and creating a potential wound infection. Consequently, the area of the proposed surgical incision must be thoroughly prepared and rendered surgically clean. Since the skin is *not* sterile, it should not be touched by the sterile gloved hand. Methods used to eliminate contamination from the skin include:

Mechanical. The skin is shaved and thoroughly washed prior to surgery.

Chemical. An antiseptic is liberally painted on the skin prior to surgery.

Draping. The surgeon drapes the skin edges except for a narrow slit through which the incision is to be made. Accessory sterile drapes are applied as soon as possible after the immediate skin edges are draped. Plastic drapes are now available for protection from contamination.

The Scrub Team's Skin. The members of the scrub team are likewise a potent source of contamination, and their skin must be thoroughly prepared prior to surgery. Methods used to prepare the skin include:

Mechanical. The hands and arms are thoroughly scrubbed with an appropriate soap or detergent.

Gowns, Gloves. Sterile gowns and gloves are donned to cover the exposed skin and outer clothing.

The Patient's Circulating Blood. Any septic process in the body is liable to be a source of contamination for the wound. This is elminated by treating any such infections prior to surgery.

The Patient's Respiratory Tract. An "ether" screen is used to segregate the patient's face and mouth from his incision. It is also advisable to have the patient wear a mask if this is feasible.

The Scrub Team's Respiratory Tracts. The surgical mask helps to reduce contamination from the respiratory trees of members of the scrub team. Limiting conversation will also help eliminate this source.

Linens, Instruments, Sutures. As these represent a potent source of contamination, all instruments, linens, sutures, et cetera, must be thoroughly sterilized prior to use.

The Circulating Air. Dust-borne bacteria are a major source of wound sepsis. To eliminate this source of contamination is most difficult. Measures include:

Thorough housecleaning and dusting frequently.

Proper ventilation within the operating room.

Ultraviolet disinfection where possible.

Reduction of traffic in and out of the operating rooms to a minimum.

Thorough cleaning of all air vents periodically.

The Patient's Gastrointestinal Tract. Surgery of the gastrointestinal tract presents a special infection hazard. The lumen of the gastrointestinal tract is a potent source of pathogenic microorganisms. This area becomes an inevitable source of contamination when the bowel is opened. Efforts to minimize contamination include mechanical and chemical disinfection of the gastrointestinal tract prior to surgery and extreme surgical care to drape off the remainder of the body when the intestinal tract is opened.

The Scrub Team's Hair. All hair must be carefully tucked under a cap or hood. Matter falling from exposed hair is heavily contaminated.

The Bronchial Tree. The threat of contamination is present whenever the bronchopulmonary tree is entered (as in a pneumonectomy). Contamination may lead to *empyema* accompanying wound infection.

SUMMARY

Chapter 3 has attempted, in concise form, to describe the entire picture of surgical sepsis and its relationship to the operating room. A great number of the actions, movements, and functions of the surgeon and his operating room team are directed solely toward the performance of aseptic surgery. A historical glimpse into surgery's past reveals the disastrous problems with sepsis, a common phenomenon less than 100 years ago. This historical summary lends perspective to the problem of surgical sepsis and acts as an added incentive for conscientious aseptic technique.

The factors predisposing to infection are legion and are poorly understood. It is obvious that contamination is not synonymous with infection. The general and local resistance of the patient, the virulence and size of inoculum of the contaminating organism, and a host of other poorly understood factors determine whether infection will occur. Nevertheless, knowledge of some of these predisposing factors will aid the nurse in anticipating the probability of surgical sepsis in her patient.

No attempt can be made in the brief summary of bacteriology given here to describe all those offending organisms responsible for surgical sepsis. Yet a brief summary of the features of the more common organisms should at least afford the nurse some idea of the widespread existence of these organisms and their damaging effect on the patient.

Finally, brief mention is made of modes and sources of contamination as this knowledge actually forms the basis of intelligent aseptic technique.

STUDY QUESTIONS

1. Much perspective can be gained by a historical analysis of surgical sepsis as outlined briefly in this chapter. As a class project, trace the works of one of the great bacteriologists or clinicians of the 19th century, such as Pasteur, Koch, or Lister.

2. List the significant advances made in aseptic technique, sterilization, and antisepsis in the past 25 years. On the whole, do you think substantial advances are still being made in the fight against surgical sepsis?

3. A 63-year-old obese diabetic female enters for vein ligation and stripping. What factors would you consider in assessing the chances of surgical sepsis developing in this patient postoperatively? What therapy should be instituted to eliminate or minimize these factors?

4. If surgical sepsis should occur in the incisions of the patient just mentioned, what organisms would you anticipate to be the most probable cause of the sepsis?

5. What is the most dangerous microorganism or family of microorganisms in surgical sepsis? Why?

6. A patient is being treated in a surgeon's office for a minor laceration. The surgeon sterilizes his instruments by placing them in boiling water for 15 minutes. Is this safe sterilization? What organisms, if present on his instruments, are liable not to be destroyed by this method?

7. What organisms are liable to be found in a surgical wound adjacent to a colostomy?

8. A 24-year-old male has suffered extensive 40 per cent second and third degree burns. On the fifth postoperative day his temperature is spiking to 103 and 104°F. A wound culture is taken. What organisms are likely to be found in the culture report?

9. What features of the burns described would lead you to believe that the dreaded pseudomonas organism has taken up residence in the burned areas?

10. Distinguish between vegetative and spore forms of bacteria.

11. Observe the scrub team carefully. Make a list of any possible breaks in aseptic technique and discuss them with your instructor.

12. Of all the sources of contamination, which one or ones is(are) the most difficult to eradicate? Why?

STERILIZATION, DISINFECTION, AND ANTISEPSIS

4

Operating room manuals are often unnecessarily crowded with sterilization data, and it is no small wonder that the student finds herself somewhat dismayed over this aspect of surgery. Much of the confusing data relate to: (1) standards of sterilization for individual items using a specific method of sterilization; (2) comparative potencies of various antiseptics and disinfectants; and, finally, (3) countless bar and line graphs demonstrating lethal effects of various agents on microorganisms.

While a certain amount of this information is necessary for clarity and completeness, it is the authors' opinion that such data should be relegated to charts and sterilization manuals kept at convenient locations within the sterilization rooms. These manuals can then be used as references for sterilization procedures.

This chapter, therefore, is not to be construed as a thesis on sterilization techniques. Nevertheless, it is hoped that a general survey of the field of sterilization, including disinfection and antisepsis, will serve to orient the student toward the important facets of this subject.

Before proceeding to the discussion of sterilization procedures, a few *definitions* are necessary:

1. *Microorganism.* As herein used, this term refers to any minute living organism, bacterial (microscopic) as well as viral (submicroscopic), including molds, yeasts, and parasites. With respect to bacteria, fungi, and yeasts, both vegetative and spore forms are included. In short, the term microorganism includes all forms of living organisms one may encounter in the operating room or on the wards.

2. *Vegetative Form.* The active phase in the life cycle of a living organism.

3. *Spore Form.* The inactive, resistant, or resting phase in the life cycle of certain organisms.

4. *Sterile.* The absence of all microorganisms, including bacteria, mold spores, and viruses.

5. *Sterilization.* The process or act of inactivating or killing all forms of microbial life; the process by which instruments, linens, or other objects are rendered sterile.

6. *Antiseptic.* A substance which, when applied to microorganisms of a pathogenic nature, either destroys or renders them innocuous by preventing or arresting their growth. The term is restricted to preparations which are applied to *living tissue* as, for example, the use of iodine as a skin antiseptic. It should be noted that antisepsis is not an absolute term such as sterility, and certain resistant forms of microscopic life may escape death or inhibition.

7. *Disinfection.* Refers to any process, chemical or physical, which results in the destruction of pathogenic organisms. A disinfectant is a chemical agent that destroys pathogenic organisms but not their spores. It is used on *inanimate objects,* e.g., the ability of formalin to disinfect a surgical instrument.

Note. Chemical disinfection differs from sterilization in its lack of sporicidal power. A few disinfectant chemicals do kill spores; however, this requires a high concentration of the chemical and many hours to do so.

8. *Surgically Clean.* This is a nebulous term referring to a surface, be it animate or inanimate, on which a *marked reduction* in the number of microorganisms has been effected by chemical, physical, or mechanical means. This reduction in the bacterial count of an object will minimize the disease-producing capabilities of the object — hence the term "surgically clean." However, it must be realized that a surgically clean area (such as the hands after a surgical scrub) is *not a sterile area,* and contact of the former with the latter is an act of *contamination.*

Sterilization, antisepsis, and disinfection can be brought about by a host of agents. New methods for achieving these desirable states for surgery are being developed constantly. The student should be familiar with the general principles of sterilization, as well as the uses and limitations of various sterilizing and disinfecting regimens. She should also be able to understand and operate the various steam sterilizers used in her hospital.

STERILIZATION BY HEAT

The Lethal Effects of Heat on Microorganisms

It is generally conceded that heat is one of the most effective and convenient methods for destroying microorganisms. The precise mechanism by which heat kills these organisms is not fully known. It may be due to denaturation (hydrogen bonds in the cell are broken by an external agent, e.g., heat or acid) of the critical genetic material in the organism. This directly results in the loss of the cell's ability to reproduce.

The death of a given bacterial or viral population subjected to heat is not a sudden event occurring at a given temperature. On the contrary, the time factor must also be taken into consideration. Thus, the longer a given bacterial population is subjected to an elevated temperature, the greater the death incidence within this population. This is known as the logarithmic order of death. It means that cells die in a geometric progression in which in each successive time interval the same number of remaining viable cells die.

Factors Determining the Thermal Resistance of Microorganisms

Several factors determine the length of time required to destroy a specific bacterial or viral population at a given temperature. A knowledge of these factors is of great practical importance in designing sterilization procedures.

Types of Heat. Steam under pressure and boiling water are forms of *moist heat.* Steam is inexpensive and sterilizes penetrable materials and exposed surfaces rapidly. This mode of sterilization is universally applied except when penetration of heat and moisture damage are factors. Steam is not toxic, is easily controlled, and requires very little operating expense. However, installation of costly equipment is necessary for routine use of this method. Suffice it to say that all living organisms can be rapidly destroyed in the presence of steam under pressure. Boiling water is not a good sterilizer because of its relatively low temperature. Its greatest advantage is its availability; but it takes an unrealistically long exposure time for microbial spores to be destroyed.

Dry heat is typically the oven type of apparatus. It is relatively slow as a sterilizer and requires higher temperatures of application. It will penetrate all kinds of materials, such as oils, petrolatum, and closed containers that are not permeable to steam. It destroys mainly by oxidation and coagulation of protein. Very little has been done in the last 10 years to improve this method of sterilization.

Temperature-Time. These two factors cannot be separated in one's thinking concerning minimal sterilizing standards. It is a false concept to consider *pressure* an essential factor. The importance of pressure is that it permits higher steam temperatures, without which no length of time would destroy certain highly resistant forms of life. But it is the *length of time at a given temperature* that determines the death of the organisms in question.

Wet Heat Destruction Variables

1. Species resistance means that certain organisms may produce cell or spore suspensions having widely different degrees of heat resistance.

2. Environmental conditions during growth and development include all conditions such as incubation temperature and the type of nutrient medium in which the cells or spores thrived.

3. Conditions present during the time of heating include variables such as level of pH, and nutrients present in the culture medium that might increase the species resistance to the heating process.

Recommended time-temperature relationships for sterilization with steam under pressure:

121°C.	15 minutes	at 15 lbs. per sq. inch on gauge
126°C.	10 minutes	at 10 lbs. per sq. inch on gauge
134°C.	3 minutes	at 29.4 lbs. per sq. inch on gauge

As a rule, then, exposure to 249°F. (120°C.) for 15 minutes is adequate for the destruction of both vegetative and spore forms of microorganisms.

Penetrating Ability of Sterilizing Agent. *Adequate sterilization can occur only when all surfaces to be sterilized come in contact with moist heat.* Consequently, the methods of packing the sterilizer to insure adequate exposure to moist heat assume major importance and will be discussed later in this chapter.

Dry Heat Destruction Variables

1. Cells or spores that are wet at the time of exposure to dry heat will only heat to the saturation temperature. This will exist as long as the cell cools itself by the process of evaporation.

2. Suspending materials give protection to spores, resulting in an increase in resistance over its nonprotected state.

3. Humidity (moisture in the environment) in the gas surrounding the cells or spores at the time of exposure to heat can affect the heat resistance of the cell. Increasing the humidity increases the resistance of the cell. An atmosphere of zero water content has greater lethal effects when combined with dry heat on the organism.

4. Death of microorganisms subjected to dry heat is based on their *loss of moisture* during the heating process. Denaturation occurs when this condition is present.

Recommended time-temperature relationships for sterilization with dry heat (Perkins, 1960):

170°C.	(340°F.)	60 minutes
160°C.	(320°F.)	120 minutes
150°C.	(300°F.)	150 minutes
140°C.	(285°F.)	180 minutes
121°C.	(250°F.)	Overnight

Principles of Steam Sterilization

Moist heat is commonly produced in the form of *saturated steam.* By pressurizing this steam, higher temperatures are possible. This saturated steam under pressure is the most dependable form of sterilization.

Initial Pressure. Steam sterilization begins when water is heated to 212°F. (100°C.), and it is converted to steam *at the same temperature.* As long as the pressure within the sterilizer remains atmospheric (normal), the temperature of the steam cannot rise above 212°F. *no matter how long the sterilizer is in use.* It would take many hours of sterilizing at this temperature to insure destruction of all forms of life (and there still would be doubts as to sterility) — very impractical in terms of operating room efficiency. This is the difficulty with boiling water sterilizers.

Increasing the Pressure. The steam is then submitted to increasing pressures within the sterilizer and this causes an increase in the temperature of the steam. Indeed, there is a quantitative and direct relationship of pressure to heat of steam. The higher the pressure in the sterilizer, the higher the temperature of the steam. In practice, this is calculated automatically on modern steam sterilizers.

Maintaining the Pressure. As steam enters the sterilizing chamber, the relatively cool air already present, being much heavier than steam, will be driven to the bottom of the chamber (Fig. 4-1).

If the air is allowed to remain in the chamber, it would eventually mix with the steam and a drop in temperature of the steam would occur. Therefore, at any given pressure, the temperature of steam mixed with cool air will be lower than if steam alone were present in the chamber. This problem is solved by an escape valve located at the bottom of the sterilizer which removes the cool air as it descends to the bottom of the chamber.

Transfer of Heat. The saturated steam permeates the material within the chamber and gives up its heat in the process. This transfer of heat from the steam to the material results in a condensation of the steam vapor back into water droplets which moisten the sterilized material. *Only those articles which are permeated and moistened by the steam will by adequately sterilized.* Here is another reason why air must be effectively and constantly eliminated from the chamber,

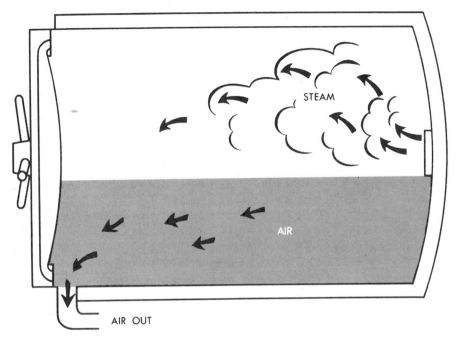

FIGURE 4–1 Under the "gravity displacement" system, steam entering under pressure at the rear of the sterilizer forces the heavier air ahead of it down and forward until it is discharged from a port at the front of the sterilizer. The system works well in the empty chamber in which minimum air-steam mixing takes place. (Courtesy Wilmot-Castle Company.)

for its presence blocks the permeation of fabrics by the steam. To be certain that the air discharge valve is functioning, a temperature-determining device is located on the air discharge valve. This temperature gauge will show increasing temperatures as the cool air is drawn out, because this air will be increasingly representative of the saturated steam being pumped into the chamber. When the drain thermometer indicates 121°C. it is assured that the chamber is at the proper temperature to sterilize.

Drying the Articles. Following sterilization, the sterilizer door is opened but the pack is left untouched for 30 minutes. This delay allows the articles to dry out, thus avoiding recontamination which would occur if the steaming pack were to contact a cool nonsterile surface.

Summary of Principles of Steam Sterilization

1. Water is heated, converting it to steam.

2. Steam is driven into a sterilizer under increasing pressures, raising the temperature of the steam to the desired levels by a proportional rise in steam pressure.

3. Cool air in the sterilizer is allowed to escape from the bottom of the chamber.

4. The temperature gauge on the air outlet valve is carefully checked to be sure it is increasing to chamber temperature levels, thus assuring that the air is being removed from the chamber.

5. Operation of the chamber is continued at the prescribed temperature and time for sterilization.

6. The sterilized articles are allowed to dry out by opening the chamber door while leaving the articles in the chamber untouched for a designated period of time.

Basic Designs and Operations of Modern Steam Sterilizers

Steam sterilizers include two types:

a. The manually operated downward or gravity displacement type, and

b. The fully automatic, high-vacuum, high-pressure sterilizer.

The standard steam pressure sterilizer for surgical supplies is the steam jacketed or double wall type. The body of the sterilizer consists of a sterilizing chamber surrounded by a steam jacket, creating, as it were, a cylinder within a cylinder.

The inner and outer chambers, the backhead, and the door are made of Monel metal welded together into a seamless unit for greater structural strength.

Pressure is first generated in the outer chamber or jacket space and is not permitted to enter the inner chamber until the proper pressure range has been obtained in the jacket. This prevents condensation from forming on the inner walls of the chamber, thus diminishing the amount of moisture contacting the material to be sterilized.

The modern sterilizer has a pressure-locked safety door which is automatically sealed when the chamber pressure is applied and which can be unlocked only by exhausting the chamber pressure.

Temperature and pressure gauges are found at convenient locations on the front of the sterilizer. The temperature of the air outflow line (usually found below the door of the sterilizer) must be maintained at 250°F. (121°C.). Jacket and chamber pressures are maintained at proper levels automatically.

Steam from the main line is admitted at the bottom of the steam jacket. In beginning operation with a cold sterilizer, steam is first admitted from the supply line to the jacket, with the connection to the chamber closed, until the jacket pressure becomes constant at 15 to 17 pounds per square inch gauge pressure. The load is placed in the chamber, and the door is locked immediately after the jacket has attained proper pressure. The operating valve is turned to "sterilize," permitting jacket steam to enter the inner chamber. The air within the chamber gravitates to the bottom and is forced out through the chamber.

The temperature will advance to 250°F. (121°C.) within 5 to 10 minutes, at which point timing of the period of sterilization begins. When the period of sterilization is complete, steam is exhausted from the chamber, the door is opened, and the materials are allowed to dry.

The high-vacuum, high-pressure sterilizer was developed in the early 1960's. It operates in this manner:

a. Air is drawn out of the sterilizer by means of a vacuum pump.

b. Steam is allowed to penetrate all portions of the load until the preset temperature is reached.

c. The sterilizer temperature (121°C. for 15 minutes; 135°C. for 3 minutes) is maintained for the determined time.

d. Venting is used to remove steam and excess moisture and to cool the load.

e. Sterile air is admitted through bacterial retentive filters.

f. The door can be opened.

One advantage of this type of sterilizer is the fast sterilizing time. Also, it can process larger volumes of materials in a period of a day than the downward displacement type, and there is less damage to materials because of the short time of exposure to high heat. There is greater assurance of sterilization with this type of sterilizer (Fig. 4–2).

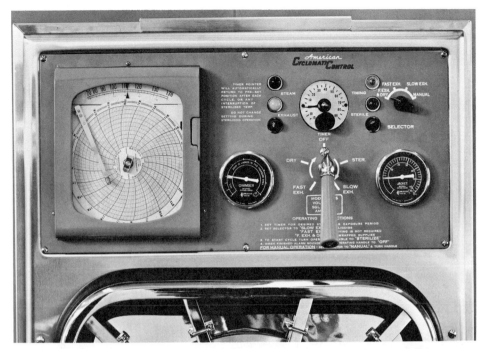

FIGURE 4–2   Control panel on a steam sterilizer. (Courtesy American Sterilizer Company.)

PREPARATION OF COMMON SURGICAL SUPPLIES FOR HEAT STERILIZATION

Dressings and Other Dry Goods

The principle of effective sterilization by moist heat depends, as was stated earlier, on *direct contact and permeation of every part* of a pack or item to be sterilized. The importance of this principle cannot be overemphasized. Its practical counterpart is this: all packs to be sterilized must be of such a *size, content, density,* and *covering* and must be *so arranged* in the sterilizer as to permit the rapid and effective flow of steam through the sterilizer. Strict adherence to this rule will insure safe and complete sterilization at the prescribed temperature-time standards.

Size of Packs. The largest pack should not exceed 12 by 12 by 30 inches for routine work. Larger packs run the risk of blocking the flow of steam from top to bottom and allowing air to diffuse out, resulting in questionable sterility of the articles.

Content and Density of Packs. The exact content of a pack depends, of course, on the purpose of the pack, and is variable from one hospital to another. Several things to remember:

1. Basins and other metallic or porcelain articles should not be included in the same pack with fabrics. The basins interfere with steam permeation of surrounding fabrics, and they also retard drying following sterilization.

2. Table drapes, gowns, and sheets are of such dense quality as to interfere with steam permeation of other articles. It is advisable to wrap these items in separate packs containing no more than two drapes or sheets each.

3. The density of the pack is determined both by its absolute size and by the arrangement of articles within it. Density can be decreased by arranging the articles in alternate layers within the pack, thus allowing "spaces" for the rapid passage of steam (Fig. 4–3).

Packaging Materials. There are three types of covers available at present:

Muslin (cloth). A covering of this type consists of two thicknesses of quality muslin. The

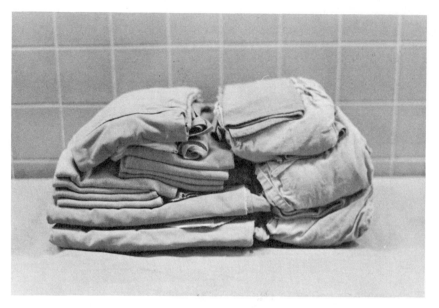

FIGURE 4–3 Standard gown and sheet pack. Note alternation of layers for better ventilation and steam penetration.

weave of the muslin permits easy steam passage, while at the same time it acts as a dust filter. The muslin must be checked for wear and tear and replaced when necessary. Cord is used to bind the pack or the corners are folded so as to make the pack self-binding. Pins should be avoided since the pinholes may result in contamination. Pressure-sensitive tape may be used on the pack to monitor sterilization; the color change on the tape will indicate that the pack has been sterilized.

Plastic. This material is used to cover the catheters and tubing. It is intended for use on large packs that are to be sterilized by heat. The edges of the plastic are rolled over and taped or vented with cotton in the spaces.

Paper. Envelopes for gloves and wrappings for some items can be made of paper. This material, if it is kept dry and is fairly dense, will provide good protection. It is porous to heat and moisture and has an adequately long shelf life.

Arrangement of Load in Sterilizer. The individual packs must be so loaded in the sterilizer as to permit rapid permeation of the steam *in and around* each pack. All packs should be resting on edge, in loose contact with each other. Large packs should be placed in the steilizer in one layer only. When upper layers are placed, they should be positioned crosswise to the lower layer. Jars and other nonporous containers are placed horizontally on edge for easy egress of air and moisture.

Drying of Load Following Sterilization. There are many methods used for drying the sterilized load. The simplest method is to open the sterilizer door after the unit has been turned off and steam has been exhausted. The moisture on the packs will then evaporate as the retained heat is dissipated. The load should not be touched for 30 minutes. A moist or damp load should never contact a nonsterile surface, as the moisture of condensation may result in contamination by capillary attraction.

Rubber Goods

Gloves. Most hospitals today have invested in pre-packaged, sterile, disposable rubber gloves. This eliminates the time-consuming and costly aspects of having personnel wash, pack, and sterilize gloves. In addition, heat has been found to be too damaging to gloves; it deteriorates the rubber. It is also most difficult to ensure steam penetration of each finger cot in the glove.

Rubber Catheters, Drains, and Tubes. As is the case with surgical gloves, most institutions now use sterile, pre-packaged, disposable rubber goods. Rubber articles are easily corroded by chemical agents. The following agents are very damaging to rubber:

1. Mineral oil, petrolatum, and other petroleum jellies.
2. Ether, acetone, benzene.
3. Acids.
4. Lysol, carbolic acid, hexachlorophene.
5. Benzalkonium chloride.

There are many others.

Surgical Instruments

Most instruments can be sterilized by heat. Exceptions are: (1) those instruments containing prisms and other lenses which are cemented in place, (2) sharp instruments, and (3) complicated instruments containing various serrated edges and complex locking devices.

Those instruments which are sterilized by heat are passed through the following routine:

1. Gross soil is removed manually or in an automatic instrument washer-sterilizer.
2. The instruments are next processed through an ultrasonic cleaner and a lubricating cycle.
3. The instruments are then packaged and passed through the main sterilizer.

High speed sterilization is often necessary in an emergency situation. So called *flash sterilizers* develop a temperature of 270°F. and sterilization occurs in 3 minutes. The substerilizing rooms found adjacent to each operating room are usually equipped with flash sterilizers. Their basic operation is similar to that of the main sterilizers.

STERILIZATION BY GAS

Ethylene oxide, a gas with a high sterilizing potential, was introduced into hospitals by 1956. It will safely sterilize endoscopes, woven catheters, ampules, polyethylene catheters, laryngoscopes, reservoir bags, face masks, suction catheters, embolectomy catheters, pacemakers, and other such items without damaging them.

Some of its *advantages* are:

a. It has good penetrating ability.
b. There is quick loss of residual gas after objects are removed from the sterilizer.
c. Objects can be wrapped loosely in paper and be sterilized.
d. As long as their depths are not too great, extraneous materials (feces, soil, or biological media) cannot be considered a hindrance to sterilization.
e. It is effective against all types of organisms.

Some *disadvantages* include:

a. It requires humidity levels of 30 per cent to sterilize rapidly.
b. Rubber goods have been found to adsorb the gas and retain it from 5 to 24 hours after the sterilization procedure. Chemical burns have occurred when these items have been handled during this post-sterilization period.
c. Recommended aeration times for various articles must be followed scrupulously.

CHEMICAL DISINFECTION OF SURGICAL MATERIALS

Disinfection by chemical means is indicated whenever materials or instruments cannot be sterilized by heat or irradiation. However, *disinfection* remains in a different category from sterilization. Disinfection can destroy bacteria, but does not have sporicidal power. A few chemicals do kill spores but it takes a high concentration of the chemical and many hours to do so. In the absence of a gas sterilizer in the hospital, some form of chemical disinfection is required.

Factors Determining Disinfecting Abilities of a Chemical

Chemicals apparently destroy or inhibit the growth of bacteria and other microorganisms by protein coagulation or enzyme inhibition. Basically, then, the same factors operative in the efficiency of heat as a sterilizing agent will be found here. These factors are:

Type of Object to be Disinfected

1. *Easiest.* A clean object with a smooth, flat, and firm surface, e.g., a scalpel blade.
2. *Most Difficult.* Grossly soiled, complicated, hinged instruments, e.g., a von Petz gastrectomy clamp, hypodermic needles, long tubing with a narrow lumen, and lensed instruments.

Type and Number of Microorganisms

1. The higher the bacterial or viral contamination, the more difficult to effectively sterilize.
2. Vegetative bacteria are relatively easy to destroy; certain viral forms cannot be destroyed, and most spores are very resistant to chemical disinfectants.

Type of Chemical. This includes the nature of the disinfectant, the concentration, and the time of disinfection.

Properties of Frequently Used Chemical Disinfectants

Mercurials. Compounds of bichloride and cyanide are the most commonly used mercurials. They are *poor disinfectants* and should not be used.

Phenols. These are fairly active germicides, but *do not kill spores.* They are bactericidal to most vegetative forms as well as to the tubercle bacillus. They may be used to disinfect feces, floors, and walls. Phenolic derivatives include cresols, Lysol, and hexachlorophene.

Chlorine Compounds

1. *Sodium Hypochlorite* (1:1000 sol.). May be used to wash furniture and floors, particularly following septic cases. It is also virucidal in its action. This substance is *highly corrosive* to instruments, and must not be used for cleaning them.
2. *Chlorinated Lime* (30 to 35 per cent calcium hypochlorite). Used on household articles in the hospital.

Formaldehyde. It is a strong, irritating, fumigant gas. The solution is known as *formalin* and is an excellent *disinfectant and a fair sporicide.* Combining formalin (20 per cent) with alcohol (70 per cent) increases its disinfecting qualities. Indeed, formalin plus alcohol is the *strongest chemical disinfectant* available, and is used mainly in the sterilization of cystoscopes, woven catheters, and other items. Time required for sterility may be 18 hours or more. Formaldehyde is highly damaging to tissues, and cannot be used as an antiseptic. This means that disinfected materials must be thoroughly rinsed before use.

Iodine. Iodine may be used both as a disinfectant and as an antiseptic. An iodine solution of 0.5 to 1.0 per cent in 70 per cent alcohol is the agent of choice in disinfection of clinical thermometers. Two per cent iodine may be sporicidal.

Alcohols. Ethyl and isopropyl alcohols are excellent germicides, destroying vegetative bacteria as well as the tubercle bacillus. They are not sporicidal. Concentrations must not go below 60 per cent in order to remain bactericidal.

Quaternary Ammonium Compounds. The best known of these substances is Zephiran chloride. In 1:750 aqueous solution, it is an excellent germicide for ordinary vegetative bacteria.

STERILIZATION, DISINFECTION, AND ANTISEPSIS 47

However, it does not affect the tubercle bacillus, and is not a sporicide. It is frequently used as a skin antiseptic in preparing the skin several days before surgery. It may also be used as an instrument disinfectant, such as for treating cystoscopes. Anti-rust substances are added to Zephiran when metal is being disinfected.

Activated Glutaraldehyde. This is an economical, noncorrosive, nonirritating agent. It is bactericidal, fungicidal, sporocidal, and virucidal. These qualities make activated glutaraldehyde an excellent disinfectant for instruments. A two per cent solution is harmless to lenses and cement mountings, and it will not interfere with electrical conductivity.

SKIN ANTISEPTICS

Disinfectants which are not irritating or corrosive to the skin may also be used as antiseptics. Some of the commonly used antiseptics and their major properties include:

Ethyl Alcohol. A 70 per cent solution is a most satisfactory skin antiseptic. It is nontoxic, inexpensive, and easy and pleasant to use. It is extremely bactericidal, even to the tubercle bacillus. It is not sporicidal.

Isopropyl alcohol disinfects the skin as well as ethyl alcohol. It should be used in concentrations of 70 to 99 per cent for bactericidal action. This increases with the concentration. It does tend to "defat" the skin and leave it dry when used repeatedly. For this reason it is not recommended as a routine hand antiseptic. It may be valuable in the preparation of the patient's skin at the time of surgery.

Zephiran. This is also a very useful and potent antiseptic. However, it has the peculiar property of being rendered ineffective if mixed with any soap or detergent. Even a thin film of residual soap will markedly reduce its bactericidal effects. Rinsing the skin with water will not guarantee the removal of residual soap. It is best to rinse the hands with alcohol, as this is the most effective soap solvent, and then apply Zephiran.

Antiseptics Containing Mercury. These are poor antiseptics and should not be used.

Iodine. One to 2 per cent iodine in 70 per cent alcohol (tincture) is an excellent skin antiseptic. Adding potassium iodide to this tincture makes it superior as an agent.

SUMMARY

Chapter 4 has surveyed the field of sterilization, disinfection, and antisepsis. It was pointed out that disinfection and antisepsis do not imply complete eradication of all forms of life, as does sterilization. Certain viruses, hardy vegetative forms (e.g., tubercle bacillus), and most spores are able to survive the germicidal powers of some disinfectants and antiseptics. Sterilization, then, is a far superior process, but has limitations in its applicability. Indeed, the various modalities of sterilization, disinfection, and antisepsis have been developed to cover certain specific situations. These may be summarized as follows:

Antisepsis **Use on Skin and Tissues**
1. Ethyl and isopropyl alcohol (70 per cent).
2. Zephiran, aqueous solution 1:750.
3. Iodine, 1 or 2 per cent solution in 70 per cent alcohol.

Disinfection   **In the Absence of a Gas Sterilizer, Use Chemical Disinfectants on**

1. Endoscopes.
2. Masks.
3. Catheters.
4. Heat-labile plastic and certain rubber goods.
5. Thermometers.
6. Floors, walls, furniture, feces et cetera.

Sterilization

Gas. May be used, if available, for all articles under "Disinfection." It may be preferable to chemical disinfection.

Steam Under Pressure. The main form of sterilization, applicable to everything else not already named.

STUDY QUESTIONS

1. Take a tour through your hospital's sterilization rooms. Give a report to your class on the types of sterilizers used, their location, and their method of operation.

2. Review your bacteriology textbook. List as many characteristics of the spore as you can. What spores are apt to be of surgical importance?

3. A surgical instrument is "sterilized" by immersing for 5 minutes in 1:750 solution of Zephiran. What organisms may still be present on this instrument, and what dangers, if any, could result from its use?

4. Describe the effects of pressure in a steam sterilizer with respect to the sterilizing ability of steam.

5. List five errors in arranging of packs in a sterilizer and how these may adversely affect its sterilizing abilities.

6. List the qualities of an ideal disinfectant. Is there such a chemical available?

7. Distinguish between a disinfectant and an antiseptic.

8. What disinfectants and antiseptics are used in your hospital? Do you think these are the best available? Explain your answer.

9. What is a gas sterilizer? List its advantages and disadvantages over the conventional steam sterilizers.

10. What, in your opinion, would be the best agent for the surgical scrub? For the skin preparation?

11. Are the agents in question 10 used in your hospital? If not, explain the advantages of the ones used in your hospital over the ones listed in question 10.

12. A 74-year-old female develops a gram negative wound infection following an elective bowel resection for carcinoma. Considering the modes and sources of contamination as described in Chapter 3, as well as the factors predisposing to wound infection, list as many sources as possible and the modes of contamination that may have led to sepsis in this case.

13. What factors predisposing to infection are actually present in the patient just described?

14. Does the presence of a *gram negative* infection lend any clues as to the source of infection in this patient?

PREPARATION OF THE PATIENT FOR SURGERY

5

PSYCHOSOMATICS AND SURGERY

Perhaps in no other field is the concept of psychosomatics — the interrelationship of body and mind — so evident as in surgery. Both before and after surgery the patient's will to survive, to cooperate, and to recover can turn an otherwise major surgical procedure into a smooth postoperative recovery and convalescence.

The mind, no less than the body, must be adequately prepared for the impending operation. Such "trivia" as an intravenous medication or a Foley catheter — trivia to the nurse and the doctor because they are accustomed to these "routine measures" — may appear to the patient as signs of a grave situation. A *simple* word of explanation may dispel these fears and offset the development of serious anxiety.

Indeed, *explanation* and *teaching* are the key words in the psychological preparation of the patient for surgery. However commonplace a procedure may appear to the medical personnel, it is strange and unknown to the patient. This unfamiliarity must be appreciated, anticipated, and resolved. Such is the prime duty of the nurse and the physician who attend the surgical patient.

The physiological preparation of the patient must be integrated with his psychological preparation. This often consists in explaining and teaching about each step, each test, and each procedure before it occurs. Tests are often complex and must be adequately understood by the nurse if she is to successfully explain them to the patient. Moreover, she must have thorough knowledge of the surgical procedure to be experienced by the patient so that she may answer his questions logically and accurately. The patient must be *taught* the information (and the procedures) that will be necessary to his successful postoperative convalescence.

INTERVIEWING THE PATIENT

The interview has several purposes:

1. To establish rapport with the patient and gain his confidence.

2. To obtain a general idea of the patient's imminent surgery. It may be that surgery is not planned for several days, and will follow an intensive diagnostic evaluation. Nevertheless, the nurse should have some idea of the sequence of events to be followed by the physician.

3. To evaluate the patient's personality, particularly with respect to his motivation to cooperate in the postoperative period.

4. To reassure the patient concerning his surgery. The patient and his family may have several questions which can be answered in general terms.

5. To determine the presence of drug allergies or allergies to other substances, such as adhesives or iodine.

6. To determine whether the patient has had any previous major illnesses or operations.

7. To determine any particular medications which the patient has taken or is now taking.

8. To determine the patient's weight and vital signs. These may be important baselines, particularly in evaluating any possible postoperative complications.

9. To determine any dietary restrictions.

A purposeful interview will go far toward determining any sort of problem that may follow the surgical procedure. More importantly, the manner in which this interview is carried out will, in large part, determine the degree of anxiety which the surgical procedure will engender in the patient. *In no area of surgical care are the nurse's services more valuable than in this subtle creation of confidence and security in the patient.*

PREOPERATIVE TEACHING

The preoperative phase allows time for the patient to ponder the circumstances which have brought him to hospitalization and to speculate on what he may feel to be an uncertain future. His lack of medical knowledge may cause him to regard his care and the people who administer it with an unrealistic perspective.

The more the nurse can teach the patient during this preoperative phase, the more she can alleviate his uneasiness in an unaccustomed situation, an uneasiness which can promote fear or even panic. The patient should be given a realistic appraisal of the events to come in an effort to reduce his preoperative and postoperative anxieties.

The patient's active cooperation and participation can be elicited provided he is given sufficient information about what is required of him in the way of responding to the nurses and doctors in the recovery area. It is to the nurse's advantage if, through skillful interviewing techniques, she can determine just how much information the patient truly wishes to know. It may be difficult prior to surgery to adequately prepare a patient physically or psychologically; there may be a lack of professional staff on the clinical unit to carry out this aspect of care, or the patient may arrive the evening before the scheduled surgery and undergo a myriad of tests in a short period of time. Alternatively, the surgeon's explanation of the operation and of the anesthesia to be administered may not be entirely adequate.

Clearly, an organized plan for teaching the patient what he will need to know is of prime importance. While the plan should be flexible enough to permit individualized teaching, certain guidelines should be followed. There should be:

1. A time set aside for discussion and explanation of the problem which has led to the need for surgery.

2. A definition and explanation of the surgical procedure.

3. A presentation of information that will ease the patient's anxiety and prepare him in the best way possible for the postoperative interval.

4. A discussion of what the patient may expect in the recovery room or intensive care unit.

5. A discussion of the patient's responsibilities in self-care upon his return to the clinical unit after surgery.

It is helpful for the patient to be told that he may not remember every detail that is presented to him. He should be assured that he will be able to recall his instructions as necessary in the course of his postoperative care.

The nurse will want to keep in mind certain points involved in teaching the patient:

1. Before beginning instruction, confer with the doctor and determine what he has told the patient.

2. Through interviewing the patient and conferring with his surgeon, determine the amount of knowledge that the patient should be given — what he wants to know and what he needs to know. Too much knowledge can increase anxiety prior to surgery. It is occasionally easier for some patients to accept aspects of postoperative care without advance knowledge of the nature of the care.

3. The patient may have difficulty in understanding your instructions if you are too technical in your use of medical jargon and unfamiliar terminology. Speak casually and clearly!

4. Provide information in small doses. Even in capsule form, it may be overwhelming.

5. In these days of hurrying and rushing, the patient may not be asked to identify his own personal fears or areas of hazy understanding. Be sure to allow ample time preoperatively for his questions. He will most often have questions about the recovery room, the intensive care unit, the surgical procedure, and how long it will take him to recover from the anesthesia.

6. What you teach the patient and what he understands and interprets may be entirely different. Question the patient to ensure that he has adequately absorbed all new explanations and demonstrations.

7. Have the patient practice new procedures and skills which you have taught him.

8. Since a high anxiety level may impede quick learning and retention of new information, you should expect to repeat your teaching and demonstration of skills more than once.

9. Do not treat all patients in the same manner; do not use the same teaching procedure for all your patients. Use variety in your teaching methods.

Ideally, the nurse who has done most of the patient's preoperative teaching should visit him every day, or at least on the first day he is in the recovery room. This will afford the patient an opportunity to relate his feelings and ask pertinent questions of the one individual who has probably best understood him or become most therapeutic to him in the preoperative phase of his care.

The nurse's preoperative preparation of the patient should involve the patient's family as well. The family should be included when preoperative teaching is in actual progress. On the day the patient undergoes surgery, the nurse should visit with the family (when possible) to answer their questions about the postoperative period. The visit by the nurse can supplement that of the doctor, and she can clarify any issues about which the family may be concerned. The nurse should be honest with the family. This will provide reassurance to the anxious family and will demonstrate an attitude of concern on the part of the nurse. The family should be kept informed of the patient's daily progress.

The quality of preoperative teaching will be reflected most of all in the postoperative situation and in the patient's responses to and degree of cooperation with those who care for him in the recovery room. The nurse's duties as a "teacher" will vary with each patient, but certain of her obligations can be readily summed up. The nurse should:

1. Highly motivate the patient to learn new concepts and/or skills.

2. Actively involve the patient in the learning process so that he is not a passive onlooker.

3. Teach at the intellectual level of the patient.

4. Begin with familiar ideas and then proceed to new material or unfamiliar ideas or skills.

5. Present information in such a way that the patient will have the use of many of his senses in the learning process. All the audiovisual materials that are available should be used.

6. Repeat instruction to the patient on a few occasions or visits.

7. Teach new skills in a step-by-step fashion (new motor skills must be mastered in a logical progression).

8. Expect a demonstration by the patient of the exact technique or skill that the nurse has taught him. The nurse must make sure that the patient knows what is expected of him.

REVIEWING THE PHYSICIAN'S HISTORY AND EXAMINATION

It is imperative that the nurse have a thorough knowledge of the past and present physical status of her patient. This requires a careful review of the physician's interview and examination of the patient. While differing in minor details, this work-up follows a definite pattern as follows.

Chief Complaint and Present Illness. This section describes the reason or reasons which prompted the patient to seek medical aid and led, finally, to his admission to the hospital. The illness may be very brief or extremely complex and chronic. Any medications or previous surgery experienced by the patient for his present illness will also be documented in this part of the work-up and will afford the nurse some idea of the gravity of the illness, its duration, and its previous treatments. This is vital information for proper management, and must be thoroughly understood by the nurse responsible for patient care.

Review of Systems. Any symptoms not directly pertinent to the present illness are recorded here. These symptoms may afford clues to other underlying diseases which could have a bearing on the postoperative course. If these symptoms appear to be significant to the physician, he will futher evaluate them with other diagnostic tests before proceeding with the operation. The nurse should be familiar with major symptom patterns and the probable organ pathology causing these symptoms. While a thorough discussion of this subject is outside the scope of this manual, certain points should be noted:

> *Cardiorespiratory Disease Patterns.* Look for cough, wheezing, shortness of breath, inability to lie flat in bed without shortness of breath (orthopnea), ankle edema, cyanosis, clubbing of fingers, history of excessive smoking, history of asthma, chest pain on exertion, and barrel chest. If one or more of these symptoms are encountered, the nurse should be on guard for postoperative cardiorespiratory difficulties.
>
> *Genitourinary Disease Patterns.* Look for frequency of urination, difficulty in voiding, burning on urination, and nocturia. In the middle-aged or elderly male these symptoms are particularly apt to suggest enlargement of the prostate which may lead to acute postoperative urinary retention or urinary tract infection.
>
> *Hematologic Disease Patterns.* Look for excessive and easy bruising, past history of excessive bleeding, and family history of excessive bleeding. If present, these symptoms should suggest the possibility of postoperative bleeding, wound hematoma formation, et cetera.
>
> *Renal Disease Patterns.* In contradistinction to urinary problems which suggest mechanical difficulty with the prostate, here one should consider previous

disease states in the kidney, such as pyelonephritis or glomerulonephritis. Look for periorbital edema, cloudy urine, ankle edema, high blood pressure, and past history of rheumatic or scarlet fever. If any of these signs or symptoms are present, close observation for postoperative renal failure is important.

Allergic Disease Patterns. Look for symptoms of hives, dermatitis, or other skin lesions, and allergies to various foods or drugs. If present, care should be taken to rule out possible allergic states to any drugs used during the patient's hospital stay.

Neurological Disease Patterns. The major symptoms and signs are severe headaches, dizzy spells, lightheadedness, ringing in the ears, unsteady gait, unequal pupils, previous convulsive states. While infrequent in patients not undergoing neurosurgery, these symptoms should be carefully sought. They may suggest extremely serious diseases which could lead to grave morbidity postoperatively.

Metabolic Disease Patterns. Except for diabetes mellitus, these conditions are rare and obscure, and will not be covered here. Diabetes should be suspected in any patient with polydipsia, polyphagia, and polyuria, particularly the elderly one with vascular problems or hypertension. Obese females and those with a family history of diabetes are also suspect.

Vascular Disease Patterns. Look for cold, pale feet, absent or diminished peripheral pulses, cyanosis or flushing of the extremities, and leg cramps on walking. Particular attention should be paid to leg and foot care in the postoperative period in any patient demonstrating one or more of these symptoms.

Gastrointestinal Disease Patterns. The major symptoms include belching, heartburn, bowel habit changes, weight loss, past history of ulcer, gastrointestinal bleeding, and jaundice. Postoperative gastrointestinal complications include bleeding ulcer, liver failure, and intestinal obstruction.

Past Social and Family History. Any significant illnesses or operative procedures in the past life of the patient or his family will be documented in this section of the examination. It is particularly important to note any drugs the patient has been taking in the past and whether he is still on these drugs. Certain medications may have an important bearing on the postoperative course. Some of them are listed here, but the list is by no means complete:

1. *For the Heart.* Digitalis or its derivatives; diuretics; antihypertensives; antispasmodics; anticoagulants.

2. *For the Lungs.* Antispasmodics; decongestants; antihistamines.

3. *Anti-inflammatory Drugs.* Specifically, steroids and their derivatives.

When in doubt as to which of these drugs should be instituted pre- or postoperatively, the matter should be discussed with the physician.

Physical Examination and Impression. Careful evaluation of this section will afford the nurse a very good idea of the present physical status of her patient. This examination and the physician's diagnostic impressions will serve to confirm or rule out any hint of pathologic change afforded by the symptom review and the past history.

Only with experience will the nurse come to appreciate the full significance of the history and physical examination and its relationship to the management of her patient both pre- and post-operatively. Only by diligent study and discussion with the physician will she be in a position to derive maximum benefit from the chart, a very important factor in adequate care of the surgical patient.

REVIEWING X–RAY, LABORATORY, AND OTHER STUDIES

No less important than the physician's history and the physical examination are the various data which will become available during the patient's preoperative evaluation. At the risk of being repetitious, it must be emphasized that here, again, the nurse must have an adequate knowledge of the significance of these studies and must avail herself of the opportunity of reviewing these studies and clearing up any vague points with the physician. Some of these studies may suggest previously unsuspected disease in vital organ systems, and will permit some degree of anticipation of postoperative difficulty. Some of the more common studies and their significance include:

White Blood Count. During the course of any acute infection, the white count is liable to be elevated. If surgery is being planned to treat an infectious condition (e.g., acute appendicitis) then an elevated white count is no contraindication to surgery. On the other hand, high white counts in patients undergoing elective procedures *may* be indicative of an unsuspected inflammatory process which could very well contraindicate surgery (e.g., an occult pneumonitis suspected by an elevated white count and confirmed by chest x-ray would require cancellation of surgery). Extremely high white counts are rarely on the basis of infection alone and may suggest a leukemic condition.

On the contrary, unusually low white counts might suggest, for example, bone marrow depression, which would again contraindicate elective surgery.

Red Blood Count. The state of the patient's blood volume may be approximately determined by a red blood count, hematocrit, or hemoglobin determination. A routine hematocrit reading, for example, may reveal an unsuspected anemia and force delay of surgery. If an anemic state is suspected, as in gastrointestinal bleeding, the hematocrit level will aid in determining the need for blood preoperatively.

Urinalysis. This is an extremely important clearance test prior to any surgical procedure. Much can be learned concerning the status of the kidneys, which frequently remain very silent in the face of serious renal disease. The nurse is responsible for seeing that a *clean* and *freshly voided* urine specimen is sent to the laboratory on each surgical patient. Specimens remaining on the ward become of decreasing diagnostic value with the passage of time. Several things can be determined by the urine study. Some of the important points to consider are:

> *Cells in Urine.* Red or white cells in the urine may suggest renal or bladder tumors as well as chronic or acute infections of the urinary system.
> *Casts.* These are oddly-shaped structures found in the urine and may be of several types. They reflect cast-off debris from various sites in the urinary tract and, depending on their type and number, may indicate severe chronic renal disease to the physician.
> *Protein.* An excessive spillage of protein into the urine is frequently associated with poor renal function secondary to chronic or acute renal disease.
> *Sugar.* Spillage of sugar into the urine may be the first clue to the presence of a diabetic state.
> *Specific Gravity.* A low specific gravity (under 1.010) may indicate poor renal function, with the kidney unable to concentrate its urine; a high specific gravity (over 1.025) may indicate a dehydrated state. Often this test has to be repeated several times to gain a valid idea as to the concentrating ability of the kidney.

Fasting Blood Sugar. This should be a routine study in all middle-aged and elderly patients, in those suspected of having diabetes, and in those with a family history of diabetes. A high fasting blood sugar is suggestive of diabetes mellitus and requires further study.

BUN or NPN. These studies reflect the amount of urea in the blood. Elevated levels may suggest poor renal ability to excrete urea and may lead one to anticipate renal failure postoperatively.

Chest X-ray. This should be a routine study on all surgical patients. Unsuspected acute and chronic pulmonary problems may manifest themselves only by chest x-ray. The nurse should read the chest x-ray report and note, particularly, the presence of emphysema, chronic bronchitis, and other such conditions which will dictate the intensity of postoperative pulmonary care which will be needed in her patient.

Electrocardiogram. This is frequently a routine test in all middle-aged and elderly patients, those suspected of having cardiac diseases, diabetics, and hypertensives. The nurse should note the cardiologist's interpretation and discuss any obscure points with the physician.

There are a great number of other studies suitable to the particular patient under investigation. Their exact significance must be understood by the nurse who should, when in doubt, seek clarification from the physician. Some of these tests will be discussed in Part II of this manual.

PSYCHOLOGICAL PREPARATION

The surgical patient, however stoic and adjusted he may seem, often harbors a great deal of anxiety concerning his impending surgery. The nurse must understand this anxiety, its causes, and its management. It is her great role in the management of the surgical patient that she supplement the physician in his attempt to allay the patient's fears.

Nature and Causes of Anxiety

Standard psychiatric textbooks should be reviewed for a thorough consideration of the nature of anxiety. It should be pointed out that anxiety is frequently occult, and may manifest itself as inappropriate humor or levity, lack of cooperation, depression, or agitation. The single most important cause of preoperative anxiety in the otherwise well-balanced patient is a *fear of the unknown.* Other causes of importance are a *fear of death or disability, fear of pain,* and *fear of a poor prognosis.* Upon a knowledge of these fears rests the management of anxiety in the surgical patient.

Management of Anxiety

Fear of the Unknown. The nurse should be able to explain every single procedure to her patient. Specific points requiring explanation include:

1. The general meaning of various x-rays and laboratory work ordered on the patient, the exact method of performing these tests, and the approximate amount of discomfort which the patient should expect.

2. A general idea as to the expected preoperative course to be experienced by the patient. The physician should be consulted to determine his plan of action.

3. The meaning of medications administered to the patient.

4. The meaning of nursing procedures carried out on the patient.

5. A general discussion of the operative procedure and what the patient can expect postoperatively.

Fear of Death or Disability. Quite frequently the patient has exaggerated ideas or even false ideas of surgical risk and disability. A simple but thorough discussion with the patient (*who frequently will not discuss these matters with his doctor*) may be all that is needed to dispel these fears. A fear of a colostomy where none is planned or even remotely considered, for example, can be the source of a deep-rooted anxiety which will completely vanish after being explained by the nurse. The patient may be particularly anxious about the nature of anesthesia because he does not understand it or because he expects to become violently ill from the gases. The nurse can do much to dispel these fears by a discussion of the safety of modern anesthetics and the lack of illness or complications following their use.

Fear of Pain.   The patient's thoughts about surgery will conjure up in him an image of his own incapacitation due to severe pain in the postoperative period. He will worry that the pain may be more than he can possibly endure. These thoughts distress him, cause psychosomatic repercussions, and increase his anxiety level considerably in the preoperative phase of care. The degree of expected postoperative pain must be explained to him honestly and reasonably by the surgeon and the nurse. His fears of being placed in a dependent role postoperatively must be discussed. The patient's worries can be quite threatening and terrifying; he may wonder if the professional personnel in the recovery area will recognize and relieve his pain when he needs such care. He must be assured that no one will allow him to suffer needlessly and endlessly before giving him medication for his pain.

Fear of a Poor Prognosis.   It is incredible, but understandable, how frequently a patient will read into his doctor's statements or gestures some omen of a poor prognosis. The nurse may, through casual but thorough interviews, uncover the cause of this gross misunderstanding and rectify the situation at once by a simple explanation of the true state of affairs. The misunderstandings surrounding cancer, for example, are too numerous and obvious to mention. These should be anticipated, diagnosed, and treated accordingly.

Spiritual Aspects

Whatever the particular religious beliefs of the physician or nurse, both must understand and appreciate the beliefs and convictions of their patient. These beliefs must not be treated lightly. Often a priest, minister, or rabbi may do more toward calming an anxious patient than all the other members of the hospital team combined.

PHYSIOLOGICAL PREPARATION

The surgical patient will undergo a more or less major physiologic upheaval secondary to the effects of anesthesia and surgery. Unless adequately prepared for the shock of these physiologic changes, disastrous results may follow. Several parameters must be considered, and these will occupy the remainder of this section.

General Medical Preparation

The patient must be in an optimal state of well-being prior to surgery. Sometimes an emergency situation offsets any plans to adequately prepare the patient for surgery; more often, however, the procedure is elective, and time can be taken for preparation. General points to consider are:

State of Nutrition.   Any patient harboring malignancy, chronic infection, or chronic gastrointestinal disease may enter the hospital in a poor state of nutrition. Under this condition, surgery is extremely hazardous as wounds fail to heal properly, anesthesia is poorly tolerated by the liver, the kidneys fail to excrete toxins adequately, blood clotting mechanisms may fail, and so forth. Every effort must be made to arrive at a state of adequate nutrition. High protein, high carbohydrate diets supplemented, when necessary, by intravenous protein-like chemicals may be ordered. If alimentation is impossible (e.g., in obstructing carcinoma of the esophagus), a feeding jejunostomy may precede more definitive surgery. The nurse must encourage the patient to eat heartily and see to it that meals are palatable, warm, and delivered at the right time.

Fluid and Electrolyte Status. Particularly in acute gastrointestinal disorders (e.g., small bowel obstruction) is there liable to be a serious imbalance of fluids and electrolytes. This must be corrected prior to surgery. The physician will depend on accurate measurements of fluid intake and output in order to help him decide on future allowances for fluids as well as the patient's response to those already administered. The nurse is responsible for complete accuracy in reporting fluid intake and output to the physician.

Blood Volume. Equally important for proper wound healing and tolerance of surgical stress is an adequate blood volume. Certain acute and chronic diseases cause serious blood volume depletion. This deficiency must be corrected, when feasible, prior to surgery.

Infection. Any chronic or acute infection must be evaluated and managed prior to surgery. When the infection is related to the reason for doing surgery, complete control is usually impossible without surgery. Nevertheless, the infection should be brought into a safe range for surgery. For example, often the chronically infected kidney must be removed. The patient is severely debilitated from the chronic kidney disease. Proper antibiotics, nutritional and blood volume management, and so forth must be undertaken prior to surgery.

Specific Organ or System Preparation

Any deficiencies alluded to in the three preceding paragraphs must now be treated prior to elective surgery.

Lungs. If there is any evidence of chronic lung disease, the nurse should:

1. Instruct the patient carefully concerning the hazards of smoking preoperatively.

2. Instruct the patient preoperatively in the methods of deep breathing, coughing, and turning.

3. Institute postural drainage exercises preoperatively after consultation with the physician.

4. Obtain culture and sensitivity studies of sputum preoperatively.

5. If aerosol sprays containing detergents and bronchodilators are ordered by the physician preoperatively, their mode of operation should be carefully reviewed with the patient.

6. If positive pressure breathing is to be used postoperatively, the patient should be instructed preoperatively.

7. Antibiotics may be prescribed preoperatively if the physician feels that an element of infection is present in the pulmonary tree.

Heart. If there is any evidence of heart disease, the nurse should:

1. Determine from the physician the nature of the condition and its probable effects on the postoperative course.

2. Institute oxygen therapy if any signs of respiratory distress or cyanosis appear.

3. Review the patient's prior medical treatment to be certain no drugs have been overlooked in the orders. When in doubt, consult the physician.

Prostate. If there are any genitourinary symptoms, the nurse should:

1. Be certain the patient empties his bladder completely on the morning of surgery. She should question the patient carefully concerning the possibility of *frequent small* voidings. This often indicates overflow incontinence of a distended obstructed bladder.

2. Report any preoperative voiding difficulties to the physician.

Hematologic. If there is any evidence of a bleeding disorder, the nurse should:

1. Be extremely careful in the skin preparation to be certain that no cuts or abrasions occur.

2. Apply firm pressure to any venipuncture and watch carefully for signs of hematoma formation.

3. Watch carefully for any signs of preoperative bleeding. This may force cancellation or deferment of surgery.

Kidney. If there is any evidence of kidney disease, the nurse should:

1. Be certain that the patient is kept adequately hydrated, provided there is no contraindication to this.

2. Be certain that the patient has voided preoperatively.

3. Keep an extremely accurate intake and output chart.

4. Inform the physician immediately of any hematuria, cloudy urine, or signs of diminished urine output.

Allergies. If any signs or history of allergy are present, the nurse should:

1. Question the patient carefully before administering any drugs that he might be allergic to.

2. Check frequently for hives or pruritus after administering any drug.

Nervous System. If any brain or spinal cord disability is present, the nurse should:

1. Watch particularly for signs of decubitus ulcers which, should they become infected, could delay surgery.

2. Check vital signs, level of mentation, and size and reaction of pupils frequently for signs of increasing brain damage.

Vascular System. If there are any signs or symptoms of peripheral vascular insufficiency, the nurse should:

1. Maintain optimum foot care for her patient.

2. Check with the physician concerning elevation of the head of the bed. This is frequently a good precautionary measure against further ischemic difficulties in the feet.

3. Check the legs and feet carefully and frequently for signs of increasing ischemia. The physician should be notified at once if there is any increasing pallor, cyanosis, pain, edema, or diminished pedal pulses. These are all suspicious signs of impending complications.

Gastrointestinal Tract. If there are any signs or symptoms suggesting gastrointestinal disease, the nurse should:

1. Check with the physician concerning any possible dietary restrictions.

2. Report any symptoms of gastrointestinal distress to the physician.

3. Observe stools for any evidence of diarrhea, bleeding, or other irregularity.

Preoperative Preparation (Figures 5–1 to 5–17)

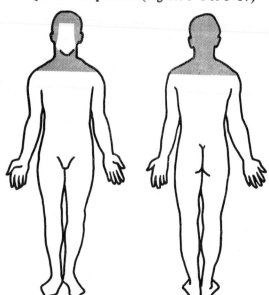

HEAD AND NECK

FIGURE 5–1 Clean the external ear canal with a cotton swab and insert a cotton plug to prevent drainage into the ear. The prepared area extends from the brow line over the head, including the ear and the anterior and posterior neck regions to the clavicular level. Facial area is excluded. (Copyright © 1968, The Purdue Frederick Company, Distributors of Betadine Surgical Scrub and Betadine Solution.)

LATERAL NECK

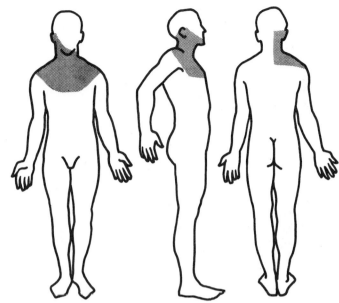

FIGURE 5-2 Ear — Clean the external canal with a cotton swab. Neck and chin — The prepared area covers the side of the face, from above the ear, and includes the chin, the anterior surface of the neck, and the upper thorax to a level just below the clavicle. Posteriorly, it extends around the neck to the spine and includes the area above the scapula. (Copyright © 1968, The Purdue Frederick Company, Distributors of Betadine Surgical Scrub and Betadine Solution.)

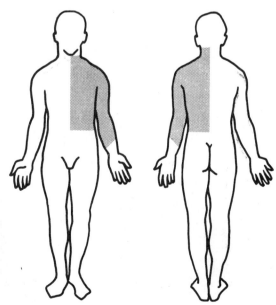

CHEST

FIGURE 5-3 The prepared area extends from the neck to the lower level of the thoracic cage and to the midline both anteriorly and posteriorly. The affected shoulder, axilla, and circumference of the arm to the midforearm are included. (Copyright © 1968, The Purdue Frederick Company, Distributors of Betadine Surgical Scrub and Betadine Solution.)

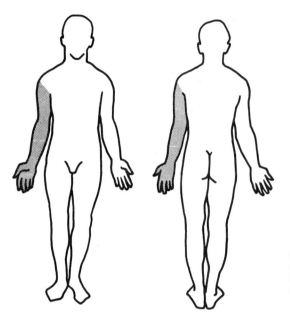

HAND AND FOREARM

FIGURE 5–4 The prepared area should include the full circumference of the arm, from the axilla to the fingertips. (Copyright © 1968, The Purdue Frederick Company, Distributors of Betadine Surgical Scrub and Betadine Solution.)

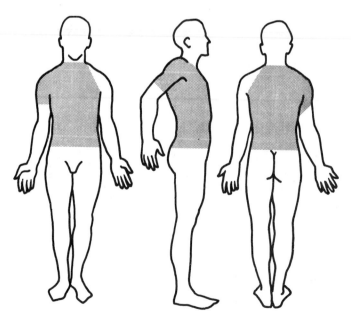

THORACO–ABDOMINAL

FIGURE 5–5 The prepared area extends anteriorly from the lower neck line to just above the pubis. Posteriorly it extends from the lower neck line to the coccyx. The affected shoulder and uppermost part of the same arm are included, and laterally it covers the circumference of the torso. (Copyright © 1968, The Purdue Frederick Company, Distributors of Betadine Surgical Scrub and Betadine Solution.)

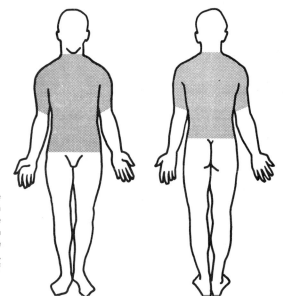

THORACO-ABDOMINAL

FIGURE 5-6 The prepared area covers the back, front, and sides of the chest and abdomen. In the front, it extends from the neck to just above the pubic symphysis. In the back, it extends from the neck to just above the gluteal fold. Arms are included almost to the elbow. (Copyright © 1968, The Purdue Frederick Company, Distributors of Betadine Surgical Scrub and Betadine Solution.)

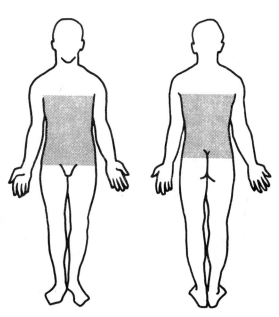

ABDOMEN

FIGURE 5-7 The prepared area extends anteriorly from the axillae to the pubis. Posteriorly, it extends from the midscapula to the midgluteal regions. Laterally, it covers the circumference of the torso. (Copyright © 1968, The Purdue Frederick Company, Distributors of Betadine Surgical Scrub and Betadine Solution.)

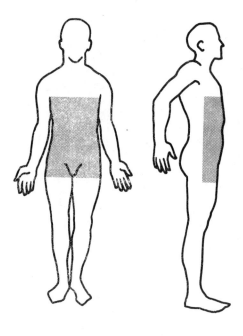

ABDOMINAL–PUBIC

FIGURE 5–8 The prepared area extends from the level of the nipple to the upper thighs, including the external genitalia. Laterally, it extends around the body to the bedline on either side. (Copyright © 1968, The Purdue Frederick Company, Distributors of Betadine Surgical Scrub and Betadine Solution.)

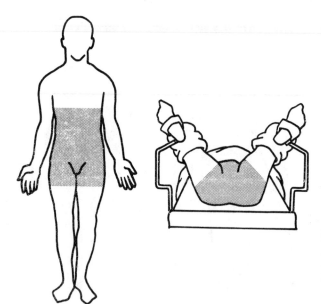

ABDOMINAL–PERINEAL

FIGURE 5–9 The prepared area extends from the level of the nipples to the upper level of the thighs. Laterally, it extends around the curvature of the body to the bedline. The external genitalia and perineal region are included. (Copyright © 1968, The Purdue Frederick Company, Distributors of Betadine Surgical Scrub and Betadine Solution.)

PERINEAL

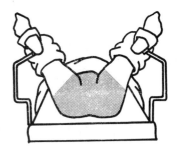

FIGURE 5–10 The prepared area covers the perineal region. Anteriorly, it extends from a point just above the pubis and posteriorly, to a point just beyond the anal region. The inner part of both thighs are included. (Copyright © 1968, The Purdue Frederick Company, Distributors of Betadine Surgical Scrub and Betadine Solution.)

THIGH

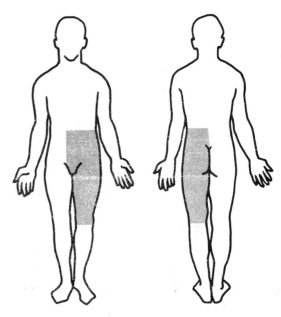

FIGURE 5–11 The prepared area extends from a level just below the umbilicus, covering the affected side of the abdomen, hip, and buttock, and the circumference of the lower extremity to below the knee. (Copyright © 1968, The Purdue Frederick Company, Distributors of Betadine Surgical Scrub and Betadine Solution.)

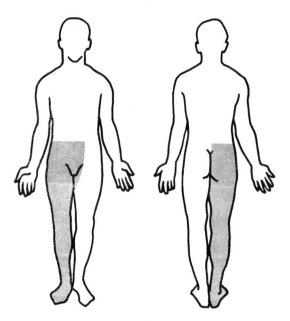

LOWER EXTREMITY

FIGURE 5–12 The prepared area extends from a level just below the umbilicus, covering the affected side of the abdomen, hip, and buttock, and the circumference of the entire lower extremity. The external genitalia should be included. (Copyright © 1968, The Purdue Frederick Company, Distributors of Betadine Surgical Scrub and Betadine Solution.)

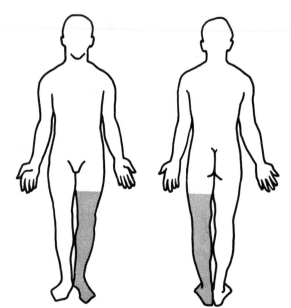

LOWER LEG

FIGURE 5–13 The prepared area should cover the circumference of the entire region from the midthigh to the distal toes. (Copyright © 1968, The Purdue Frederick Company, Distributors of Betadine Surgical Scrub and Betadine Solution.)

SACRO–PERINEAL

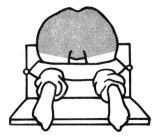

FIGURE 5–14 The prepared area includes the buttocks from the level of the iliac crest to the upper third of the thigh, including the anal region. (Copyright © 1968, The Purdue Frederick Company, Distributors of Betadine Surgical Scrub and Betadine Solution.)

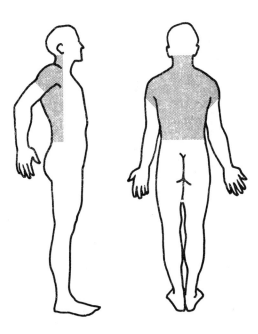

UPPER BACK

FIGURE 5–15 The prepared area extends from the hairline to the waistline, including the shoulders and axillae. Laterally, it extends to the bedline. (Copyright © 1968, The Purdue Frederick Company, Distributors of Betadine Surgical Scrub and Betadine Solution.)

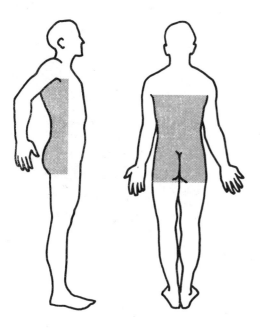

LOWER BACK

FIGURE 5–16 The prepared area extends from the level of the axillae downward to include the buttocks and anal region. Laterally, it extends to the bedline. (Copyright © 1968, The Purdue Frederick Company, Distributors of Betadine Surgical Scrub and Betadine Solution.)

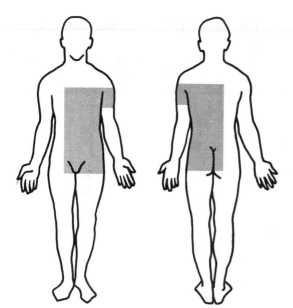

FLANK

FIGURE 5–17 The prepared area extends anteriorly from above the level of the nipple to the upper thigh and includes the external genitalia. On the back it extends from the midscapula to the midgluteal regions. Laterally, the sternum and spine should be covered. (Copyright © 1968, The Purdue Frederick Company, Distributors of Betadine Surgical Scrub and Betadine Solution.)

The Skin. There is a good deal of variation in the details of skin preparation as practiced at different hospitals. Consequently, a detailed description seems pointless. Nevertheless, several general principles may be listed.

Extent of Prep. This must usually be wider than the proposed incision would seem to require because of the possibility of an unexpected extension of the incision. Generally speaking, preps should be as follows:

> *Head.* Extent of prep and its timing should be discussed with the neurosurgeon. Often this is done by the surgeon in the operating room.
>
> *Neck.* Prep from chin to nipple line anteriorly; extend prep laterally to hairline.
>
> *Face.* Patient should shave himself; no further prep should be done until specifically ordered by surgeon. *Never shave the eyebrows.*
>
> *Chest.* For posterolateral thoracotomies, prep skin from vertebral column posteriorly to midsternal area anteriorly, including entire axilla on side of surgery. For anterior thoracotomies, include entire anterior chest to umbilicus.
>
> *Flank.* Prep from vertebral column on side of surgery to umbilicus anteriorly; prep anterior chest on side of surgery.
>
> *Abdomen.* Prep the entire abdomen from the nipple line to and including the pubis.
>
> *Inguinal area.* Prep lower abdomen from umbilicus to and including pubis; prep scrotum; prep upper thigh on side of surgery.
>
> *Perineum.* Prep scrotal region; prep perianal region and buttock to level of coccyx.
>
> *Extremity.* Always prep the entire extremity.

Method and Timing of Prep. A sharp straight or safety razor should be used, and good lighting is necessary. Shaving must be *against the grain* of the hair shaft to effect a clean close shave. Every precaution must be used to prevent nicking of the skin, as this allows infection to start preoperatively. The prep is usually done on the evening prior to surgery. In the case of orthopedic and neurosurgical procedures, many surgeons prefer to prep in the operating room on the day of surgery.

Regardless of who on the clinical unit is designated to do the prep, the head nurse or nurse in charge is ultimately responsible for its adequacy. Each prep must be supervised or "checked out" by the head nurse.

The Gastrointestinal Tract. Regardless of the type of surgery planned, it is wise to have the stomach as empty as possible to prevent aspiration while the patient is under anesthesia. Consequently, the patient is ordered "n.p.o." after midnight. Some surgeons also prefer to have a Levin tube inserted while the patient is still on the ward. This should be done by the house physician or a specially trained nurse. There is hazard associated with insertion of these tubes.

If there is to be a day or two of forced bed rest following surgery, it is probably wise to empty the lower gastrointestinal tract so as to prevent an uncomfortable degree of constipation postoperatively. Furthermore, under the relaxing influence of anesthesia, the rectum is apt to become incontinent of feces if these are not removed preoperatively. Therefore, most surgeons request some form of enema before surgery.

The Urinary Bladder. To prevent early distention postoperatively, it is wise to have the patient void while on the ward just before surgery. Some surgical procedures may require insertion of a urinary retention catheter prior to surgery. If premedications have been given and the patient is to be ambulated to void prior to surgery, care must be taken to avoid injury that might result from syncope.

Premedications. The exact routine of premedications may differ somewhat according to the nature of the surgical procedure planned, the particular wishes of the surgeon or anesthetist, and the type of anesthesia to be given. Whatever medications are used, the nurse must know their dosages, routes of administration, duration of effect, and possible immediate side effects.

In general, three types of medications are used:

Drying and Vagolytic Agents. These agents decrease pulmonary and oropharyngeal secretions, thus minimizing operative and postoperative secretions. In addition, they obliterate vagal reflexes which, often induced during anesthesia and surgery, could cause serious and even fatal heart rhythms. *Examples:* atropine; scopolamine.

Sedatives and Tranquilizers. These agents allay the patient's anxieties, reduce the pulse and blood pressure, and, in general, make for a smoother, more efficient induction of anesthesia. *Examples:* Nembutal; Seconal, Valium.

Analgesics. These drugs also have a sedating effect and generally seem to relax the patient prior to induction. *Examples:* morphine, Demerol. Analgesics must be administered at the time requested by the surgeon or the anesthetist. Should this be overlooked, the surgeon or anesthetist should be notified at once.

Other Medications and Special Procedures. These depend on the nature of the surgery, and will be described in Part II of this text.

Charting. This must include the signing and witnessing of the operative consent form, all laboratory and other diagnostic data, all medications given and time administered, and the patient's preoperative temperatures, vital signs, and weight. It should be noted here that vital signs on the preoperative check list may be totally inaccurate owing to anxiety and fear on the patient's part. For this reason there should be a succession of vital signs charted on the graphic sheet to illustrate the range of these physiological indices. The nurse who prepares and sends the patient to the operating room from the clinical unit on the day of surgery should write a progress note on the patient's chart specifying the date and time that he is taken to surgery. The nurse should also indicate the patient's personality type (as far as can be determined from observation during the preoperative period), his idiosyncrasies, and any handicaps which may be present, such as hearing loss or poor eyesight.

Final Check List

1. Skin prep done and checked out by the nurse. Any abnormal skin condition noted.
2. Jewelry, hair pins, contact lenses, prostheses, and dentures removed and stored.
3. Urinary bladder emptied and time noted.
4. Premedications given and charted (on medication sheet) and checked off (on doctor's order sheet).
5. Regular medications (i.e., those administered daily or as necessary) given and charted.
6. Vital signs (temperature, pulse, respiration, blood pressure) charted.
7. Weight and height noted and charted (especially for patients undergoing special or complex procedures).
8. Operative permit signed, witnessed, and on chart.
9. All laboratory and other diagnostic data noted on chart.
10. Doctor's order sheet, additional order sheet, progress note sheets, and nursing care plan included on chart.
11. Any special orders (e.g., Levin tube inserted) checked and carried out.
12. Results of preoperative enema charted.
13. Family notified of surgery.
14. Spiritual desires of patient satisfied.

15. Valuables removed from unit and handled according to hospital policy.
16. Hospital gown donned by patient.
17. Identification band placed on wrist and/or ankle.
18. Record assembled to include all necessary charge vouchers and forms.
19. Any necessary equipment readied and sent to the operating room with the patient.
20. Any allergies the patient may have noted and marked on chart where appropriate.

With the completion of the check list the patient is now psychologically, physiologically, and spiritually prepared for surgery, and the nurse awaits the return of her patient for the postoperative recovery and convalescence phase of his illness.

SUMMARY

Chapter 5 has attempted to describe the entire preoperative preparation of the surgical patient for his impending surgery.

It has been repeatedly emphasized that the psychological and physiological facets of this preparation must be considered simultaneously since the two components are integral parts of every patient. Any attempt to neglect one aspect at the expense of the other may lead to disastrous results.

A second emphasis has been an attempt to orient the nurse toward a closer working relationship with the physician and his investigation of the patient's illness. The physical examination, the laboratory and x-ray data, the medical progress of the patient should all be thoroughly understood and followed by the surgical nurse, who must consider herself an active participating member of the surgical team.

The general nature of the psychospiritual as well as the physiological preparation of the patient is discussed. In Part II, more specific steps will be described.

STUDY QUESTIONS

1. While interviewing a patient, you have learned that he has been on long-term cortisone medication for rheumatoid arthritis. The physician's chart makes no mention of this and, presumably, the physician is unaware of this history. What complications, if any, may occur during or after surgery if cortisone is withheld from this patient?

2. List several other commonly used drugs that a patient may be taking, the reason for his taking these drugs, and the complications that may be expected postoperatively if the drugs are inadvertently withheld.

3. In view of your answers to these questions, do you think it is an important aspect of surgical nursing for the nurse to interview the patient and review the chart, x-ray, laboratory data, et cetera? Or, on the contrary, do you think these are solely the physician's responsibilities? Be able to defend your point of view in a class discussion with your instructor.

4. Review a preoperative patient's chart and note any abnormal findings, x-rays, or laboratory data. Relate these findings to the postoperative course of this patient in terms of possible complications.

5. How would you initiate an interview with a patient? What type of questions would you have in mind during this interview?

6. Design a teaching plan that would cover a patient who is scheduled for surgery in 3 days.

7. Review a patient's laboratory data. Define each test and relate its significance to the surgical patient.

8. List several specific causes of anxiety in the preoperative patient. Have you come in contact with patients harboring any of these causes of anxiety? Discuss these patients with your class and describe your way of handling them.

9. How does an adequate nutritional balance affect the postoperative course of a surgical patient? List specific complications that may arise in the malnourished surgical patient.

10. What are the psychological benefits of adequate preoperative preparation of the patient?

6   WOUNDS AND WOUND HEALING

The painful, inflamed surgical wound is the most obvious characteristic of surgery. Indeed, it accounts for a good deal of the depression, apathy, and physical discomfort of the patient. A firm knowledge of wounds and wound healing is fundamental to sound nursing care of the surgical patient.

A great deal has been written about the biochemistry of a wound and the exact metabolic events that take place between the moment of wounding and the development of a firm, painless, and well-healed incision. These complex chemical reactions will not be described here. Rather, this chapter will describe the clinical aspects of wound healing, including normal events, complications, and management.

TYPES OF WOUNDS

Wounds vary in severity from the simple, superficial, clean wound (e.g., a thyroidectomy incision), to the vastly more serious deep, contaminated wound used in a laparotomy for septic peritonitis. The severity of the wound will determine the time of healing, degree of pain, probability of wound complications, presence or absence of tubes, drains or suction devices, and so forth. Proper management of the wound assumes a knowledge of the fundamental principles of wound healing as it exists in all wounds, as well as the more specific events that arise in different types of wounds.

Wounds may be conveniently divided into several categories as follows:

1. *Superficial or Deep*
a. *Superficial:* involving only skin, subcutaneous tissue, and sometimes fascia (e.g., thyroidectomy incision, or hernioplasty incision).
b. *Deep:* penetrating a serous cavity, entering a joint space, or undermining major muscle groups (e.g., thoracotomy incision, arthrotomy incision, or reduction of compound fracture incision).
2. *Clean or Contaminated*
a. *Clean:* involving elective surgery where the incision is placed through uncontaminated skin in a relatively clean area of the body and where no contaminated viscus has been entered and there has been no known break in aseptic surgical technique (e.g., a hernioplasty incision).
b. *Contaminated:* involving elective or emergency surgery where the incision is placed through contaminated skin or placed in a relatively contaminated area of the body. Where a contaminated viscus has been entered or where there has been a break in aseptic surgical technique the wound is also considered to be contaminated (e.g., any surgery in the presence of furunculosis; anal or vaginal surgery; or large bowel surgery).
3. *Open or Closed*
a. *Open:* whenever an incision is left partially or completely open to encourage drainage and minimize sepsis. Such an incision will close secondarily or will be closed secondarily by the surgeon. Open incisions are used when there has been gross contamination of the wound (e.g., most war wounds are left open; wounds massively contaminated by spillage of bowel contents).
b. *Closed:* the vast majority of incisions are closed primarily with or without drains or other catheters.
4. *Traumatic or Surgical*
a. *Traumatic:* always considered contaminated; frequently left open or drained.
b. *Surgical:* see all previous subdivisions.

The prototype of the superficial clean wound might be a thyroidectomy incision. It is considered superficial since it does not enter a body cavity. It is usually a clean or noncontaminated wound performed for nonseptic diseases of the thyroid gland in a relatively clean area of the body and under elective circumstances. This wound should heal *per primam* and without sepsis in 97 to 99 per cent of cases. It will not cause a great deal of pain, since motion of the neck is easily limited by the patient. A minimal amount of bloody drainage will occur for 12 to 24 hours, followed by a serous discharge for an additional day or two. Other than cellulitis, few serious complications are to be expected. One or two small rubber drains are placed at the time of surgery to ensure easy egress of blood and serum. These drains are removed a day or two after surgery. Since there is very little motion of the neck, sutures may be removed in about three days. This minimizes any "cross marks" and yields a cosmetically acceptable incision. If one were to remove the sutures one day postoperatively and gently spread the incision with a forceps, the edges would separate easily because they are held together in a very loose bind by coagulated blood and serum. There is essentially no tensile strength to the incision at this stage of wound healing. By the third postoperative day some tensile strength has developed as fibrin begins to "glue" the edges of the wound together. It is still rather easy to spread the edges apart but one is now aware of a definite binding effect going on within the depths of the wound. Between the third and the tenth postoperative days fibroblasts have begun to lay down a dense collagen network within the wound and tensile strength increases rapidly. It would become difficult and painful to separate the wound edges seven to ten days after surgery.

Management of the simple, clean, superficial wound is minimal. After the drains have been removed, no dressing is necessary. While it is not advisable to handle the wound, it is highly unlikely that exogenous infection could be introduced as early as 24 hours postoperatively. The use of complicated "dressing techniques" is ritualistic and adds nothing to the proper care of the patient. Sterile instruments are used to change dressings, when present, and to remove sutures. Masks, gloves and antiseptic solutions are of doubtful value.

Significant edema and excess wound pain may signal the beginning of wound sepsis or cellulitis. Should a definite zone of erythema form around the wound edges, antibiotics and warm, moist compresses may be used. Any drainage should be cultured and appropriate antibiotics started when the bacteriology report is available. Cellulitis usually means a streptococcal infection, whereas an abscess or purulent drainage may be due to staphylococcus. Penicillin is probably the drug of choice as an initial antibiotic, pending culture reports. The patient is kept in bed to immobilize the wound until sepsis is brought under control.

While some wound separation can occur in this type of incision, dehiscence and evisceration are not problems here. Wound separation is best treated with splinting of the neck, to avoid excess movement, and cross tapes or "butterflies" for 2 to 3 days.

Unless infection or serum collection is a problem, incisional pain is usually controlled rather easily with oral analgesics, such as codeine. More potent narcotics are not usually indicated. The need for repeated doses of morphine should raise the suspicion of impending wound infection or some underlying emotional cause.

The prototype of a deep, clean, simple wound might be a thoracotomy incision made for cardiac or pulmonary surgery. This wound is considered simple, since it does not carry with it the more complicated ramifications and consequences of an extensive laparotomy incision. If pulmonary tissue is resected, the wound must be considered at least *potentially contaminated,* since respiratory organisms can escape at the time of bronchial transection. Nevertheless, when done for elective cardiac or pulmonary surgery, this wound may be expected to heal *per primam* and without sepsis in 95 to 97 per cent of cases. Bonding of the wound follows the same timing and sequence of events as with more superficial wounds. Thoracotomy tubes usually exit from the chest at some distance from the incision and have no influence on wound healing.

Thoracotomy wound sutures are removed 7 to 10 days postoperatively. Serious wound complications are uncommon in chest surgery although an occasional empyema may evacuate through the wound. Cellulitis is also quite uncommon and usually responds well to adequate antibiotic therapy. Wound pain, however, may be very intense following a thoracotomy and is partially related to the continuous motion of the chest during each respiration. The pain may be quite prolonged, requiring a great deal of narcotics for control. Because of this pain, the patient consciously and unconsciously "splints" his chest on the side of the surgery. This predisposes to pulmonary complications such as atelectasis and pneumonia. While too much narcosis may depress respirations and lead to respiratory complications, too little pain relief may set the stage for equally severe problems. Intermittent positive pressure breathing devices are very useful here in effectively preventing under-ventilation due to "splinting."

The abdominal wound is potentially the most troublesome. It may be the cause of serious and critical complications. It is often a contaminated wound either because the surgeon has purposefully entered the gastrointestinal tract or because septic conditions arising within the abdomen have required an abdominal incision. This incision is therefore far more prone to postoperative infection. In addition, the abdominal incision is subject to the most serious of all wound complications — dehiscence and evisceration.

GENERAL PRINCIPLES OF WOUND MANAGEMENT

Most incisions are initially covered with a secure sterile dressing of gauze and tape. If the wound has been sutured *per primam* and if no drains have been used, the dressing may be safely removed as early as 24 hours postoperatively. The exposed incision is sealed to any surface bacteria, and wound sepsis from exogenous sources should not be a problem. The *exposure technique* actually minimizes wound infection by eliminating the warm, moist environment of a blood-soaked, hermetically sealed dressing. Furthermore, the exposed incision is more easily examined at frequent intervals without subjecting the patient to painful dressing changes. There are aesthetic objections to the exposure technique, however, and most patients seem to prefer a covered wound.

When the surgical patient has returned to the ward, the first order of business is attention to the vital signs, level of consciousness, perusal of surgeon's orders, and so forth. Once these critical areas have been evaluated, the nurse should concern herself with the wound and its dressing. Several questions should come immediately to mind:

What Type of Wound and Where Located? By familiarizing herself with the different types of wounds and their management, which will be discussed later in this chapter, the nurse is better able to anticipate problems and handle them intelligently. The location of a wound is particularly important in the early postoperative period: edema or hematoma in a neck wound, for example, may lead to fatal airway obstruction if not anticipated and managed early; upper abdominal incisions lead frequently to splinting of the chest cage, with diminished respiratory excursions and serious atelectasis.

Have Any Wound Drains or Suction Catheters Been Used? The number and type of drains and tubes, when used, are usually recorded on the surgeon's note and the anesthesiologist's chart. Staining of the dressing may be due to a drainage tube in place. In addition, should the dressing fall off or be pulled off by the restless patient, the nurse can note whether the drains remain in place or whether they have been inadvertently removed. If suction catheters have been used, are they adequately secured to the dressing? Does the surgeon wish them attached to gravity drainage or negative pressure? Are they to be irrigated? Are they functioning adequately or do they appear to have clotted? Are they lying twisted or kinked under the patient?

Is Hemostasis Adequate? Beware of the bulky dressing with several layers of tape. It may mask brisk and rather significant hemorrhage before staining through. If there is any doubt, loosen one edge of the dressing and observe for any telltale dripping of fresh blood along the skin surface. Circle small areas of blood stains on the dressing and watch for expansion of the stain in the early postoperative period. A wound that has been drained may stain through even the bulkiest of dressings. However, if there is any doubt in your mind about adequacy of hemostasis, notify the surgeon immediately. He may wish to change the dressing or to have you reinforce it. *It is never wise to change this first dressing yourself!* Any dislodgment of drains or tubes will invariably be ascribed to faulty dressing technique and any subsequent wound infection will raise surgical eyebrows in *your* direction. Should the surgeon request such a dressing change, it would be well to check local policy first with your supervisor.

Has a Wound Binder Been Ordered by the Surgeon? Some surgeons swear by them and others are opposed to their use. If no order exists, check first with the surgeon. Do not apply a binder unless so ordered or unless it is routine in your hospital. If an abdominal binder is to be used, be certain that it fits snugly but does not interfere with respirations. Check also that it does not compress any suction tubes or T-tubes. In the early postoperative period the binder will have to be removed often for estimating hemostasis.

Late wound management consists of checking for signs of early infection or more serious sequelae such as dehiscence and evisceration. Sepsis should be suspected when unexplained fever sets in 3 to 7 days after surgery. Inspection of the wound in adequate lighting may reveal unusual swelling of the wound edges or a tense, rounded, shiny wound. Sometimes a barely perceptible erythematous hue may be the only clue to beginning sepsis. Light palpation may reveal unusual tenderness in certain areas of the wound and a soft, fluctuant, or boggy sensation so characteristic of a subcutaneous abscess. Do not hesitate to make such observations, record them succinctly in your notes, and report them to the surgeon. This is sound surgical management and well within the prerogatives of a professional nurse.

Wound dehiscence and evisceration are the most serious complications of an incision. They are limited almost exclusively to abdominal incisions. Dehiscence represents a total disintegration of the mechanical bonding of the wound brought about by influences not totally understood. Evisceration implies an extrusion of abdominal contents onto the surface of the abdomen. This latter event is frequently fatal due to shock and sepsis. Awareness of these complications, a high index of suspicion in certain cases, and careful and frequent scrutiny of the wound can lead to early diagnosis of wound disruption and may indeed be life-saving.

Factors Predisposing to Dehiscence

While no abdominal incision is completely immune to dehiscence, certain predisposing factors, when present, should alert the nurse to the possibility of dehiscence and evisceration. These factors are related to:

> The type of patient.
> The type of incision.
> The type of wound closure.
> The postoperative course of the patient.

Some *patients* are good candidates for a wound dehiscence. Obesity, malignancy, malnutrition, bronchitis and emphysema, advanced age, and a host of related factors that set the stage for poor healing must always put one on the alert for dehiscence in the early postoperative period. Typically, these patients look chronically ill before surgery, either because of their disease or because of their poor state of nutrition. It is far less usual for major dehiscence to occur in the young, thin, well-nourished, muscular individual with a firm abdominal wall and obviously good healing powers. Dehiscence is also closely related to the *type of incision* used. A short, transverse incision is far less likely to dehisce than the lengthy, vertical one. In general, transverse incisions always heal more rapidly and with far less difficulty. This is related to the direction of stress occurring during acts of coughing, defecating, straining to urinate, and so forth. These lines of stress are from side to side, tending to separate the longitudinal incisions while approximating the transverse incisions.

The *type of wound closure* used must also be considered. Large stay sutures of wire or nylon placed through full thickness of the abdominal wall to include peritoneum are far less likely to permit frank dehiscence and evisceration than a closure of absorbable suture material incorporating small "bites" of peritoneum and fascia. The nurse should review the operative note to determine the type of closure used. Whenever there is doubt about the healing capabilities of a patient, and particularly when long, vertical incisions have been used, the surgeon will frequently reinforce his closure with stay sutures. Failure to do so may invite dehiscence.

The *postoperative course* of the patient has a great deal of influence on wound healing. Significant abdominal distention as a result of untreated paralytic ileus, excess vomiting, urinary retention, atelectasis, and pneumonia all place undue stresses on an incision when its tensile strength is not sufficient to withstand great and prolonged increases in intra-abdominal pressures. Wound hematomas, seromas, and infection are also likely to interfere with good wound healing and set the stage for dehiscence.

To summarize: While wound dehiscence can occur in *any* patient under *any* circumstances, one should be on the alert for this event in the following situations:

Type of Patient: obesity
                      malignancy
                      malnutrition

diabetes
bronchitis and emphysema
advanced age
cirrhosis with ascites
Type of Incision: long, vertical incisions
Type of Wound Closure: hasty closures, as in emergencies
closures not incorporating stay sutures
closures relying on absorbable suture material
Postoperative Course: prolonged paralytic ileus
atelectasis and pneumonia
wound hematoma and sepsis
chronic urinary retention

Early Warning Signs of Dehiscence

Unexplained Fever. Low-grade fever persisting or developing after the third or fourth postoperative day and without obvious cause suggests (a) occult wound infection, (b) thrombophlebitis, (c) occult wound dehiscence. Every effort should be made to arrive at a diagnosis as rapidly as possible. This is not always easy to do. Repeated wound examinations are in order until the fever resolves or an adequate explanation is found.

Unexplained Tachycardia. Significant wound dehiscence is often accompanied by tachycardia and occasional hypotension. Again, wound infection, wound dehiscence, and thrombophlebitis represent the most common explanations of a late tachycardia.

Unusual Wound Pain. After 3 or 4 days postoperatively, the patient usually feels a gradual lessening of wound pain. Prolonged wound pain, increasing wound pain, or severe wound pain often signals the beginning of sepsis or dehiscence.

Prolonged Paralytic Ileus. Ileus is a normal, physiological counterpart of major abdominal surgery. Its precise etiology has not yet been discovered but, of itself, ileus is of no consequence. When ileus lasts more than 3 or 4 days after surgery, and when it is accompanied by increasing abdominal distention, one must suspect complications. Intra-abdominal sepsis, wound infection, and occult wound dehiscence are three common causes of prolonged and intractable paralytic ileus.

Diagnosis and Management of Wound Dehiscence

Wound dehiscence may present in a very obvious way with the sudden gush of large quantities of serosanguineous fluid from a previously dry and seemingly innocent wound. This gush of fluid indicates a separation of the peritoneal and fascial edges with loss of intra-abdominal fluid. The saturated wound dressing is usually accompanied by exacerbation of wound pain, a rise in the pulse rate, and, if left untreated, the development of hypotension. When these events occur, the dressing should be removed and the wound inspected. A heavy dressing with a binder should be applied, the patient instructed to remain very still, and the surgeon notified at once. It takes only *one cough* at this stage to cause evisceration, a grave complication. When the surgeon arrives he will confirm the diagnosis and return the patient to the operating room immediately for resuturing of the incision.

Before the surgeon arrives, it is mandatory that the nurse remain with the patient at all times, seeing to it that evisceration does not occur. A heavy dressing with a binder, as well as supporting the wound with hands may be necessary while awaiting the arrival of the surgeon. The operating room staff should be alerted and an intravenous line prepared for the patient.

At times dehiscence occurs in a far more subtle fashion. There may be only early warning signs as listed above. The wound should be inspected frequently. Any serous drainage should be brought to the surgeon's attention immediately. He may need to remove several skin sutures and palpate the recesses of the wound with his gloved finger in order to diagnose wound dehiscence.

The earlier wound dehiscence is detected, the lower the subsequent mortality. A high index of suspicion and a careful scrutiny of any suspicious wound are the key factors in arriving at an early diagnosis.

SUMMARY OF SPECIFIC WOUNDS AND THEIR CARE

Wounds of the Head and Neck Region

Craniotomy Incision. This is usually an oval, flap incision made through skin, muscle, and galea, and with a corresponding oval cut-out in the cranial bone. The skin and muscle flap is sutured with fine silk or twisted wire, and the incision is not drained unless gross contamination has occurred, as from a severe head trauma. In the early postoperative period, a compression dressing is left in place to encourage hemostasis. Once this has been accomplished, no dressing is necessary. Twisted wire sutures offer the advantage that they may be tightened or loosened by the surgeon simply by a twist of each suture. The sutures are removed in 4 to 7 days. Healing is excellent because of the excellent blood supply of the scalp. Sepsis is rarely a problem. Occasionally hematomas form and are aspirated with a syringe and large needle. The aspirated blood or serum should be cultured. Craniotomy incisions may be classified as simple, clean, and superficial. They require very little care and should cause very few complications. Should there be any significant bloody drainage through the dressing in the first few hours after surgery, the nurse should reinforce the dressing and report this problem to the attending surgeon.

Thyroidectomy Incision. This was discussed previously.

Radical Neck Dissection. This incision is used for primary or metastatic neck cancer. Like any *radical* dissection it is characterized by (a) the development of relatively thin, wide skin flaps; (b) resection of a great deal of tissue bulk, which leaves dead space; and (c) the need for some form of negative pressure catheters for evacuating fluid exudate.

Wound complications are directly related to these three characteristics and will be discussed in that order.

Thin Skin Flaps and Their Complications. A radical dissection for cancer must attempt to remove all overlying subdermal lymphatics within which tumor cells may be found. The surgeon attempts to include all these subdermal lymphatics in his dissection while still sparing the blood supply to these thin skin flaps. At times the dissection removes the blood supply from a portion of the skin flap and ischemic necrosis develops. This will eventually result in an area of skin slough, which, if it is large enough, will require secondary skin grafting. When sloughing occurs over the carotid vessels, there is a distinct hazard of massive hemorrhage as necrosis invades the wall of these large vessels. Every effort is made at the time of surgery to cover the neck vessels with healthy muscle but this is not always possible or successful.

Creation of Dead Space. Radical dissection results in the removal of muscle, fascia, fat, lymphatics, and loose areolar tissue. A large dead space results into which tissue exudates will flow. This causes hematomas and seromas to form, and these, in turn, impede healing and predispose to wound sepsis. In addition, since microscopic lymphatics are transected during the operative procedure, a great quantity of lymph also exudes into the wound, bringing with it the threat of fluid collection and sepsis formation.

Need for Suction Catheters. Fluid formation and dead space must be minimized if one is to avoid later sepsis and other wound complications. At one time bulky compression dressings and multiple soft drains were used in a desperate effort to combat fluid exudation and dead space formation. These bulky dressings were uncomfortable, difficult to manage, and did not effectively prevent seromas, hematomas, and sepsis. Indeed, many of these radical incisions became infected, gathered large collections of fluids, and required multiple aspirations. In recent years surgeons have come to rely on suction catheters and minimal dressings for radical dissections. These catheters not only evacuate wound exudate but actually pull the skin flaps snugly against the underlying tissue, thus obliterating dead space. A very light dressing is used for a day or two. If the skin flaps are healing well, no further dressing is necessary. When working effectively, these catheters greatly improve the healing rates of radical incisions. There are many types of catheters commercially available, although they can be fashioned from any sort of available rubber tubing. They all suffer from the inherent weakness of early failure due to clot formation within the catheters. The surgeon may request that these catheters be irrigated to maintain patency. This should be carried out with diligent aseptic technique. The junction of catheter and suction tube should be thoroughly prepared with an iodine-based antiseptic. Sterile gloves should be used and a small amount of saline instilled through the catheters. As soon as they are patent, they are immediatley reconnected to low suction so as to reestablish negative pressure and encourage proper functioning of the catheters.

The sutures are removed 5 to 10 days postoperatively. If there has been no flap necrosis and no sepsis, the wound should be well healed by this time and should offer no further complications. Partial flap necrosis must be observed very carefully. Particular attention should be paid to the location of the area of necrosis in relation to the carotid artery. In good lighting, and with the patient's neck hyperextended and rotated away from the incision, the nurse can observe the pulsations of the carotid artery and the distance from the area of skin necrosis. Should any bleeding occur from the depths of a necrotic area near the carotid vessel, the surgeon should be notified at once. A trickle of blood may be the first warning sign of an impending massive hemorrhage.

Wounds of the Chest (Thoracotomy Incisions)

These have been described above. In general, few complications are to be expected in these incisions, which heal rapidly and without sepsis. Management of chest tubes is described in another section of this book.

Wounds of the Abdomen (Laparotomy Incisions)

Appendectomy. Usually a McBurney or a small, vertical incision is made; very few problems are encountered in this operation; dehiscence and evisceration occur only rarely; superficial wound infection is frequent in cases of a ruptured appendix; sutures are removed in 5 to 7 days.

Inguinal Hernia Repair. Usually an oblique incision in the inguinal area is made; healing without sepsis is expected in 98 per cent of cases; sutures are removed in 7 to 10 days; no dressing is required.

Cholecystectomy. Usually a right subcostal or a right paramedian incision is made; dehiscence is a possibility with either incision but more frequent with the paramedian incision; an intra-abdominal drain is always used in biliary tract surgery and is removed in 6 to 8 days following surgery. If the common bile duct has been explored, a t-tube will also be used. If dressings need to be changed, care must be taken to avoid dislodgment of drain or t-tube. Sutures are removed in 7 to 10 days. Some surgeons use large *stay sutures.* These may be left in for two weeks.

Gastric Surgery. Usually a left paramedian or a midline incision is made. There is a higher sepsis rate because of entrance into the stomach, although the acid secretions usually result in a rather surgically clean wound. These upper abdominal incisions are quite painful and often lead to chest splinting and pulmonary atelectasis. These incisions are only rarely drained. Sutures are removed in 7 to 10 days. Dehiscence is a definite possibility here.

Colon Surgery. Usually a left paramedian incision is made, although some surgeons prefer the stronger transverse incision. There is a higher incidence of sepsis and dehiscence in these incisions than in any other abdominal incision. Stay sutures are frequently used and left in for two weeks. Drains may be used if contamination has occurred. The wound may be left open above the fascia for secondary closure if the surgeon expects infection.

Surgery of the Extremities

These incisions heal very well and with a very low incidence of infection, or seroma or hematoma formation. They are usually not drained. Sutures are left in for 7 to 10 days. Stay sutures are not used. Dressings are not necessary after 1 to 2 days.

Perineal Surgery

This is a highly contaminated area. Absorbable catgut only is used. There is always a great deal of exudate and erythema around these incisions, which heal very slowly and are accompanied by a great deal of local discomfort. Sitz baths are very helpful. Drains are usually not used. Occasional abscesses form but these are usually not of great consequence.

THE PATIENT AND HIS WOUND

The senior author has been particularly impressed with the great deal of mystique attributed to the wound by the majority of surgical patients. A significant amount of anxiety is generated in the patient's mind both preoperatively and postoperatively as he whiles away his time imagining a host of terrible things that can happen to his wound if he moves, coughs, breathes, or in any way disturbs the status quo. Although "bursting" of a wound is a real thing, it is, fortunately, very uncommon and probably not at all related to the patient's postoperative activities. Indeed, if a patient were to lie perfectly still for fear of bursting his wound, far greater complications could ensue (e.g., pneumonia, phlebitis). The nurse should discuss the wound with her patient, determine his "concepts" of a wound, and try to eliminate false ideas that serve no useful purpose and frequently may lead to complications.

SURGICAL DRAINS, TUBES, AND CATHETERS

7

The surgical nurse is responsible for the proper management of many types of drains, catheters, and other devices employed by the surgeon in the course of his operative procedure. The subject is complex because of the wide variety of devices available and their many uses. The considerable rate of progress in the development of new and better equipment and the not infrequent custom of many surgeons of insisting on the special merits of particular drains — and the rituals surrounding their management — further complicate the matter.

In order to simplify matters somewhat, this chapter will concern itself only with drainage problems affecting the abdominal cavity and its contents. The emphasis will be on the general principles of drainage and will avoid, where possible, descriptions of the various types of tubes, catheters, drains, and other products on today's surgical market. These principles will be found valid for all other types of surgery, and more specific discussion will be found in the appropriate chapters of Part II.

PURPOSES

The fundamental purpose of all surgical drains, tubes, and catheters is to permit or encourage the escape of body fluids from the body when it would be detrimental for these fluids to accumulate within body cavities. These fluids include blood, lymph, pancreatic juice, intestinal juice, bile, and pus. To bring about this escape of fluids, some type of drain or tube of appropriate construction is arranged with one end placed near or in the organ or cavity to be drained and the other end passed through the body wall and either left bound within a dressing or attached to a drainage or suction system.

Since the use of drains and tubes is never completely without risk, the surgeon must weigh the hazards of drainage against the dangers of not draining. This is not always a clear-cut decision, for there are many controversies surrounding the questions of *when* to drain, *what type* of drain to use, *when to remove* a drain, and so on. Some surgeons (the "drainers") are very liberal in their use of drains. They tend to discount or minimize the alleged dangers of drains and feel that the potential risks of undrained collections of body fluids far outweigh any theoretical dangers associated with drains. Other surgeons (the "non-drainers") are quite impressed with the hazards of drains and use them only when the indications for their use are unquestionable, as determined by convention and long surgical experience.

This chapter will not attempt to enter into these controversies except by way of emphasizing both the risks and the safety features of properly used drains. Simply put, there are *six situations* which arise in abdominal surgery and which merit serious consideration for the use of some form of drainage.

Situation One: Abscess Cavity. Whenever the surgeon encounters a thick-walled abscess cavity, such as may be present in a chronic subphrenic abscess, he will place drains in the cavity to ensure that the cavity will remain collapsed after surgical drainage of pus and will heal from the deepest portion outward. Failure to keep the cavity open with some form of drainage invites a reaccumulation of pus under pressure and a recurrent abscess. The surgeon usually employs a Penrose or cigarette drain for this purpose and he leaves it in place for 5 or 6 days. The drain is removed gradually by advancing it about an inch at a time beginning on the fourth or fifth day after the operation.

Examples of this type of abdominal situation requiring a drain include:

a. Chronic subphrenic abscess.

b. Pelvic abscess due to a ruptured appendix or a ruptured diverticulum.

Situation Two: Insecure Closure of the Gastrointestinal Tract. At times, owing to poor blood supply, infection, malnutrition, or excess tension on a suture line, the surgeon anticipates delayed leakage from an anastomosis or from a closure of the gastrointestinal tract. Such leakage, if unvented to the outside, could result in postoperative abscess or generalized peritonitis. A drain or sump catheter is placed near the site of surgery to collect any intestinal contents which might begin to leak and to alert the surgeon that a leak has started. Since leakage is not likely to occur for several days after surgery, this drain or catheter must be left in place 7 to 10 days and then gradually removed.

This type of situation can occur:

a. *After a Gastrectomy.* The duodenal closure may be insecure because of severe inflammation from ulcer disease.

b. *After a Low Anterior Rectal Resection.* The bowel wall is very weak because it lacks a serosal layer, and many anastomoses will leak for a short period of time.

Situation Three: Anticipated Leakage. Experience indicates that surgery performed on certain organs carries a high risk of leakage of juices found in these organs, regardless of how smooth the operative procedure or how secure the operative field happens to be. Some form of drainage is used in anticipation of leakage and is usually removed in about 6 days if drainage is negligible.

This type of situation can occur:

a. *After Gallbladder Surgery.* Cholecystectomy often leads to leakage of bile from minute biliary ducts which traverse the liver bed to enter the gallbladder. Bile will leak from the liver bed for several days after surgery, and a drain is necessary to encourage escape of this bile from the abdomen.

b. *After Pancreatic Surgery.* There is a high likelihood that some pancreatic juice will leak after pancreatic resection irrespective of how securely the pancreas is sutured. This juice can be lethal if not properly drained, and appropriate suction must be used in order to prevent destruction of the abdominal wall.

Situation Four: Trauma. Drains are used whenever abdominal trauma has occurred, particularly when the trauma is massive and is associated with devitalized tissue and contaminated debris, two factors which can lead to abscess formation.

Situation Five: Decompression of the Gastrointestinal Tract. Catheters are used to decompress the gastrointestinal tract when it is anticipated that a temporary dysfunction may result in a build-up of intestinal fluids which could threaten leakage from the tract at the site of surgery.

This type of situation can occur in surgery involving:

a. *The Common Bile Duct.* Whenever surgery is performed on the common bile duct, a T-tube is sutured into the duct and the end brought out through the abdominal wall and attached to drainage. The use of the decompressing T-tube is necessitated by the possibility that temporary dysfunction of the ampulla of Vater could result in pressure build-up within the common bile duct. The T-tube is removed only after a postoperative cholangiogram has determined that bile is flowing freely through the ampulla of Vater into the duodenum. This may occur on the tenth or eleventh day after surgery.

b. *The Duodenum.* Occasionally the surgeon may doubt the security of his closure of the duodenum after gastrectomy. This will usually prompt him to leave a Penrose drain adjacent to the duodenum. However, if closure of the duodenum is unusually difficult and would require excessive tension on the suture line, the surgeon may choose to close the duodenum over a catheter, using the latter as a decompressing device to prevent build-up of duodenal juices and subsequent leakage. The tube is brought out through the abdomen and placed either on dependent drainage or on low suction. It will be left in place for 12 to 14 days until a secure tract of fibrous tissue has formed between the duodenum and the abdominal wall.

Situation Six: Following Radical Surgery. Radical surgery for carcinoma usually requires extensive dissection and laying open of large tissue plains which exude lymph and blood for several days after surgery. It is impossible to control this type of exudation in the operating room. Large collections of lymph, serum, or blood can lead to troublesome infection postoperatively and should be prevented by an appropriate type of tube. A suction catheter will effectively remove serum and blood, and is left in place until no longer functioning. This usually takes about 3 to 5 days.

This type of situation can occur after:
a. Surgery for a large incisional hernia.
b. Perineal surgery performed as part of abdominoperineal resection.
c. Radical mastectomy.
d. Radical neck dissection.
e. Radical groin dissection.

TYPES OF DRAINS

The student is referred to operating room instrument manuals supplied by surgical manufacturers for a complete description of the myriad drains, tubes, and catheters available to the surgeon. Often the individual preference and experience of the surgeon will dictate the exact drain he will use rather than some "hard" scientific principle. Nevertheless, there is some rationale behind the basic choice of drains; the following is a simplified discussion of the types of drains and for what reasons they are chosen for use in surgery.

The basic drain used for abscess cavities and for situations in which leakage of body fluids is anticipated is the *Penrose drain.* This is a soft rubber drain that will not damage nearby organs and causes very little tissue reaction. It acts primarily by capillary action, drawing any pus or fluid along its surfaces and through an aperture or "stab wound" made adjacent to the main incision. It was first used by surgeons in 1859 and remains the most widely used drain today. It is employed to drain skin and subcutaneous abscesses, intra-abdominal abscesses, and collections of blood, lymph, and serum. It is often placed near an intestinal anastomosis thought to be insecure.

Gauze was used a hundred years ago as a draining substance because of its absorption powers and good capillary action. To avoid adhesions to surrounding tissues, it is now placed inside a Penrose drain, forming the so-called *cigarette drain.* Like the Penrose drain, the cigarette drain is widely used, and in fact is employed in much the same way and for the same purposes as the Penrose drain. Some surgeons insist that it is more effective than the Penrose drain; others feel that it has no particular advantages over the simpler Penrose design.

The *Foley catheter* is often used to drain the gallbladder when tube cholecystostomy is indicated. It may also be used rather effectively for tube gastrostomy. The catheter's balloon acts to prevent accidental extrusion from the gallbladder or stomach.

The *sump catheter* (See Fig. 7–1) is a double-lumen device that prevents adjacent tissue from clogging the apertures in the suction tube by means of an outer "screen" of perforated tubing. It is usually attached to low suction, either continuous or intermittent, and is particularly useful where high volume fluid outputs are anticipated (e.g., intestinal fistulae, pancreatitis).

COMPLICATIONS OF DRAINS

Hemorrhage.   The "stab wound" used for exit of the drain may begin to bleed in the early postoperative period. Hemorrhage from unsuspected vessel damage at the time of fashioning the stab wound may be profuse; however, this is a rare event. Firm tubes, such as sump catheters, may lodge against large intra-abdominal vessels and cause delayed hemorrhage several days after surgery.

Sepsis.   Retrograde contamination of the abdomen by bacteria passing inward along a drain or catheter is a real possibility. Indeed, many studies of postoperative intra-abdominal sepsis point to the drain as the offending device. Since the drain is frequently used *because* of intra-abdominal sepsis, this drain complication is often underestimated by surgeons who are too liberal in their use.

Bowel Herniation.   The stab wound is a potential weak area in the abdominal wall and, if too large, may lead to postoperative herniation of intestines with secondary incarceration and small bowel obstruction.

Loss of Drain.   If the drain has not been sutured securely to the skin, postoperative abdominal distention may cause the drain to recede into the abdominal cavity, and a second laparotomy may be necessary to retrieve it.

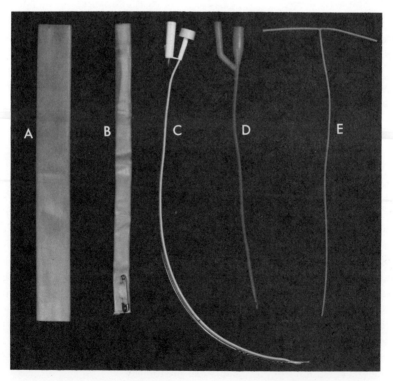

FIGURE 7–1   A = Penrose drain; B = cigarette drain; C = sump catheter; D = Foley catheter; E = T-tube.

Accidental Loss of Intraluminal Catheter. The restless patient may inadvertently pull out a T-tube or a catheter duodenostomy. If this accident occurs early in the postoperative period — before a fibrous tract has formed to seal the defect in the common bile duct or duodenum from the general abdominal cavity — a fatality may occur.

THE NURSE'S ROLE IN THE MANAGEMENT OF DRAINS AND CATHETERS

The nurse's responsibility for the care of drains, tubes, and catheters begins as soon as the patient returns to the surgical ward. It is essential that the nurse become aware immediately of any such devices used by the surgeon. She must know why each drain or tube was used and what should be anticipated as the drains begin to function. The surgeon's detailed operative report may not be charted for two or three days after the operation. Often he will write a brief operative note in the clinical progress notes, and this can be a source of information about the types of drains that have been used. In many cases the anesthesiologist's notes or the operative nurse's notes will record any drains or tubes that have been used. If none of these sources make mention of drains, the surgical nurse should contact the surgeon to find out about these important details. Only by properly understanding these drains and their specific purposes and possible complications can the nurse undertake an intelligent plan for their management.

This plan need not be complicated if the nurse recognizes the purpose of each type of tube. Bearing in mind that the fundamental purpose of all surgical drains and tubes is to permit easy egress of body fluids, several important observations should be kept in mind when managing these tubes:

Is the Tube or Drain Functioning Properly?

Most Penrose and cigarette drains are buried under the surgical dressing, and their function cannot be adequately judged in the immediate postoperative period. A few days after the surgery, however, careful observation around the drain site will indicate how well the drains are functioning. If pus is to be drained, for example, then pus should be passing out around the drain site! If the drain is malfunctioning, the pus will reaccumulate in the abdomen or in the wound, which can result in fever, increasing abdominal or wound pain, and a general "failure to do well." The drain may have to be twisted or advanced to break up any adhesions which have caused it to function improperly.

Tubes and catheters are usually placed on dependent drainage or are attached to some form of continuous or intermittent suction. Not infrequently the senior author has discovered a patient lying on a kinked catheter which should have been positioned better. The *kinked catheter* is an obstructed catheter and will not work correctly. The nurse should be certain that the catheter is taped correctly to the dressing in order to avoid any such kinks. Suction machines frequently fail to function properly, and such failures also may lead to malfunction of the tube. When there is doubt that the suction is working, the suction tubing should be disconnected from the surgical drain and its suctioning power tested with a basin of sterile saline.

Body fluids usually drain at about the same rate over any given 8-hour time period. A good rule of thumb to follow is to compare the amount of drainage in one 8-hour period with that in another. If there has been a substantial decrease during your work shift, there is a good possibility that the tubing is *now* malfunctioning.

Is the Tube or Drain Secured Adequately?

A drain left unsecured can create a dangerous and potentially fatal situation. Penrose and cigarette drains must be sutured to the skin and a safety pin passed through them as an added precaution. If this has not been done, the nurse must notify the surgeon of it *at once.* Failure to secure the drain may lead to the retraction of the drain into the abdominal cavity, necessitating a second operation. Should a drain inadvertently fall out during a dressing change, it should be noted in the nurse's report and the surgeon notified.

The restless patient may accidently pull out an intraluminal catheter. This is not an uncommon experience on a busy surgical ward and may be disastrous. The patient should be restrained and a secure dressing or binder placed over the tube to ensure against any dislodgement.

What is the Nature and Volume of the Drainage?

The nurse should note at least every 8 hours (or more frequently) the nature and volume of drainage from any catheter or tube used by the surgeon. The data should be entered in an *appropriate* column on the intake/output chart. The nurse's clinical notes should include a description of the color, consistency, and volume of the discharge, as well as any *change* in the quality of the discharge that he or she observes. Marked discrepancies in volume output, for instance, may indicate malfunctioning of the drainage system (as we have noted) or a change in the physiological status of the organ being drained. *Example:* A gastrostomy tube inserted 4 days ago for drainage after gastrectomy has drained approximately 300 cc's per 8-hour shift for the past 2 days. Suddenly a marked increase in drainage is noted — up to 1000 cc's in one 8-hour shift. This suggests a distal obstruction at or beyond the gastrojejunostomy, with back-up of gastric juices through the gastrostomy tube.

SUMMARY

The surgical drain has a long and complicated history. In its various forms, it has been used almost from the beginning of modern surgery. Its use is basic to surgery and will probably remain so for many decades to come. Although drains have many functions and a variety of forms, fundamentally they are put to use to permit the escape of body fluids from the body when this is thought necessary by the surgeon. A proper understanding of this basic principle and its many facets will aid the nurse in the management of the various drainage devices, regardless of the area of the body in which they are used or the type of surgery for which they have been employed.

8 ANESTHESIA AND THE PATIENT

Anesthesiology is a highly specialized and complex study. A nurse must spend two to three years beyond her actual nursing study to become an anesthetist. Thus it is almost impossible for the nurse who is versed only in her own field of surgical nursing to master the entire field of anesthesia. Nevertheless, she must have a general knowledge of anesthesia, the various anesthetics used in surgery, their methods of administration, their possible side effects, and the complications arising from their use. In this way she can anticipate the problems of the surgical patient in undergoing and recovering from anesthesia. This chapter will briefly present the aspects of anesthesia that are important for the surgical nurse to know.

THE PREOPERATIVE VISIT

All patients undergoing surgery will have a history and physical examination performed by the operating surgeon. The anesthesiologist will also spend some time with the patient preoperatively in order to accomplish several important tasks. In essence, the anesthesiologist works out a medical and emotional assessment of the patient, fosters the establishment of rapport, provides patient education, and makes the selection of the premedications and anesthetic technique to be employed.

The surgical nurse will have a very significant role in these preoperative functions, for she has a more prolonged contact with the patient during the preoperative phase than does the anesthesiologist. Just as the surgical nurse must communicate with the surgeon in order to understand his goals and relate them to her own in the care of the patient, she ought also to make rounds with the anesthesiologist in an effort to understand the specific goals and plans he has in mind for the patient.

Patient Assessment

It is assumed that a complete history and physical examination have already been performed when the anesthesiologist begins his routine. He will repeat in depth the aspects of the history relevant to anesthesia. He will particularly want to know what happened during any previous operations and anesthesias and what complications, if any, the patient experienced. A knowledge of the patient's smoking and drinking habits, the presence of any pulmonary, hepatic, renal, or cardiovascular disease will influence the selection of the type of anesthesia to be administered.

The smoker will require a greater depth of anesthesia to obtund the cough reflex and will be much more susceptible to postoperative pulmonary complications. The regular drinker will require larger narcotic dosages because of a cross-tolerance to narcotic drugs.

It is important to know what allergies the patient may have so that allergenic drugs (and similar drugs as well) may be avoided. Medications that are being taken by the patient may alter the choice of anesthetic agents to be used. Certain antibiotics may potentiate the effects of muscle relaxants, for example. A patient on digitalis should not receive a large dose of atropine as part of the premedication regimen.

If the patient has taken steroids for longer than a week during the previous year, it may be considered desirable to give some steroids with the premedication to counterbalance a residual pituitary-adrenal axis depression. The surgical nurse may help in all this by obtaining a complete list of the drugs currently being used by the patient, his previous drug allergies or reactions and so forth.

Should the examination of the patient indicate areas of pathology, it may be necessary to have special investigations performed, such as a chest x-ray, an electrocardiogram, liver function tests, pulmonary function studies, and tests of arterial blood gases. (*Note:* In most cases, the majority of these tests are now done routinely.)

Because the prime consideration in the preoperative phase is to *prepare* the patient for surgery, investigations must determine not only what abnormalities are present but whether the patient is in as healthy a state as possible. Are there any correctible disorders? If there is electrolyte imbalance, anemia, uncontrolled diabetes, or congestive heart failure, then these should be corrected, as far as is possible, before undertaking elective surgery. Even a patient with a "runny" nose should be required to wait until he has recovered before anesthesia is administered for elective surgery.

When the surgery is urgent, the risks of waiting until the non-surgical abnormality has been corrected should be weighed against the risks of delaying the surgery. Obviously, the patient who has ruptured an abdominal aortic aneurysm and is rapidly losing blood requires immediate surgery, other abnormalities notwithstanding. However, the patient who has an acute intestinal obstruction would be less of a risk if his surgery were delayed two or three hours while an attempt is made to correct the fluid and electrolyte imbalance consequent to his disease.

Patient Education and Reassurance

Within the limits of the patient's ability to comprehend — and within the limits of what he wants to know — the nurse should provide a detailed description of what will happen to him under anesthesia. Some patients want to know merely that they will be asleep before the surgeon operates; others may want to know the exact mode of action of the anesthetic (e.g., a very short-acting barbiturate) that may be used. Patients have a right to know and a right *not to know;* both rights must be understood and granted to each patient.

The establishment of rapport with the patient involves the creation of trust in the doctor and nurse by not withholding any information that the patient may wish to know. An explanation of what will happen will do more to assuage the patient's fears than the narcotic premedication, and will reduce the dose required. Many of the cardiac arrhythmias which pose problems during anesthetic induction are the result of secretions of endogenous epinephrine due to fear. If this fear is diminished, so too will be the incidence of arrhythmias. The surgical nurse can contribute significantly in this respect and should spend some time, when possible, with the anesthesiologist as he makes his preoperative rounds so that she becomes familiar with the responses of the patient to the anesthesiologist's questions and explanations. A great many patients will ask the same questions a few hours later. Both the patient and the nurse will find it disconcerting if her answers differ significantly from those of the anesthesiologist.

Selection of Anesthetic Technique

Throughout the preoperative visit, the anesthesiologist will be making a judgment as to what anesthetic technique should be employed to best suit *the operation and the patient.* The selection will depend on the physical and emotional state of the patient and the requirements of the surgery and the operating surgeon. These factors will be discussed in greater detail later in the chapter.

At the end of the preoperative visit the anesthesiologist will write the orders for premedication in the chart.

PREMEDICATION

The premedication is an integral part of the anesthetic technique. The various drugs used for premedication have four major pharmacological effects. Some patients may be judged to require only one of these effects, while others may need all four. The premedication is usually administered intramuscularly about one hour prior to the induction of anesthesia. The aim is to have the drug reach its peak effect as the anesthesia is begun. The timing is important. If the patient is called to the operating room unexpectedly early, it may be more advantageous if the anesthesiologist administers the premedications intravenously in the operating room. The nurse must note carefully on a preoperative check sheet the time of administration of the premedication. If there is some delay in the time of the operation, the anesthesiologist may need to repeat some portion of the premedication before inducing anesthesia.

The four functions of premedications are as follows:

Emotional Sedation. This is a highly variable requirement in terms of drug dosage. A young, healthy person with a tendency to neurotic anxiety will require a generous dose, whereas a frail, elderly patient, whose personality is well-adjusted and who is obviously confident in the abilities of his medical attendants may need none at all. The more effective the rapport between patient and doctor, the less the sedative action will be required. The rapport between a nurse and her patient is no less important.

Basal Narcosis. This involves the administration of a drug that will provide a degree of long-lasting analgesia designed as a base for the rest of the anesthetic routine. This is now regarded as a relatively unimportant part of the premedication. It is more efficient to administer small intravenous doses during the anesthetic routine as clinical indications warrant.

Parasympatholytic Actions. Drugs with parasympatholytic actions have two useful effects. First, they prevent the bradycardia and possible cardiac asystole that may be brought on by vagal hyperactivity, which may occur, for example, during (a) the administration of succinylcholine, (b) endotracheal intubation, (c) the use of vagal-stimulating anesthetics such as halothane, or (d) incision or traction of the peritoneum. Second, they reduce the secretions of saliva and respiratory tract mucus. These secretions would otherwise increase during anesthesia and contribute to obstruction of the airway and the likelihood of pulmonary complications, such as atelectasis.

Anti-nausea Effect. Until recent times many drugs used in premedications and general anesthesia caused nausea and vomiting in up to 50 per cent of all patients. It therefore became necessary to use drugs which would have an anti-emetic effect. Today, most anesthetic agents contain anti-nausea components. Nevertheless, it is still useful to employ premedications that are specifically anti-emetic.

DRUGS USED AS PREMEDICATIONS

Some of the drugs used to premedicate patients are:

Barbiturates: These drugs are almost purely hypnotic in action and have no analgesic effect. They have the disadvantage that in a significant number of children and elderly patients, they will produce excitement and disorientation rather than sedation. Although there are more reliable sedatives available, barbiturates are still used frequently as premedications.

Demerol: Demerol, when used alone, is almost purely an analgesic, and therefore has no sedative effect in the patient who is experiencing no pain. Because it may produce nausea or even vomiting, it is usually combined with a drug such as Phenergan, a sedative and anti-emetic which produces in combination with Demerol a degree of emotional sedation that neither drug produces alone.

Morphine: This drug produces excellent analgesia and emotional sedation, but it may cause some nausea. A large dose may provoke significantly dangerous hypoventilation in a susceptible patient.

Papaveretum: Exhibiting all the properties of morphine plus an anti-emetic effect, papaveretum is almost ideal in fulfilling three of the four requirements of premedication, provided it is given in carefully judged dosages.

Phenothiazines: These drugs (and similar compounds, such as Thorazine, Sparine, Valium, and Phenergan) are all emotional sedatives with anti-nausea effects. However, they lower the pain threshold and produce a degree of vasodilatation which could be dangerous in a hypovolemic patient.

Atropine: This drug produces a vagolytic effect and has some *anti*-sedative action. Many patients find the drug's effects (especially dry mouth) uncomfortable, and the increase in pulse rate produced by the drug can be dangerous in a digitalized patient or a patient with thyrotoxicosis, for example. For these reasons it is often given intravenously by the anesthesiologist immediately before induction of anesthesia.

Scopolamine: Like atropine, this drug reduces parasympathetic acitivity, but it also produces some amnesia and sedation. In combination with drugs like papaveretum, it has been used for many years in the induction of "twilight sleep."

"Neuroleptanalgesic" Agents: In recent years, combinations of such drugs as the analgesic Phenoperidine with a sedative have been used to produce a state of emotional detachment in which the patient becomes apathetic. The most commonly used "neuroleptanalgesic" agent is *Innovar.* The drug incidentally has a strong anti-nausea effect.

TYPES OF ANESTHETICS

AGENTS THAT BLOCK THE PERIPHERAL STIMULUS AT ITS ORIGIN

These agents afford local anesthesia within minutes, are relatively harmless, and do not cause any general loss of sensation. They cause little or no relaxation of tissues and do not allay anxiety. The agents block the peripheral nerve endings of the mucous membranes, skin, and periosteum, and induce anesthesia when directly introduced into the proposed surgical site by means of *topical application* or *local infiltration.*

Topical Application

Mucous membranes readily absorb certain anesthetic agents, affording short-term local anesthesia for minor procedures. These agents are sprayed or dropped on mucous membranes such as those of the nasopharynx, the rectum, the vagina, and the buccal mucosa. Xylocaine, the most popular such agent, is rapidly effective and does not entail the complications encountered with other agents, such as cocaine or butacaine.

Uses

1. To anesthetize the nasopharynx and larynx prior to bronchoscopic or laryngoscopic examination.

2. To anesthetize a painful rectal lesion prior to rectal examination.

Administration. The agent is usually kept in an aerosol spray container and is directly applied to the mucous membrane as a fine mist. Several sprays or applications may be necessary in order to completely anesthetize the area, and the effects are of a very short duration.

Complications. Very rarely, patients may react to topical anesthetics with an anaphylactic shock state, usually the result of prior sensitization to the drug. The condition is treated with cortisone and adrenalin. A careful history of drug allergy should be taken prior to the use of topical anesthetics.

Local Infiltration

The surgical site may be injected intracutaneously and subcutaneously, thereby blocking peripheral nerve impulses. Xylocaine, again, with or without adrenalin, is used almost exclusively as the drug of choice.

Uses. All types of minor procedures, including excision of small skin lesions, suturing of lacerations, extraction of teeth, and excision of external hemorrhoids.

Administration. A hypodermic syringe is used to inject the agent directly into the surgical site. In the case of skin anesthesia, a no. 25 bore needle is used to raise a small skin wheal, following which a larger needle (no. 19 or no. 20) may be used to produce a wider and deeper area of local anesthesia. Anesthesia is obtained in 2 to 5 minutes and will last for several minutes. The duration of anesthesia may be lengthened by adding a vasoconstrictor (adrenalin) to the anesthetic. Local vasoconstriction enhances the length of anesthesia by permitting the drug to remain at its site of injection for a longer period of time.

Complications. Allergic reactions, again rare, may result in anaphylactic shock. Toxic blood levels of the local anesthetic and/or the added adrenalin can cause periods of excitement and confusion progressing to loss of consciousness, convulsions, and respiratory and circulatory arrest.

AGENTS THAT BLOCK THE TRANSMISSION OF PAIN IMPULSES ALONG AFFERENT NERVES FROM THE SURGICAL SITE

Local anesthetics such as xylocaine or Marcaine may also be injected *regionally* — that is, at a certain distance from the proposed surgical site. Such procedures are able to afford a *greater* surface area of block than local anesthesia, as the afferent nerves from a wide area may be blocked by merely injecting the large nerve bundles emanating from a given area.

Uses and Examples of Regional Block Anesthesia

Digital Block. To obtain anesthesia of an entire finger for treatment of injury or infection.

Ulnar and Radial Block. May be used to anesthetize the entire hand.

Brachial Plexus Block (Axillary or Supraclavicular). The entire arm is rendered insensitive so that soft tissue and orthopedic procedures may be performed.

Special Form of Regional Block (Intravenous Block). This block involves the filling of veins of the arm with xylocaine after a tourniquet has been applied to the upper arm. This block may also be used for soft tissue or orthopedic procedures on the arm or hand.

Administration. Regional blocks (with the exception of intravenous block) require a high degree of knowledge of the regional anatomy relative to the particular location of major afferent nerve bundles that affect sensation from the proposed surgical site. The anesthetic agent is injected around the nerve bundles and anesthesia is brought about in the surgical site within 10 to 30 minutes, depending upon the size of the nerve bundles and their distance from the surgical site. The anesthetic effect will last 30 to 60 minutes.

Complications. Absorption of an anesthetic agent into the blood stream, with all its potential hazards, is more likely to occur with regional anesthesia than with local anesthesia simply because the needle usually penetrates deeper into highly vascular tissues such as muscles. The great care that must be taken to avoid such an occurrence involves withdrawing the syringe before each injection of anesthetic agent.

Injecting an anesthetic agent around the base of a digit to produce digital anesthesia is usually quite safe. However, vasoconstricting agents should be steadfastly avoided, as gangrene of the digit can occur from prolonged total ischemia.

There are specific complications associated with certain regional blocks:

Brachial Plexus and Supraclavicular Blocks. The needle tip is very near the apex of the lung at the time of infiltration of an anesthetic agent. A small tear in the pleura may lead to a pneumothorax. This occurs in about one per cent of supraclavicular blocks. It is usually innocuous when unilateral but may be very dangerous when bilateral. All patients who have had this type of block should have frequent examinations of their breath sounds for 24 hours and, if there is any asymmetry of breath sounds, a chest x-ray should be ordered.

Deep Cervical Nerve Blocks.   In performing such blocks, there is a risk that an anesthetic agent may be injected into a vertebral artery, resulting in loss of consciousness, apnea, and, possibly, a convulsion.

Intravenous Block with Tourniquet.   A systemic toxic effect can occur from leakage of anesthetic material through a faulty tourniquet or from rapidly decompressing the tourniquet. A sudden discharge of large amounts of xylocaine into the general circulation can result in cardiac arrhythmias or cardiac arrest.

AGENTS THAT BLOCK THE CONDUCTING PATHWAYS IN AND AROUND THE SPINAL CORD

Local anesthetic agents may be injected extradurally (epidural block anesthesia) or intradurally (spinal anesthesia), depending on the type of operative procedure to be carried out and the preference of the anesthesiologist. Epidural anesthesia avoids the complications of arachnoiditis and spinal headaches, both of which occur occasionally from spinal anesthesia.

Uses.   Epidural and spinal anesthesia are very versatile techniques and can be used for a variety of surgical, obstetrical, and neurological procedures.

Administration.   The actual techniques of these procedures need not be described here. The student is referred to textbooks of anesthesia for a complete description.

Complications.   Epidural anesthesia is remarkably free from serious side effects. Occasionally there is an extensive anesthetic block of preganglionic sympathetic nerve fibers, resulting in serious hypotension. Spinal anesthesia, on the other hand, may lead to arachnoiditis, meningitis, and prolonged, rather severe post-spinal headaches. Subarachnoiditis, a rare complication, may result in varying degrees of paralysis, which is usually permanent.

AGENTS THAT BLOCK THE "AWARENESS CENTERS" IN THE BRAIN

These agents are the "general anesthetics" — those agents that render the patient relaxed and calm and produce varying degrees of loss of sensation, including total loss. A complete discussion of all the complex areas of general anesthesia is outside the scope of this book, but certain points should be outlined. The wide variety of gases and liquids that serve as general anesthetics can be analyzed in terms of their route of administration: whether the agent is administered directly into the lungs, intravenously, or rectally. Accordingly, there are three types of general anesthesia: inhalational, intravenous, and rectal.

Inhalational Anesthesia

Inhalational anesthesia is induced by various gases and liquids administered directly into the lungs by means of a mask-breathing technique or through an endotracheal tube. The agents are inhaled by the patient and rapidly gain entrance into the circulatory system at the capillary-alveolar site, from which they pass to the central nervous system. Here they block all sensory pathways to the brain and render the patient unconscious.

Some of the more commonly used inhalational anesthetics are:

Nitrous Oxide.   This analgesic gas is probably the most commonly used inhalational anesthetic today. It is not a very potent anesthetic and is often combined with a narcotic, a muscle relaxant, or a volatile agent such as halothane. It is frequently used as an analgesic to lessen uterine pain occurring during labor.

Cyclopropane. This potent anesthetic agent is seldom used today, principally because it is highly explosive. It is capable of producing deep anesthesia and good muscle relaxation. Newer and safer agents, particularly halothane and penthrane, along with the excellent muscle relaxants that are now available, have all but eliminated cyclopropane from general use. However, when strong circulatory support is needed, as in the patient in shock, it remains an excellent drug.

Halothane. This volatile liquid is a very popular anesthetic with a wide spectrum of use today. The induction of halothane is rapid, and pleasant, with few side effects. Because of evidence (of a rather tenuous nature) incriminating halothane as an immunological hepatotoxin, it is usually avoided in the jaundiced patient or the patient with known or suspected liver disease, past or present.

Penthrane. This is a longer-acting agent than halothane but is less of a relaxant. It may be nephrotoxic, depending on the dosage employed. It is often used in obstetrics to produce basal analgesia.

Uses of Inhalational Anesthetics. General inhalational anesthesia is standard for most major operations of the head, neck, thorax, and upper abdomen. It is the only anesthetic method that fulfills the *three main objectives of anesthesia:*

1. *Prevention of pain:* Since inhalational anesthesia renders the patient unconscious, prevention is complete.

2. *Relaxation of tissues:* Some general anesthetics cause excellent relaxation (e.g., cyclopropane) at safe dosage levels. Others (e.g., halothane) require muscle relaxants as supplements.

3. *Allaying of anxiety:* The patient is fully asleep at all times.

Complications of Inhalational Anesthesia. The induction of anesthesia is far safer nowadays than it was only 30 years ago. Nevertheless, with the advances in surgery and the development of more and more complex surgical procedures, medicine has necessarily developed more and more potent anesthetics, muscle relaxants, and so forth. Some of these agents, in unskilled hands, are extremely toxic. Complications are generally of a cardiopulmonary, hepatic, or cardiorenal nature, with many metabolic counterparts.

Most complications of general anesthesia occur on the induction of or emergence from anesthesia. The operating room nurse must give her whole attention to the anesthesiologist and the patient at these times.

Cardiopulmonary Complications

Cardiac Arrhythmias and Cardiac Arrest. The chemical environment that surrounds the myocardium and helps sustain the normal cardiac rhythm is quite sensitive to many disturbing stimuli, particularly anoxia. Under anesthesia, retention of carbon dioxide and the development of acidosis and anoxia may set the stage for a cardiac arrest, often heralded by a variety of complex cardiac arrhythmias. Careful monitoring of the respirations and the patient's color and vital signs, along with a thorough knowledge of *lethal* combinations (e.g., hyperkalemia plus anoxia), will go far toward preventing a great number of these operative disasters.

Should cardiac arrest occur in the operating room, the scrub nurse and circulating nurse have several immediate duties. Chief among these are:

1. Note the time of the cardiac arrest; if special stop clocks are present in the operating room, these should be started at once.

2. An electrocardiogram, defibrillator, and cardiac pacemaker are made available at once.

3. The circulating nurse is to assist the anesthetist by obtaining special drugs, aiding with intravenous lines, and so on.

4. The scrub nurse prepares a knife, rib spreaders, sponges, and other materials appropriate for opening of the chest (should this be necessary).

Bronchospasm and Laryngospasm. The irritating effects of certain anesthetic agents, as well as their possible allergenic effect on the laryngeal and bronchial mucosa, can result in acute bronchospasm and laryngospasm. Such spasms are particularly apt to occur in the heavy smoker, the patient with chronic lung disease, or the patient with an overt acute upper respiratory infection. If a spasm goes unchecked, anoxia follows, leading to cerebral edema or cardiac arrest. One of the great advantages of an endotracheal tube is that it prevents obstructive respiratory disease mechanisms such as laryngospasm. It also prevents pulmonary aspiration of gastric contents during vomiting.

Vomiting and Aspiration. Anesthetics act to abolish certain protective reflexes surrounding the opening of the laryngotracheal area. When this effect is combined with the irritating actions of certain anesthetics on the gastrointestinal tract, vomiting of gastric contents may occur, with aspiration into the tracheobronchial tree. Such an event can lead to acute anoxia and death. In other cases, aspiration may lead to postoperative pulmonary edema and chemical pneumonitis, a combination which itself may prove fatal. This tragic complication is avoidable if the stomach is kept empty prior to induction of anesthesia and if the induction is carried out skillfully and rapidly. When in doubt about the contents of the stomach, it is wise to insert a Levin tube preoperatively and aspirate the organ. However, there is still *no guarantee* that there is no retained food or fluid in the stomach, and the administration of anesthesia remains, under these circumstances, an extremely hazardous procedure. A skilled anesthetist, aware of the dangers, may elect to "crash induce" with rapid intubation or prior intubation of the awake patient in order to avoid possible complications.

Respiratory Obstruction and Failure. In addition to physiological obstruction (laryngospasm and bronchospasm), mechanical obstruction of the airway may occur shortly before or during anesthesia. The relaxed tongue may obstruct the larynx; excessive mucus may act as a mechanical block to the tracheobronchial tree; foreign bodies, such as a tooth, may dislodge and implant in the airway. Edema of the larynx (caused by tumor or inflammation) and large, substernal thyroid tumors are also possible causes of obstruction.

Respiratory failure is usually due to overdosage of respiration-depressing drugs given during induction or during maintenance of anesthesia. It may also be due to cerebral edema, breath-holding during the induction period, carotid body stimulation, or traction on the mesentery.

Shock and Hypotension. The normal physiological mechanisms that support blood pressure are a complex group of neurophysiological, chemical and endocrine mechanisms that complement and supplement each other in the maintenance of cardiovascular homeostasis under varying conditions. The assorted premedications and powerful anesthetic agents used today, combined with blood loss, surgical trauma, anoxia, and the like, are strong noxious stimuli which tend to derange the mechanisms supporting blood pressure.

Possibly the most common and direct cause of significant operative shock is blood loss. In a sense, this shock is not directly due to the anesthesia, and perhaps should not be considered as a complication of anesthesia. However, since the normal reflexes to shock are depressed by anesthetic agents, and since the anesthetist is responsible for recognizing and treating blood loss shock occurring in the operating room, it is best considered here.

Surgeons tend to underestimate blood loss. It is the function of the anesthetist to keep a running account of blood loss by whatever method he feels is most effective. Weighing of surgical sponges soaked with blood, monitoring of vital signs and central venous pressure, determinations of blood volume, and many other methods have been suggested for estimating the amount of blood lost in a given procedure. Each method has its advocates, and perhaps no method is completely reliable. The senior author has been impressed, over the years, with the accuracy of the anesthetist's estimates; in addition, in the majority of cases involving large blood losses and replacements, serial postoperative hematocrits and blood volume determinations have been close to the mark.

The circulating nurse shares in the responsibility of counting and weighing blood-soaked sponges, should this be the method chosen to estimate blood loss.

Other causes of operative shock include:

1. Dehydration.
2. Vasodilator effect of certain anesthetic agents (e.g., halothane).
3. "Neurogenic shock," secondary to inadequate anesthesia, producing vasodilation in response to pain.
4. Traction on mesentery.
5. Occult cerebrovascular accidents which may not be fully realized until after surgery.
6. Cardiac arrhythmias or arrest
7. Respiratory failure with peripheral anoxia.
8. Acute adrenal insufficiency.

Cerebral Complications

Cerebrovascular Accidents. These may occur during the induction period, operatively, or as the patient is recovering from anesthesia. More often occurring in the elderly, arteriosclerotic patient, this complication may be fatal during or shortly after surgery. The carotid pulses should be checked preoperatively. Murmurs or diminished pulsations should be noted. Hypotension superimposed on carotid artery insufficiency may be a disastrous combination.

Convulsions. These are often secondary to anoxia and excessive buildup of carbon dioxide in the circulating blood due to poor ventilation.

Emergence Delirium. This is a state of severe excitement during recovery from certain anesthetics, particularly cyclopropane.

Renal Complications

Renal ischemia secondary to operative hypotension, superimposed on an already injured or chronically damaged kidney, may result in acute tubular necrosis, with postoperative renal failure. The initial phase may not be recognized until long after recovery from anesthesia, but it should be understood as a complication related to the anesthetized state. The patient should be kept well oxygenated and well hydrated during any operation, but these requirements are particularly urgent if he is known to have had any previous renal disease.

"Minor" Complications

These include corneal abrasion, injuries to the lips and tongue, damaged teeth, impairment of vocal cords, peripheral nerve injury from improper positioning, fires and explosions, and a host of other problems which begin as "simple" incidents. "Little" oversights and "brief" periods of inattention may lead to tragic conclusions. The law that "if something *can* go wrong it *will* go wrong" applies as strongly in the operating room as anywhere else. The circulating nurses and the scrub nurses, along with all personnel attending the patient, share a common goal: to *get the patient through* safely and efficiently.

Postoperative Complications

These are covered in detail in the chapter on recovery room management and will not be repeated here.

Intravenous Anesthetics

These agents afford a very simple and extremely rapid means of pleasantly inducing anesthesia in the surgical patient.

Thiopental sodium and Brevital are the most commonly used of the intravenous anesthetics. They are injected via a secure intravenous catheter placed in the upper extremity. The dosages must be carefully judged according to the patient's size, age, and state of health. At low doses, they are sufficient to cause sleep, but pain reflexes are not abolished. Consequently, these agents must be supplemented with some other general anesthetic to produce enough analgesia and relaxation for surgery.

Intravenous anesthetics depress respirations. Large doses are toxic, resulting in respiratory arrest and death. Small doses may, at times, cause severe bronchospasm, which can be fatal. Careful monitoring of respiration and the presence of easily accessible endotracheal tubes make these complications rare occurrences in a modern surgical suite.

Uses. Intravenous anesthetics find their most common use in the production of unconsciousness prior to the use of more powerful anesthetics. As mentioned, sleep is induced smoothly, rapidly, and quite pleasantly, thereby obviating any need for the patient to experience noxious, malodorous anesthetic gases while awake.

Used alone, intravenous anesthetics may provide sufficient analgesia for dental extractions, uterine dilatations and curettages, pelvic examinations, endoscopic examinations, and other minor procedures.

Rectal Anesthetics

Anesthetic agents such as pentothal may be administered rectally, although this is very rare today. The rectal mucosa rapidly absorbs the anesthetic, which is then delivered via the circulation to the central nervous system. Loss of consciousness is never complete, so that a *basal narcosis* occurs — a state that must always be supplemented by other agents if surgery is planned. Hypnotic effects appear about 5 minutes after rectal administration and last for 1 to 2 hours.

MISCELLANEOUS ANESTHETICS

Cryothermia

Marked reduction in surface temperature diminishes pain reflexes. Under extreme conditions, when life is threatened and the patient can not tolerate conventional anesthesia, it is possible to cool the affected part with ice and operate. However, this procedure — cryothermia — probably has no role in modern surgery because of the use of a wide variety of more effective, safer techniques.

Hypnoanesthesia

Carefully selected patients may be hypnotized and rendered pain-free by autosuggestion. It has been used in obstetrics where fetal safety is a necessity and in certain dental procedures. The difficulties of the procedure are related to the selection of subjects, some of whom are resistant, and to the posthypnotic aftereffects, which are especially likely to occur in the neurotic patient who might be the best candidate for suggestion in the first place. By and large, hypnoanesthesia has no place in the everyday practice of surgery.

Acupuncture

So little is known about this procedure, at least in this country, that it is mentioned merely for the sake of completeness. It is possible that acquisition of more knowledge of its potential and action will result in its addition to the anesthesiologist's armamentarium.

FACTORS DETERMINING THE CHOICE OF ANESTHETIC

NATURE OF THE PROCEDURE

Minor Procedures. Most minor procedures can be safely carried out with local infiltrative or regional block anesthesia. The excessively nervous patient may also be given a basal narcotic or sedative to relax him and make the experience less traumatic.

Major Procedures. Basically, the choice is between general anesthesia or some type of block anesthesia. General anesthesia is used for all major head, neck, thoracic, and upper abdominal surgery. The choice of general anesthetic agent will depend on:

1. *Whether relaxation is necessary.* Generally speaking, agents causing relaxation are more potent and dangerous than agents merely causing analgesia. When possible, therefore, the relaxant agents are avoided. Facial and neck surgery, for example, require very little relaxation, and relaxants are therefore avoided.

2. *Whether an explosive agent is acceptable.* Any work requiring electrocautery or fulguration contraindicates use of explosive agents.

Spinal anesthesia, as a form of block anesthesia, can be used for lower abdominal, pelvic, perineal, and lower extremity surgery. It should be avoided in disc and other back surgery, and in upper abdominal surgery as well.

PHYSICAL CONDITION OF THE PATIENT

Those with Severe Cardiac Disease. Agents which are known to cause cardiac arrhythmias (e.g., cyclopropane) should be avoided or used with caution in such patients. Spinal anesthesia is often hazardous, as severe hypotension, leading to myocardial infarction, may occur.

Those with Chronic Pulmonary Disease. Agents causing severe irritation of the tracheo-bronchial tree (e.g., ether) should be avoided.

Those with Known Bleeding Disorders. Spinal anesthesia is contraindicated here, as an epidural hemorrhage may occur, leading to paraplegia. Likewise, and for the same reason, patients receiving anticoagulants should not undergo spinal anesthesia.

Those with Central Nervous System or Nerve Root Disease. Spinal anesthesia is contraindicated.

Those with Jaundice or Hepatic Disorders. Halothane is contraindicated.

SUMMARY

The nurse plays an important and active role in all phases of modern anesthesiology, and it behooves her to understand the uses, dangers, complications, and pharmacological actions of anesthetic agents.

Preoperatively, the surgical nurse, like other members of the surgical team, is called upon to aid in the total assessment of surgical and anesthetic risk factors, previous drug experiences of the patient, known underlying disease states, and so forth. She is more than a *confidante.* The nurse should evaluate the patient's condition by looking for cardiac problems, carotid murmurs, renal symptoms, and a multitude of often subtle risk factors that may escape other members of the surgical team. She should review the medical chart and the data as they become available. Any discrepancy, any clue to some unexpected or unnoted problem, should be called to the surgeon's and anesthesiologist's attention. It is *never safe to assume* that someone else knows the problem.

During surgery — and especially during induction of and emergence from the anesthetic state — the circulating nurse must be acutely aware of the important physiological and pharmacological events that are transpiring. She must watch for details: Is the IV fluid flowing? What is the time on the clock? Are the nail beds cyanotic? Is the patient positioned on the table to minimize nerve trauma? Is the patient strapped in position correctly? The list of these details, so important to the well-being of the patient, lengthens as the surgical nurse gains experience in the care of the operative patient.

Postoperatively, the surgical nurse begins the important task of anticipating anesthetic and surgical complications. A firm theoretical knowledge must be supplemented by experience and hard work so that the nurse may continually assess and reassess the patient in the particularly precarious period as he emerges from the anesthetic and enters the recovery room phase.

9   THE OPERATING ROOM EXPERIENCE

The student is gradually introduced to operating room activities. Each experience must be mastered thoroughly before a new one becomes safe and instructive. This chapter will attempt to follow the student's progressive introduction to the operating room. Each operating room instructor approaches this educational task differently. The precise chronology of the student's experiences may be at variance with what is outlined here. Nevertheless, the *general principles* and experiences described will aid the student in orienting herself to *any* operating room environment and will afford her added insight into the rationale of each experience. Details of procedure are minimized, as they serve only to confuse the student who must learn them through individual instruction.

THE ROLE OF THE OPERATING ROOM TEAM

Surgery is a complex field requiring a *coordinated team* effort. In Chapter 1, the three objectives of surgical patient care were noted, and it is well to repeat them here:

1. The delivery of a psychologically and physiologically prepared patient to surgery.
2. The safe, efficient, and sound alleviation of the patient's problem.
3. The careful guidance of the patient's immediate postoperative course.

These objectives are partially fulfilled in the clinical unit preoperatively and in the recovery room postoperatively. But it is in the operating room itself that the operative team must fully coordinate its work if the surgery is to have a successful outcome.

As the student first approaches the operating room, she should strive to form a *general picture* of the operative team. This picture should define the *duties* of each member of the team and depict these members in actual function as they carry out their duties. Such an over-all concept will aid the student immensely when she later assumes the role of scrub nurse or circulating nurse.

ROLE OF THE ANESTHESIOLOGIST AND ANESTHETIST

The general well-being of the patient is the responsibility of the anesthesiologist and his anesthetist. By relieving the surgeon of this responsibility they permit him to concentrate on the technical aspects of the operation.

In addition to their general responsibilities of evaluating the patient preoperatively, anesthetizing the patient, and keeping him at adequate but safe levels for surgery, the anesthesiologist and anesthetist:

1. Infuse whatever drugs are required by them or the surgeon.
2. Transfuse blood or blood products as necessary.
3. Alert the surgeon to any impending difficulties and treat these as they arise.
4. Supervise the recovery room management of the patient.

PROFESSIONAL NURSING IN THE OPERATING ROOM*

Definition

Professional nursing in the operating room involves the identification of the physiological, psychological, and sociological needs of the patient; to meet these needs, programs of nursing care that are individualized to each patient must be instituted. All programs must be based on a thorough knowledge of the natural and behavioral sciences, and of course must be designed to maintain the health and welfare of the patient before, during, and after surgical intervention.

Clinical Practice

The paramount objective in the clinical practice of professional operating room nursing is to provide a standard of excellence in the care of the patient that will extend from the preoperative period through the actual surgery to the postoperative period. This objective is achieved by:

1. Identification of the needs of the patient.
2. Development and implementation of an individualized plan of nursing care that meets the identified needs of the patient.
3. Coordination of the individualized plan with the responsibilities of the other members of the health team, thereby promoting continuity in the nursing care for each patient.
4. Application of the principles of asepsis and technical knowledge so that a safe environment for the welfare of the patient may be ensured.
5. Guidance of other professional and allied technical personnel in the nursing care of the patient by teaching and supervising them (and by evaluating their performance as well).
6. Initiation of or cooperation with research projects designed to develop a body of scientific knowledge relative to the care and coordination components of professional operating room nursing.

---

*The material in the following two sections (i.e., "Definition" and "Clinical Practice") has been adapted from "Definition and Objective for Clinical Practice of Professional Operating Room Nursing," AORN Journal, November, 1969, 10:43–47.

ROLE OF THE CIRCULATING NURSE

The more experienced or senior nurse usually assumes the role of circulating nurse. As the only nonscrubbed member of the surgical team, the circulating nurse represents the connecting link between the scrub team and all other departments which may be called upon to assist the surgeon. She is, as it were, instructor, supervisor, and manager in the room assigned to her.

A list of some of the general duties of the circulating nurse will aid the student in appreciating the importance and versatility of this member of the surgical team.

Duties Relating to the Operating Room

1. Checks the room for general cleanliness and orderliness prior to each case.
2. Checks operating room lights, suction and oxygen machines, and other pieces of equipment, making certain they are all available and properly functioning.
3. Adjusts lights, stands, stools, and other equipment as it is used in each case.
4. Checks proper functioning of sterilizer.
5. Rearranges and supervises the preparation of the room after each case in anticipation of the following case.

Duties Relating Directly to the Patient

1. Receives and identifies patient from the receiving area.
2. Introduces herself to the patient and attempts to develop rapport and confidence.
3. Aids in transferring patient to operating room table.
4. Positions and secures patient on table and confirms position with surgeon.
5. Covers patient's hair with a cap.
6. Rearranges draw sheets, cover sheets, and anesthesia screen to be certain nothing will interfere with the operation.
7. Initiates skin prep according to routine of hospital and surgeon.

Duties Relating to Operating Room Personnel

1. Helps to gown all members of the scrub team.
2. Keeps a constant vigilance on proper dress, movements, and techniques of all personnel to insure no break in aseptic technique.
3. Checks to be certain scrub nurse has everything she needs to begin the operation.
4. Is available to the scrub nurse for advice and for obtaining any special equipment deemed necessary as the case proceeds.
5. Checks with the surgeon concerning any special equipment or suture material he may require.
6. Supervises and aids in sponge, needle, and instrument counts.
7. Calls x-ray or laboratory technicians at the surgeon's request.
8. Calls pathologist at the surgeon's request.
9. Keeps room as clean and orderly as possible during the case.
10. Is available to the anesthesia team for obtaining special drugs, aiding with initiation of intravenous fluids, and so forth.

11. Accepts, labels, and records all specimens received from the surgeon.

12. At conclusion of case, she assists in transferring patient to litter for trip to recovery room.

ROLE OF THE SCRUB NURSE

Becoming an efficient scrub nurse requires, above 'all else, *experience.* This must be intelligent experience, based on a thorough understanding of each proposed surgical procedure and a careful observation and anticipation of each step in the operation.

THOROUGH UNDERSTANDING OF THE PROCEDURE

The scrub nurse must:

1. Read the schedule, noting type of case, estimated length, and type of anesthesia to be used.

2. Review basic anatomy, physiology, and operative technique books if she is not already thoroughly familiar with the type of case.

3. Check all types of instruments to be used in the case. If there are any special instruments that may be needed, she should discuss these with the surgeon to obtain some idea of his preferences.

4. Discuss any questions about the nature of the case with the surgeon.

5. Have available all the types of sutures that will probably be used in the case. She should discuss with the surgeon any preferences he may have.

Observation and Anticipation of Each Step in the Procedure

The scrub nurse must:

1. Observe the skin incision, for example, from the viewpoint of how much bleeding is occurring. She may be able to anticipate the need for hemostatic clamps and ligatures to control this bleeding.

2. Observe the progress of the dissection and isolation of tissues. With experience, she will be able to anticipate the need for special retractors, sponges, abdominal packs, and the like.

3. Observe the surgical field. She should try to keep it free from all unnecessary instruments, sponges, and free suture ends. Neatness is a major factor in safe, efficient surgery.

4. Anticipate special problems. For example, if a ruptured appendix is found at laparotomy, she will properly anticipate the need for suction apparatus, culture swabs, and drains, and will advise the circulating nurse accordingly.

5. Observe all members of the operating team for possible breaks in aseptic technique. It is her responsibility, as it is that of any member of the team, to announce such breaks in technique.

6. Watch the surgeon's hand signals carefully. With practice, she will understand many of the unspoken signals for instruments.

The scrub nurse's duties are manifold and include:

1. Aiding the surgeon and assistants in gowning and gloving.

2. Aiding the surgeon or assistant in draping the patient.

3. Handing instruments, sponges, sutures, etc. to the surgeon and his assistant as needed.

4. Holding retractors, if necessary.

5. Aiding in the sponge, needle, and instrument count.

6. Observing the team for breaks in aseptic technique.

ROLE OF THE SURGEON AND HIS ASSISTANT

The surgeon performs the operation with the help of his assistant. The assistant is responsible for *exposing* the operative site for the surgeon. This requires that he *retract* nearby tissues away from the operative site and *sponge* or *suction* blood and serum as it accumulates and obscures the local anatomy. Should small venous or arterial bleeders be found in the operative site, often it is the assistant who grasps them with hemostats preparatory to ligating them with suture. Either the surgeon or his assistant will ligate these "bleeders."

It is important that the scrub nurse understand the various functions of the surgeon and his assistant or assistants. In this way she can better anticipate which instruments each is likely to request of her. Although the situation is extremely variable in each case, some of the specific functions of surgeon and assistant, and the instruments or materials required, are as follows:

Laparotomy

	Technique	*Material Required*
Surgeon:	Incision of skin, sub-cutaneous tissue.	Skin knife and deep knife.
	Incisions of deep fascia and peritoneum	Metzenbaum or Mayo scissors; toothed forceps.
	Dissection and exposure of local pathological conditions.	Smooth dressing forceps and Metzenbaum scissors.
Assistant:	Controls subcutaneous "bleeders."	Small straight or curved hemostats; 4 by 4 sponges; fine cotton, silk, or catgut ties.
	Exposure of deeper tissues.	Retractors; "lap" pads; long dressing forceps and suction.

The nurse would do well to make a mental list of this progression and the instruments required as she observes several cases.

ROLE OF THE SURGICAL TECHNICIAN

The surgical technician should be a skilled worker qualified by his grasp of theory and his clinical experience to provide services in the operating room under the direction of the operating room supervisor. The technician is a part of the operating room team and is responsible for medical asepsis, safety measures, and overall efficient performance in the operating room. His knowledge of and experience with aseptic technique entitle him to prepare materials and supplies for use at the time of the operation and to assist during surgical procedures in the same fashion as a scrub nurse.

ROLE OF OTHER DEPARTMENTS

Pathologist. He is often called upon by the surgeon to identify the pathologic process discovered by the surgeon. This often occurs in the form of the "frozen section," a rapid microscopic analysis of tissue handed to the pathologist.

X-ray Technician. Occasionally the surgeon may require an x-ray in the operating room. The circulating nurse is responsible for notifying the x-ray technician. Certain situations frequently require the help of the x-ray department:

1. Operative cholangiograms: to determine presence or absence of stones in the common bile duct.

2. Plain film of abdomen to determine location of a missing sponge.

3. Arteriogram: to determine patency or obstruction of a blood vessel.

The x-ray technician must, of course, exercise aseptic technique in the operating room. The circulating nurse must see to it that no breaks in aseptic technique occur while the x-ray is being taken. The x-ray tube must be properly shielded from the operative site with a sterile towel. The machine itself must not contact the operating table. Finally, the technician must exercise care so as not to contact sterile equipment in the operating room.

With this general picture of the specific roles of various members of the operating room team in mind, the student nurse will begin her progressive experience in the operating room.

OPERATING ROOM EXPERIENCES

Assignment One: Follow a Patient through His Surgery to the Recovery Room

Purposes
To learn the proper dress of an operating room nurse.

To become acquainted with the physical nature of the operating room suite.

To learn the fundamental principles of safe conduct and aseptic technique in the operating room.

To observe the various members of the surgical team as they carry out their functions.

PROCEDURES

Acquaint yourself thoroughly with the patient's general condition and the reason for his impending surgery. This should include a survey of the chart, the preparation of the patient for surgery, and a brief informal interview with the patient.

Review the surgical anatomy and surgical steps to be undertaken.

Be certain *you* have no cutaneous or respiratory infections. If in doubt, consult your instructor or supervisor before appearing in the operating room suite.

Operating Room Dress, Cap, and Mask

You will then be conducted to the nurses' dressing room and assigned a uniform.

1. Undergarments must be *safe* with respect to static electricity.

2. The *scrub dress* must be form-fitting so as to eliminate chances of its brushing against a sterile surface.

3. The *cap* must completely cover your hair, as the latter is a source of contamination from airborne bacteria.

4. The *mask* must cover your nose and mouth and fit firmly below your chin.

Conductive shoes. Special shoes or shoe covers must be worn to insure proper conductivity of static electricity into the floor. Once you have put on your shoes, conductivity should be tested on the *conductometer* which you will find in the operating room or in the corridor (Fig. 9–1).

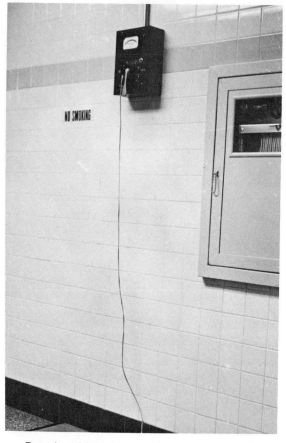

NO SMOKING

FIGURE 9–1 A typical conductometer located in the main operating room corridor.

Remain with your patient in the corridor at all times. Quiet conversation with him will do much to calm his fears. Be extremely prudent when answering any of his questions.

While awaiting the scrub team and circulating nurse, you have an opportunity to study the physical nature of the operating room suite as described in Chapter 2. You should compare the nature of your operating suite with the description given in this manual.

Safety Precautions with Regard to Anesthetic Gases

1. You have already tested your own conductivity on the conductometer. This is a most important safety precaution.

2. Although the operating room tables, stands, and stools are all equipped with conductive chains or casters, any unnecessary scraping of these articles along the floor is dangerous, as this may generate static electricity.

3. Smoking is allowed only in specific lounges with doors closed.

Fundamental Principles of Aseptic Technique

In Chapter 3, the modes and sources of contamination were encountered. It is well to repeat them here:

Modes of Contamination

1. Direct contact between a nonsterile and a sterile surface.

2. Nonsterile moisture droplets falling on a sterile surface.
3. Nonsterile air circulating over a sterile surface.
4. Hematogenous: from the patient's circulation.

Sources of Contamination

1. The scrub team's skin.
2. The scrub team's respiratory tracts.
3. The patient's respiratory tract.
4. The patient's circulation.
5. Linens, instruments, sutures, and other equipment.
6. The circulating air.
7. The patient's skin.
8. The patient's gastrointestinal tract.
9. The scrub team's hair.
10. The bronchial tree.

Briefly, aseptic technique consists in eliminating or minimizing all modes and sources of contamination, for *where there is no contamination, there can be no sepsis.*

Sources 1 and 2 are eliminated or minimized by the surgical scrub and by masking, gowning, and gloving. The weakest link in this area is the escape of bacteria through the surgical mask, which is relatively permeable to finely dispersed moisture droplets on which bacteria cling. To diminish this source of contamination, *all unnecessary conversation* in the operating room is prohibited. Masks should be changed between cases or, in exceptionally long cases, a second mask may be put on after 2 or 3 hours have passed. Improved, chemically treated masks are now available and seem to lessen the chances of droplet contamination. When you are not in the operating room suite, you should not let the surgical mask hang from your neck; discard the original mask and take a new one when you return to the operating room.

Source 3 is minimized by the use of an anesthesia screen, when feasible, to separate the patient's nose and mouth from the operative site. Some hospitals also mask the patient.

Source 4 is minimized by the preoperative eradication of any known respiratory or other infections in the patient.

Sources 5 and 6 will be discussed in this section of the manual.

Sources 7, 8, 9, and 10 will be covered in other sections.

Linens, instruments, sutures, and other surgical equipment are *initially* sterile when the surgery begins. They can become contaminated by contact with a nonsterile surface, article, or person, or from the circulating air, and then, in turn, become sources of contamination. *Aseptic technique* consists in observing all the "rules" or principles laid down to positively prevent contamination of these articles during the course of the operation. These principles of aseptic technique are as follows:

1. All articles of doubtful sterility are to be considered nonsterile, *however remote the doubt.*
2. Any article whose sterile pack has been found unfastened is considered nonsterile.
3. Any linen which is moistened becomes permeable to organisms. If one of its surfaces is in contact with a nonsterile area, then its other surface is considered contaminated.
4. Sterile instruments, sutures, and linens must be passed to the scrub nurse. They are not to be dropped on a sterile table. Nor is the circulating nurse to reach over a sterile table with her hands.
5. A nonsterile person is to remain in a nonsterile area of the operating room, and must not lean over or reach over a sterile area.
6. Likewise, a sterile person is to remain in a sterile area, and must not lean over or reach over a nonsterile area. The sterile area of the sterile table ends at the level of the table, below this level being theoretically unsterile even though apparently draped. The theoretical sterile area of a gown extends, in front, from shoulder to waist, including sleeves. The arms and hands must never

reach above or below these levels. When passing instruments to the surgeon, one must be particularly careful to keep the hand and arm down low at the level of the operating table, avoiding a possible contact with the surgeon's mask or face.

7. The lip of a sterile container is nonsterile. When pouring from it, a few drops should be dispensed into a catch basin before pouring the sterile solution into sterile basins.

8. The edge of a pack or paper container is nonsterile, and must not contaminate the enclosed articles.

9. Measures used to minimize the circulating air as a source of contamination:
   a. *Frequent and Thorough Housecleaning.* The entire operating room suite must be kept uncluttered and as dust-free as possible. Germicidal agents are used according to a definite prescribed routine by well-trained personnel.
   b. *Proper Ventilation.* The ventilators must be of adequate size and checked periodically for proper function.
   c. The doors to the operating room are kept closed at all times.
   d. All unnecessary traffic to and from the operating room is forbidden.
   e. All unnecessary motion in the operating room is forbidden, e.g., dirty linens carefully placed into appropriate catch basins, *never thrown.*
   f. Conversation is kept at a minimum.
   g. All personnel not necessary for the proper course of the operation are forbidden in the operating room.
   h. Ultraviolet disinfection of circulating air is used in some hospitals.

Increasing Your Learning Power in the Operating Room

If you are to obtain maximal benefit from your operating room experiences, a proper viewpoint is necessary. Too often the student nurse stands at a great distance from the operating area so that it is impossible to observe the scrub team properly. Use a foot stand and position yourself at the table, near the anesthesiologist. This will keep you outside the sterile field and yet close enough to observe the procedure.

This manual should guide you as to the surgical procedure being done. Be certain you have reviewed the steps of the procedure carefully before the surgery begins.

With proper preparation you will be in a position to ask intelligent questions of the surgeon as he performs the surgery.

Observe the scrub nurse carefully. Note:
1. Arrangement of instruments and sutures on the Mayo stand.
2. How she hands instruments to the surgeon.
3. How she continually cleans the operative field of old sponges and suture ends.
4. Arrangement of instruments and basins on the reserve table.
5. How she aids surgeon in gowning and gloving.
6. Arranging of drapes and suction.
7. How she cleans instruments as she receives them back from the surgeon.
8. How she works with the circulating nurse.

Observe the circulating nurse carefully. Note:
1. How she transfers patient to operating table and positions and straps him in place.
2. How she adjusts the operating table and rearranges sheets so as not to obstruct the proposed surgical area.
3. The skin prepping procedure.
4. How she aids surgeon in gowning and adjusts surgical lights.

    5. How she observes and instructs scrub nurse.

    6. How she keeps room tidy.

Observe the anesthesiologist. Note:

    1. Induction of anesthesia.

    2. Method of giving spinal anesthesia.

Observe the surgeon and his assistants. Note:

    1. Progress of surgery.

    2. Hand signals for instruments and sutures.

    3. Use of instruments in sequence.

Learning in the Recovery Room

Know major problems to be anticipated in each type of case.

Know general procedures carried out in the recovery room.

Note patient's signs of recovery from anesthetic agents.

Ask questions of doctors and nurses in the recovery room.

SUMMARY OF ASSIGNMENT ONE

The most important thing you should have learned thus far is the importance of team function. Each member of the operative team has complex but specific duties which he or she must carry out effectively and efficiently. Very little conversation is necessary, as the team appears to function automatically. This comes only with experience and practice, intelligently applied.

You should also have observed something of the physical nature of the operating room suite referred to in Chapter 2 as the "surgical environment."

Finally, you should have learned the proper dress of a nonsterile member and proper, safe, and aseptic conduct in the operating room.

A careful self-review will help you determine how effectively you have used this operating room experience. With each trip to the operating room you should keep the purposes of these experiences fresh in your mind and try to achieve perfection before you proceed to the next step:

Assignment Two: Scrub in on a Case and Assist the Scrub Nurse

Purposes

To learn how to scrub.

To learn gowning and gloving procedures.

To observe the scrub nurse's duties at close range.

PROCEDURES

The Surgical Scrub

The hands and arms are teeming with microorganisms, both saprophytic and pathogenic. These organisms may be the source of surgical sepsis should the surgical gloves be punctured during the operation. Some of these organisms (transient flora) are acquired by daily contact with articles, other people, et cetera. These are easily removed by simple soap and water rinsing. Others (resident flora) have adapted to a particular individual's skin environment and are very persistent in their desire to remain with the individual. These, and a third group (deep flora) which reside around and in sebaceous glands, are not removed by ordinary soap and water rinses. Indeed, even a lengthy mechanical scrub with antiseptics will fail to remove all microorganisms from the hands and arms. *It is impossible to render the skin sterile.* Nevertheless, a sharp reduction in transient, resident, and deep flora of the hands and arms can be effected by a properly planned surgical scrub, rendering the hands *surgically clean but not sterile.*

Several points should be stated before you proceed to the technique for the surgical scrub:

The hands and arms can never be rendered sterile, no matter how long the scrub or how strong the antiseptic.

The undersurface of the fingernails is a most difficult area to clean. Hence the nails should be neatly trimmed each day.

The number of resident and deep flora is reduced by frequent scrubs. Conversely, there is a sharp increase in the number of these organisms when the surgical scrub is carried out only occasionally.

The resident flora is sharply increased in the presence of a wound or a burn. Since it is uncomfortable to scrub these areas vigorously, the nurse should not scrub in until the wound or burn is completely healed.

Microorganisms proliferate rapidly under the surgical gloves during a case. Therefore, a surgical scrub must be carried out between all operations, clean or septic, regardless of whether or not contamination has occurred during glove and gown changing.

The surgical scrub, to be effective and thorough, must be a conscious effort. It cannot be carried out properly while the nurse is distracted or conversing with other members of the operating team.

The student should have her scrubbing technique "checked out" with her supervisor or instructor before entering the operating room.

The actual scrub procedure will vary from hospital to hospital, and depends on the antiseptics or detergents used. Figures 9–2 to 9–6 show basic scrubbing principles and are self-explanatory.

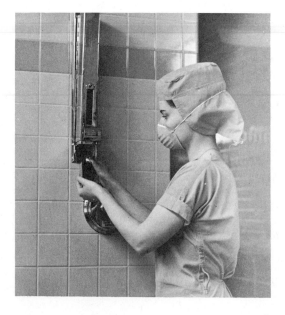

FIGURE 9–2 A sterile brush is taken from the automatic brush dispenser.

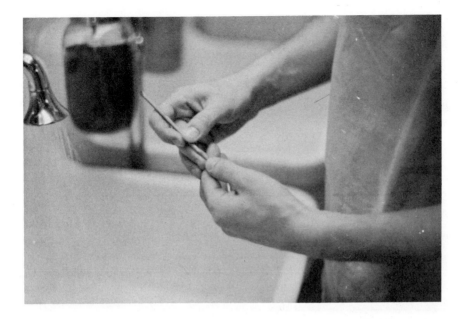

FIGURE 9–3 The undersurface of the nails harbors an abundance of microorganisms. A pointed wooden stick or metal file is used to remove excess dirt from below the nails prior to the scrub.

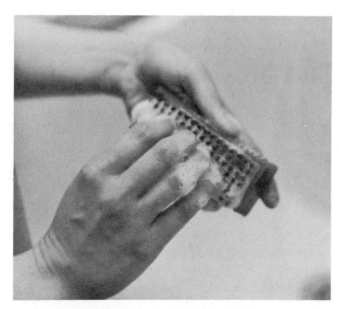

FIGURE 9–4 The nails are held perpendicular to the brush and scrubbed vigorously.

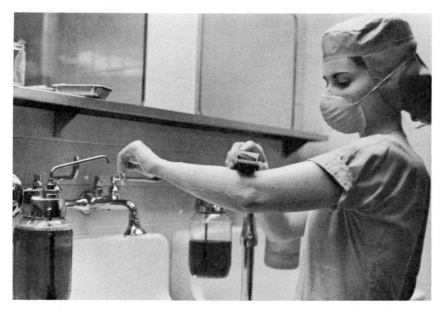

FIGURE 9-5 The arms are scrubbed up to and including the elbows. Note that the hand is held higher than the elbow to avoid contamination from dirty water dripping down the arm. Note also that the arms are kept at a good distance from the body.

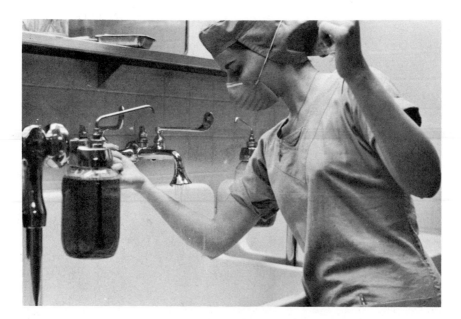

FIGURE 9-6 The arms are rinsed from the hands to the elbows and, again, the hands are held higher than the elbows.

Gowning and Gloving

The skin of the hands and arms, as well as the nonsterile scrub suit or dress, must be covered with sterile gloves and gown in order to prevent contamination of surgical supplies and linens. A precise aseptic routine has been developed which permits gowning and gloving without contamination. This routine must be understood and mastered until it is done confidently and simply.

Drying the Hands after a Surgical Scrub

1. A sterile hand towel is taken from a separate table.
2. The arms and elbows are held above the waist and away from the body to avoid contaminating the towel (see Figures 9–7 and 9–8).
3. One corner of the towel is used to dry the hands.
4. The other end of the towel is then grasped for drying the elbows, avoiding any contacting with hands against area of towel used to dry elbows.

Gowning. There are several points in aseptic technique that must be borne in mind concerning the gown:

1. When donning a gown, care must be taken to avoid contamination of the outstretched sleeves of the gown.
2. The back of a gowned member of the team is nonsterile.
3. A wet sleeve is no longer sterile.
4. The outside of a gown must not be touched with the hands.
5. A torn gown must be removed by the circulating nurse.

The gown is taken from the gown and glove table, with only the inner side being touched (see Figures 9–9 to 9–11). It is held by its upper half, away from the body, and allowed to unfold. It is then opened *from inside* and the arms are inserted into the sleeves. The circulating nurse then completes the gowning and ties the strings behind the scrub nurse. If the gown has a double back, there is a double tie at the front, which the scrub nurse unties. To the end of one of the ties she clamps a sterile snap, which is handed to the circulating nurse. The scrub nurse then pirouettes and accepts the tie after it is released from the snap. She can then tie herself in.

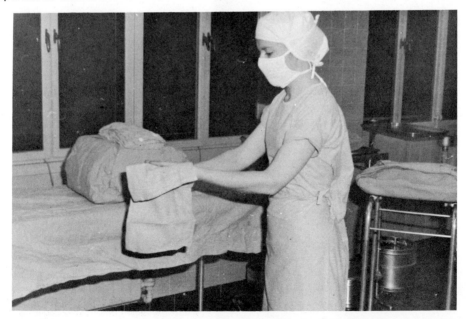

FIGURE 9–7 Correct method of holding drying towel. Note the distance between the free edge of the towel and the scrub dress.

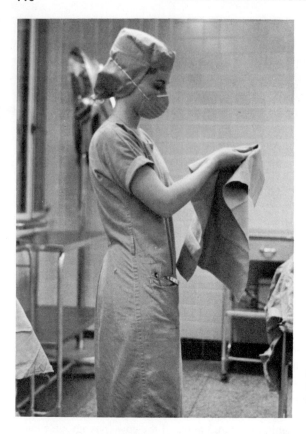

FIGURE 9–8   Incorrect method of holding drying towel. Note contamination of lower end of towel with scrub dress. This is a very common source of contamination.

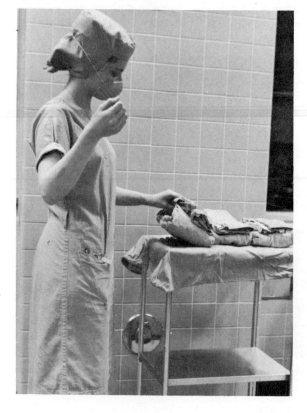

FIGURE 9–9   The sterile gown is removed from the gown and glove table. Note the position of the free arm.

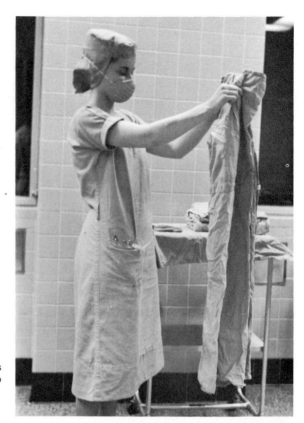

FIGURE 9-10 The gown is held by its upper end, away from the body, and allowed to unfold.

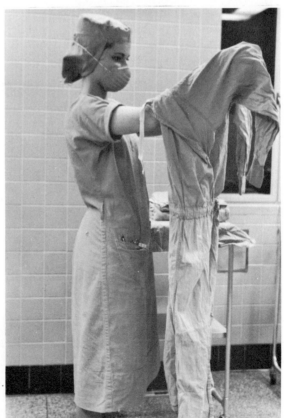

FIGURE 9-11 The arms are inserted into the gown. The remainder of gowning is done by the circulating nurse.

Gloving.   There are two methods of applying gloves (see Figures 9–12 to 9–16).

Open Method.   The inner lip of the glove is grasped with one hand and the other hand partially inserted into the glove. Using this partially gloved hand, the remaining glove is placed on the other hand, grasping the glove *within the cuff,* that is, remaining on the outer side of the glove. Finally, the cuff of the first glove is unfolded and pulled up on the sterile sleeve of the gown.

Closed Method.   In this method, the sleeves cover the hands, and gloves are applied with the sterile tips of the sleeves. This method requires more dexterity and is not as fast as the open method. Neither method has any significant advantage over the other, provided one is adept with each method.

Observing Scrub Nurse's Duties

This operating room experience will give you an opportunity, at closer range, to reexamine the scrub nurse's duties and, perhaps, to assist her (see next section).

SUMMARY OF ASSIGNMENT TWO

A review of this section will make it obvious that the most important lessons to be learned here concern methods and procedures developed to prevent contamination and surgical sepsis. Scrubbing, gowning, and gloving techniques have this one purpose in mind.

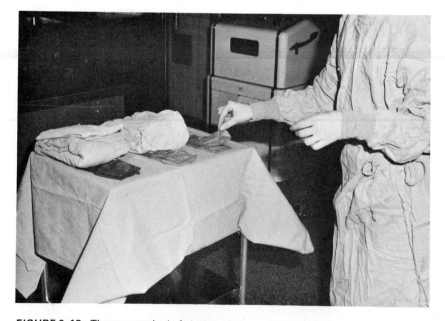

FIGURE 9–12   The open method of gloving: the inner cuff is used to apply the first glove.

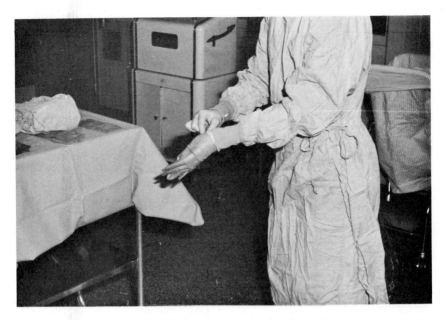

FIGURE 9–13 The open method of gloving: the first glove is being pulled over the cuff of the gown. Note that only the inner cuff of the glove is touched by the scrub nurse.

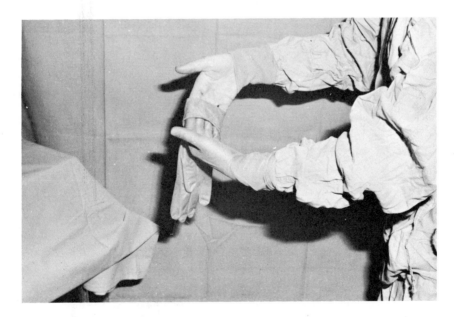

FIGURE 9–14 The open method of gloving: the second glove is grasped by the gloved hand, which is inserted on the outer side of the out-turned cuff.

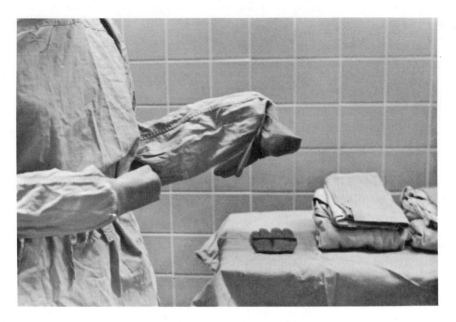

FIGURE 9–15 The closed method of gloving: the first glove is grasped with the sterile cuff of the surgical gown.

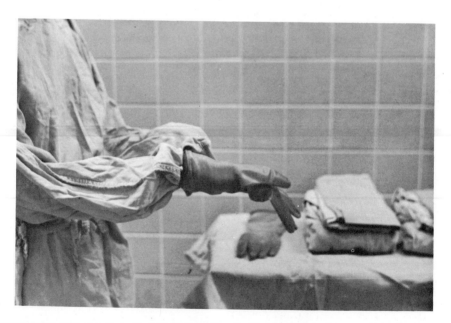

FIGURE 9–16 The closed method of gloving: the glove is placed over the opposite cuff and worked on. The procedure is then repeated with the other glove.

Assignment Three: Scrub Nurse

Purpose

To learn the various functions of a scrub nurse. (Many schools of nursing do not include this experience as part of the nurse's curriculum. This trend away from actual scrub nursing is open to serious question.)

PROCEDURES

The setting up and assisting at an operation are best illustrated by keeping in mind an actual operation. The following is a description of the major activities of a scrub nurse on an *exploratory laparotomy*. This is brief and general. Details are avoided.

Preliminary Steps

The nurse does a complete surgical scrub.

The *major laparotomy pack* has been partially opened by the circulating nurse. The scrub nurse completes the opening of this pack and dries her hands with a towel found on top of the "lap" pack (Figs. 9–17, 9–18). She then gowns from the "lap" pack and receives her gloves directly from the circulating nurse.

She then drapes and prepares the stands and tables.

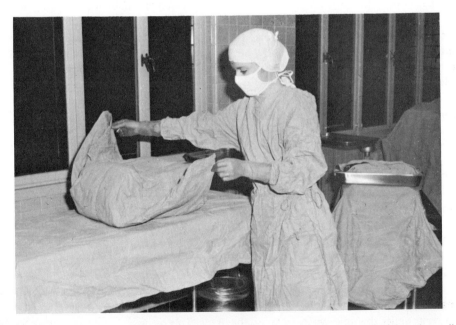

FIGURE 9–17 The scrub nurse opens the outer layer of the sterile laparotomy pack. Note the sterile sheet covering the table. This was the outermost layer of the lap pack which was opened by the circulating nurse (see Figures 9–27 and 9–28).

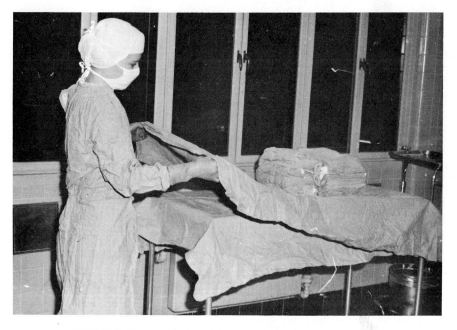

FIGURE 9–18   Completion of the opening of the laparotomy pack.

Draping

A drape in the operating room consists of a sterile covering purposely used as a barrier against surface bacteria. It is utilized to decrease contamination of the patient's surgical wound and to render all surfaces in close proximity to the patient and instruments "sterile" by covering both with suitable sterilized materials. Sheets, towels, and surgical drape sheets are used for this purpose. Drapes come in (1) textile, (2) plastic, and (3) waterproof materials. Some of the two latter types are disposable. Self-adhering, thin plastic drape sheets are applied to the skin after an adhesive has been sprayed on it. This material (the plastic) then adheres to the skin and seals it from contamination.

Double thickness drapes are used for instrument tables and patient coverings. This thickness reduces the risk of possible contamination by moisture. Bacteria can move through and contaminate a textile when it becomes moist or wet. The process by which this occurs is called "capillary attraction." The drape is then considered "unsterile" and is removed.

Important Points to Remember When Using Drapes

1. If antiseptics are used on the skin in order to render it surgically clean, the area must be allowed to dry sufficiently before the skin is draped with a sterile, double-thickness cloth drape.

2. When drapes are being placed by the doctor or nurse, the drape itself must shield the sterile gloved hand of the individual performing this service. Keep the sterile gloved hand behind the drape; this is accomplished by putting a fold on the outer edge of the drape and keeping the gloved hand under this fold when applying the drape. This maneuver will reduce the likelihood of an unsterile surface coming into contact with the sterile gloved hand or hands as the drape is laid on the stand, table, or patient. Beware of contact with lights, floor, and undraped furniture.

3. "Fanning" the air with a drape facilitates airborne contamination. Therefore, move the drape quietly and slowly. Do not "whip" it through the air. Allow plenty of space so that the drape may be unfolded conveniently without rendering it unsterile by contacting an undraped surface.

4. Drapes that are covering a surface are only considered to be sterile on the top of such a surface. Sides and bottom of the drape are not considered sterile when it has been placed on an object or on the patient, since the range of human vision cannot always be counted on to notice breaks in technique and resulting contamination of the drape.

Glove Table. Separate glove packs are opened by the circulating nurse and the gloves removed by the scrub nurse, who places them, along with the surgical gowns found in the laparotomy pack, on the glove table. These will be used by the surgeon and his assistant(s).

Two Basin Stands. The large basins will contain warm sterile saline for use by the surgeon and his assistant in cleansing their gloves of blood and debris periodically during the operation.

Mayo Stand. This is draped with a special coverall drape and placed over the patient's sterile drapes for convenient use by the scrub nurse. It contains: sponges, sutures, and needles; hemostats; Kelly clamps; straight and curved scissors; suture scissors; scalpels and blades; smooth and toothed forceps; needle holders; and Allis forceps.

Instrument Reserve Table. This is kept to the side of the operating table in an easily accessible spot but safe from contamination by the backs of the scrub team. It will contain additional gloves and gowns, drapes and towels, special instruments and basins, skin towels, extra sponges, and "lap" pads (Fig. 9–20).

The scrub nurse aids in gowning and gloving the surgeon and his assistant(s).

She does a sponge count with the circulating nurse. This involves a double verbal count of all sponges and larger abdominal packs with a confirming simultaneous count by the circulating nurse. The circulating nurse will then record the number of packs in use in an easily visible place.

She aids the surgeon or his assistant in draping the patient.

She then adjusts the Mayo stand to proper level, sets down an instrument towel on the sterile drapes overlying the patient, and passes the suction equipment to the surgeon for attachment at the head of the table.

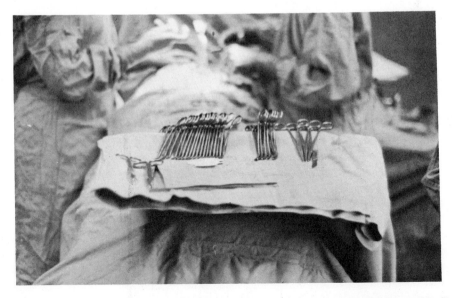

FIGURE 9–19 The Mayo stand in place. Note its location with respect to the operating table. Note also that it is kept free of clutter.

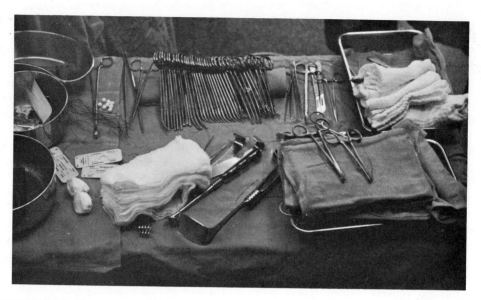

FIGURE 9–20   The instrument reserve table. It contains most of the instruments and equipment that will be used as the operation proceeds.

Sutures and Needles

In Chapter 1 it was stated that incision of tissues was an essential act of surgery. The incised tissue will separate and will bleed. *Reapproximation* of this tissue and *control of bleeding* (hemostasis) are necessary for firm rapid healing. These, then, are also essential acts of surgery and are accomplished, for the most part, with sutures and needles.

The Surgeon's Use of Sutures and Needles

Ligating Bleeding Vessels. From the moment of the skin incision, small arteries and veins will begin to bleed. This bleeding will obscure the dissection and render the procedure hazardous and time-consuming. The surgeon and his assistant will therefore clamp these "bleeders" with hemostats and then ligate them with appropriate suture material. Usually this will be accomplished with the *free-hand tie,* using suture material without a needle. Occasionally this is not possible or the vessel is quite large, in which case a *suture ligature* is used. This consists of a suture attached to a needle, and the surgeon actually penetrates the surrounding tissue with the needle and then ties the suture around the bleeder.

The surgeon will use the smallest suture consistent with safety. This, in turn, is dependent on the size of the vessel being ligated. Whether he uses absorbable gut or nonabsorbable silk or cotton depends, in the final analysis, on his judgment as to the advantages and disadvantages of each for a given situation.

Suturing Tissues. The reconstruction of dissected tissues, as well as the closure of the wound at the termination of the procedure, will depend on the use of various types of sutures with attached needles. Here, again, no simple rules can be set down to help in deciding which sutures a particular surgeon will use. The nurse should discuss the surgeon's general preferences with him prior to surgery and have these sutures and needles available. She should bear in mind that he may have to alter his choice depending on the local conditions encountered. More will be said on the choice of suture materials in this section and under each specific operation in Part II of this manual.

The Scrub Nurse's Responsibilities

There are four basic responsibilities.

Check Sutures and Needles. *Know the kinds of sutures and needles generally used* by each surgeon prior to his handling of the case. Reference to the surgeon's suture card (kept on file), as well as confirmation of this with the surgeon while he is scrubbing, will avoid unnecessary delays. It is often very difficult for the surgeon to anticipate every type of suture or needle he may need during a case, and the scrub nurse must learn to be adaptable and to open only a sufficient number of sutures and needles needed *at any given time.*

Have Sutures Ready. *Set out the sutures in advance,* and try to keep one or two sutures ahead of the surgeon to avoid delays.

Anticipate Surgeon's Needs. As the case proceeds, the scrub nurse will save a good deal of operating time by carefully observing the progress of suturing, thereby anticipating the needs of the surgeon for more suture material. It is often wise to ask the surgeon if he will need more of a certain type of suture that he is currently using. *It is better to waste one or two sutures by opening too many than to waste operating time by falling behind the surgeon with sutures.*

Keep Track of Needles. The surgeon is often distracted by the procedure and cannot remain aware of each and every needle he uses. It is the nurse's responsibility to see to it that each needle she hands the surgeon is returned to her before handing him another. If she fails to receive a needle, she should ask the surgeon if he has placed it somewhere else. Under no circumstance should the surgeon receive a new needle until the previously used needle has been returned to the nurse.

TYPES OF SUTURES AND NEEDLES

There are countless types of sutures and needles, in all sizes. A complete enumeration would serve only to confuse. The nurse should be aware of the commonly used types, what determines the use of each, and the advantages and disadvantages of each. A few points on each of these considerations are in order.

Sutures

Basically, there are two kinds of sutures:

Absorbable. These are digested and absorbed by the body tissues after a certain period of time. Among the commonly used absorbable sutures are *plain catgut,* having a rapid absorption time; *chromic catgut* (coated with chromic acid), having a slower absorption time; and *polyglycolic synthetic suture.*

Nonabsorbable. These sutures remain permanently in the body tissues (except when used on the skin), and include silk, cotton, Nylon, wire and Mersilene.

There are several advantages and disadvantages of absorbable over nonabsorbable sutures. Basically, catgut causes an initially more severe foreign body reaction than any of the nonabsorbable sutures. Its main advantage is that is is eventually absorbed, and hence the foreign body reaction is a limited one. On the other hand, surgical gut is notorious for its *knot slippage,* and must be tied very firmly and carefully to avoid the hazards of a knot untying. Knot slippage is less of a problem with some nonabsorbable sutures.

Perhaps the main advantage of absorbable gut is in the presence of infection (e.g., a ruptured appendix). The presence of nonabsorbable suture material could lead to chronic draining sinuses in the presence of infection, whereas gut would be rapidly absorbed and no further reaction would occur.

Catgut is supplied in various lengths, the most common being 54 inches. Its size or caliber is measured in units beginning with very fine, 6–0, up to no. 4, the heaviest. Hence, the sizes range as follows:

6–0, 5–0, 4–0, 3–0, 2–0, 0, 1, 2, 3, 4, in increasing diameter.

Silk is available in many different forms, as free ties from 6–0 to no. 5, on spools, swaged on to various types of needles, and so forth.

It is difficult to categorize uses of various types of sutures. The following examples are generally accepted uses for various sutures:

Skin Closures

Type: Nonabsorbable (either silk, cotton, Nylon, or wire).

Size: Varies with the area of the body and the cosmetic results sought (e.g., abdomen, 2–0 to 4–0 silk or cotton, and face, 4–0 to 5–0 Nylon or silk).

Subcutaneous Bleeders

Type: Either, depending on the surgeon's preference and the presence or absence of infection.

Size: Fine, such as 3–0 or 4–0.

Deep Fascia

Type: Either, depending on the surgeon's preference and the presence or absence of infection.

Size: Heavy, such as 2–0 or 0.

Peritoneum

Type: Usually absorbable chromic gut.

Size: Heavy, usually 0.

Gastrointestinal Anastomoses

Inner Mucosal Layer

Type: Absorbable chromic gut.

Size: 3–0 or 2–0.

Outer Seromuscular Layer

Type: Nonabsorbable, silk or cotton.

Size: 2–0 or 3–0.

Needles

Again, there are innumerable types of needles. Basically, needles may be curved or straight, and the point may be round (noncutting) or have a cutting edge (cutting). Further, the needle may have an open eye for the insertion of suture material, or the suture material may be swaged on to the back end of the needle. The advantages of the swaged-on suture are two: there is no eye to enlarge or tear the opening made in tissue, and the suture does not slip off the needle. The major disadvantage is its higher cost. In general, the following uses are made of the various types of needles:

Straight Needles (such as Keith): Skin closure; some surgeons also prefer them for gastrointestinal anastomoses.

Cutting Needles: Used on any durable tissue in which a blunt or round needle would make penetration very difficult, e.g., skin, tendon, galea, cartilage, periosteum, cervic uteri.

Round or Noncutting Needles: Used on all other types of tissues, including viscera, subcutaneous tissue, muscle, peritoneum.

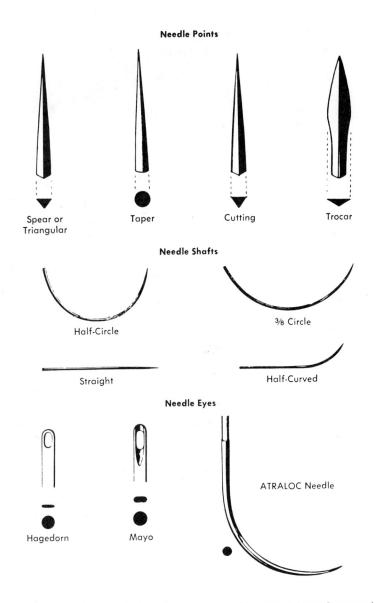

FIGURE 9-21 Basic surgical needle components. (Courtesy Ethicon Company.)

Much time can be saved by learning the proper methods for threading a suture on a needle, grasping the needle with the needle holder, and handing the suture and holder to the surgeon. From the surgeon's viewpoint, several important points should be stressed:

Threading Suture on a Needle

The short end of the suture should be about one-third the length of the long end. If it is shorter, it will tend to slip out of the eye of the needle while the surgeon is suturing. If longer, it will tend to be bound up in the tissue after the surgeon has passed the needle through the tissue.

Avoid "locking" the suture in the nose of the needle holder, as this weakens sutures.

Check each suture for knots before handing to surgeon. A knot can destroy the suture line of an important anastomosis by widening the aperture through which the suture has passed.

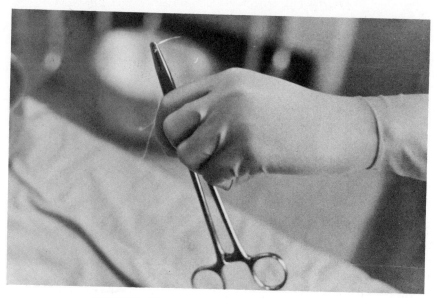

FIGURE 9-22 Correct position of needle on holder.

Pass the suture through the eye of the needle from the inner or concave side of the needle. This tends to reduce loss of suture from needle (see Figure 9–23).

Grasping the Needle with the Needle Holder

Grasp the needle with the holder just below the flattened eye of the needle. There must be enough length to the needle so that the surgeon can complete his suturing "arc" through tissue.

Be certain that the needle is grasped perpendicular to the needle holder, unless directed otherwise by the surgeon for suturing under special conditions.

Check the grasping power of each holder by attempting to pivot the needle in the jaws of a clasped holder. If the needle is unstable or pivots easily, the holder should be discarded from the case.

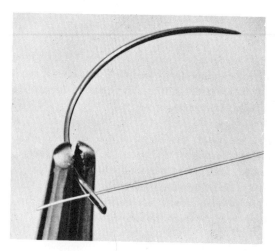

FIGURE 9-23 The needle is grasped at its flattened surface by the needle holder. The suture is passed from the inner, concave side of the eyelet to minimize loss of suture from needle. (Courtesy Ethicon Company.)

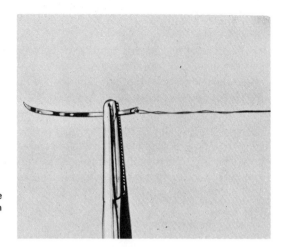

FIGURE 9–24 Note correct distance of needle on both sides of needle holder. (Courtesy Ethicon Company.)

Handing Suture and Holder to Surgeon

Hand any instrument to the surgeon firmly so that he will know by tactile sensation alone that the instrument is in his hand.

Hand the suture and holder to the surgeon in its functional position (Figure 9–25).

Be certain that the suture ends are not wrapped around the handle of the suture holder, as this will invariably catch on the hand or fingers of the surgeon. The suture ends should be hanging completely free from the handle of the holder.

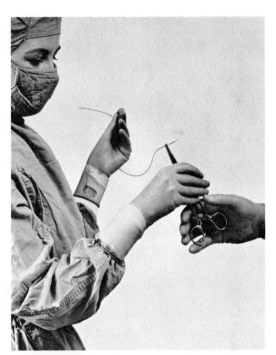

FIGURE 9–25 Suture is handed to surgeon in its functional position. The free end of the suture is held by the nurse to avoid its being caught up in the handle of the suture holder. (Courtesy Ethicon Company.)

Special Instruments

Many cases will require the use of highly specialized and complex instruments. These include, for example, the von Petz gastrointestinal clamp, the Bovie hemostatic machine, the nerve stimulator, and a host of others. These special instruments will be described when indicated in Part II. The scrub nurse should review the mechanism and function of these instruments when used in the case she is to scrub on. If they are sterile instruments, as, for example, the von Petz clamp, the scrub nurse should be certain the instrument is in working condition before handing it to the surgeon. These special instruments are handed to the scrub nurse by the circulating nurse either before surgery starts or during surgery as the situation arises. The sterile special instruments are kept on the instrument reserve table until called for by the surgeon.

Assisting the Surgeon

Ultimately, the major function of the scrub nurse consists of preparing and making available the proper equipment for a case, presenting this equipment to the surgeon as he requests it, and helping the surgeon toward achieving an aseptic technique on his patient. *Reasoned speed* is of the essence in good surgery and good assisting. In all things she does, the scrub nurse must *waste no time* and keep a steady flow of equipment going as required by the surgeon.

There are several general points that can be made regarding the assisting of the surgeon:

Observe the operative field closely and *anticipate* the surgeon's needs.

Be adept at handing instruments to the surgeon. Observe him closely for silent hand signals.

Keep the operative field neat at all times.

Watch for breaks in aseptic technique.

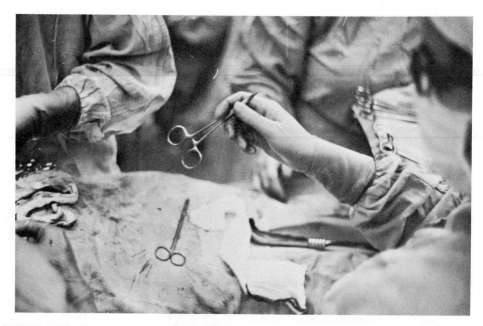

FIGURE 9-26 The nurse anticipates the surgeon's need for hemostats and keeps one ready for immediate use.

Typical Laparotomy

A laparotomy might proceed somewhat as follows:

The Incision. The skin and subcutaneous tissue is incised with a sterile blade which is immediately discarded.

Hemostasis. Subcutaneous bleeders are clamped with curved hemostats and ligated with fine ties of catgut, silk, or cotton. The area is periodically sponged by the assistant to aid in visualizing further sources of bleeding.

Isolation of Skin Edges. Many surgeons will now attach skin towels to the edges of an incision, using towel clips to isolate the wound edges.

Incising Fascia and Peritoneum. A clean knife or curved cutting scissors is used to incise the deep fascia and the peritoneum. Toothed forceps are used to elevate the peritoneum prior to incising it, as this will prevent inadvertent damage to the underlying bowel.

Exploration. Prior to definitive surgery, the entire abdomen is explored. However, in the case of an acutely inflamed organ, e.g., acute appendicitis, the surgeon will wisely avoid contamination and will not perform a general exploration. For exploration, the assistant will often require a large right-angled retractor to elevate the abdominal wall while the surgeon is performing his exploration.

Packing Organs Adjacent to Operative Site. Very frequently the operative site is obscured by surrounding viscera, e.g., the stomach, duodenum, and large bowel may obscure the biliary tree, making cholecystectomy hazardous; or the lung might obscure the pulmonary vessels, making their dissection dangerous. In these cases, the surgeon will use large packs and properly placed retractors to obtain the maximum *exposure* possible.

Adjusting Lights. Part of good exposure requires frequent adjustment of light sources. This is actually the duty of the circulating nurse, but the scrub nurse, being closer to the surgical site, can often guide the circulating nurse in the proper placement of the lights.

Surgical Dissection. Depending on the local anatomy, each surgical procedure will require a certain amount of dissection of surrounding tissues and a certain set of instruments. For most abdominal and thoracic cases, Metzenbaum or long Metzenbaum scissors, smooth dressing forceps, so-called "peanuts" or "pushers," and plenty of sponges are usually required. Each type of case will require different types of instruments. Also, each surgeon usually has his preferences. These selections of instruments will be anticipated by the scrub nurse only with experience.

Excision or Reconstruction. The actual essence of the operation consists, frequently, of excision of an entire organ, resection of a part of an organ, reconstruction of an organ, or both resection and reconstruction. These acts of surgery frequently require specialized instruments, and their description will be deferred for Part II.

Closure. The scrub nurse anticipates the closure and begins her first sponge count with the circulating nurse. In the case of a laparotomy, Kocher clamps will be used to grasp the edges of the peritoneum. The peritoneum, fascia, and skin will be closed serially by the surgeon using his preference for suture material. A second sponge count must be done before completion of the closure.

Dressing the Wound. This is done by the surgeon and his assistant, or may be delegated to the scrub nurse.

Cleaning Up. This is a joint responsibility of the scrub nurse and circulating nurse.

SUMMARY OF ASSIGNMENT THREE

It takes a great deal of practice and intelligent experience to become a good scrub nurse. Speed, efficiency, and ability to anticipate and to make versatile judgments must be developed in the scrub nurse, and this takes time.

Certain prerequisites of the good scrub nurse are:

1. Thorough familiarity with the anatomy, pathology, and surgical technique of each case she scrubs in on.

2. A working knowledge of the names, mechanisms, and uses of all the instruments she might use in a given case.

3. A thorough familiarity with the preferences of each surgeon. This will require a knowledge of his suture and instrument preferences, his general mode of operation, his basic speed, et cetera.

Assignment Four: Circulating Nurse

Purpose

To learn the various functions of the circulating nurse.

PROCEDURES

The circulating nurse is responsible for total coordination of her room. Her duties begin long before the operation starts and are not finished until the room is in readiness for the case to follow.

Again using an exploratory laparotomy as a sample case, the functions of the circulating nurse are briefly outlined.

Preliminary Steps

The circulating nurse is responsible for assuring that the operating room is clean and in order prior to the case assigned to her. She must check the lights, suction and oxygen units, substerilizer, and other pieces of equipment, making certain that they are all available and properly functioning.

She then obtains a major laparotomy pack and a basic instrument set, along with any special instruments as listed on the doctor's preference card.

The outer wrap of the laparotomy pack is opened by the circulating nurse (Figs. 9–27, 9–28).

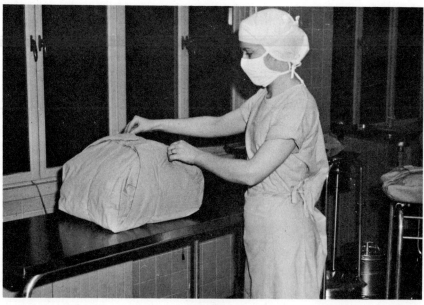

9–27

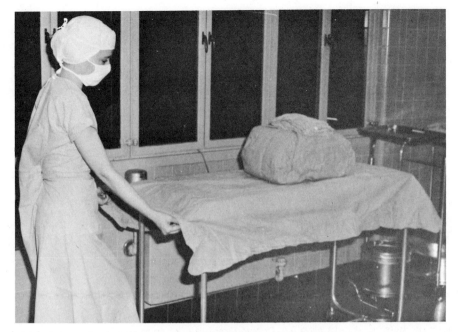

9–28

FIGURES 9–27 and 9–28   The circulating nurse opens the outer sheet of the laparotomy pack.

The patient is greeted, properly identified, and then transferred to the operating table. The nurse then positions and secures the patient on the table and *confirms position with the surgeon.*

After the scrub nurse has opened the laparotomy pack and draped all her tables, the circulating nurse hands her any special instruments to be used, as well as sutures, knife blades, sterile warm saline, and so forth.

The circulating nurse ties the gowns of all members of the scrub team, including the scrub nurse.

The Skin Prep

The skin prep table is a small, movable stand on casters, and usually is supplied with a wash basin, sterile gloves, sterile 4 by 4 sponges, and cotton-swab prep sticks for cleansing the umbilicus (Fig. 9–29).

In most hospitals, the initial skin prep is performed on the wards. The surgical area is therefore cleanly shaven prior to delivery of the patient to the operating room. The circulating nurse should *check for adequacy of this prep.* If in doubt, it is better to reshave the area, getting as close a shave as is possible. The nurse should also check for any signs of infection (e.g., furuncles). If found, these should be pointed out to the surgeon, as their presence may contraindicate proceeding with the operation.

The type of skin prep used will vary with each hospital. It may consist of an initial soap and water prep, followed by application of an antiseptic. The soap and water prep is usually done by the circulating nurse. Perhaps more important than the type of detergent used is a vigorous mechanical scrub. There is no place here for a "feather-light" touch. The timing and extent of the prep also vary with each hospital. Generally a 3 to 5 minute prep is considered adequate, particularly if the surgeon has instructed his patient to take daily baths at home prior to surgery.

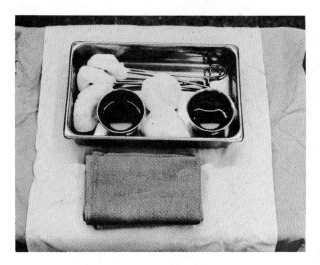

FIGURE 9-29 The skin prep kit and
its contents. (Courtesy Ethicon Company.)

The extent of the prep should always be considerably wider than the intended site of incision, as circumstances may require extending the incision in any direction. The prep always proceeds in a concentric, circular fashion *from the incision site outward.* In the case of an abdominal prep, the umbilicus is initially cleansed with swabs, removing all imbedded dirt. Following the initial scrub, the soap must be removed with clear sterile saline, removing all traces of soap. The chemical prep that follows is performed by the surgeon or his assistant. Many chemical antiseptics are available today. Iodine-based antiseptics are gaining wide popularity.

Special prep situations (e.g., cancer of the breast; around colostomies) will be described in appropriate sections of Part II.

Progress of Case

Since the circulating nurse represents the only nonscrubbed member of the operating team, it is imperative that she remain in constant contact with the team and remain fully aware of the progress of the case. A good deal of unnecessary delay occurs when the circulating nurse loses contact with her case. She must therefore stay in the room as much as is possible, leaving only to obtain necessary equipment. Should she require a break, a substitute nurse should be adequately apprised as to the progress of the case.

The circulating nurse has several responsibilities during this stage of the case:

Maintain a tidy room.
Keep the scrub nurse equipped with adequate numbers of sponges, sutures, et cetera.
Adjust lights frequently as required by the surgeon.
Observe all members of the team for breaks in aseptic technique and inform them immediately when a break occurs.
Accept, label, and record all specimens received from the surgeon.
Call x-ray or laboratory technician at the surgeon's request.
Call pathologist at the surgeon's request.

Conclusion of Case

The circulating nurse assists in transferring the patient to the litter for delivery to recovery room. She then cleans and prepares the room for the following case.

SUMMARY OF ASSIGNMENT FOUR

The circulating nurse is truly the coordinator of the operating room team. Her various duties before, during, and after a case have been described in general so that the student may have an idea of the extent of the circulating nurse's role. The long list of specific duties, the subtle points in aseptic technique, and the wide scope of her judgment cannot be described in a brief operative manual.

SUMMARY

Operating room nursing is a complicated and highly responsible position. The health and life of the patient are in the hands of the surgical team. One break in aseptic technique could spell the difference between a successful, clean case and one destroyed by sepsis. Such responsibility cannot be delegated lightly. Only highly trained and experienced personnel can share in the satisfying work of the operating room. It is for this reason that the student is advanced slowly and progressively in her surgical experiences.

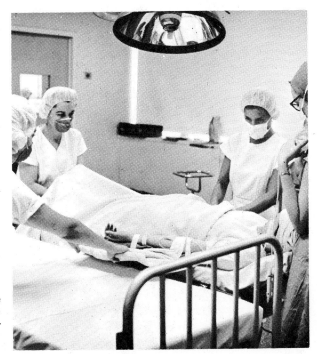

FIGURE 9–30 The circulating nurse aids in transferring the patient from the operating table. (Courtesy Ethicon Company.)

This chapter has attempted to describe, in general terms, this increasing responsibility delegated to the student under the guidance of her nursing instructors and the operating room supervisor. This manual cannot be construed as a short cut to operating room training. Such an interpretation could be disastrous, as there is no substitute for *guided experience.* Nevertheless, careful consideration of the principles in this chapter will serve as a *guide* and a *review* of surgical nursing.

STUDY QUESTIONS

1. List several principles of aseptic technique as used by the scrub nurse, the circulating nurse, and the surgeon. Keep a list of several possible breaks in aseptic technique you have seen in the operating room and discuss these with your instructor.

2. What is the purpose of the sponge count? Be able to describe the details of this procedure to your class.

3. Why is it important for the scrub nurse to familiarize herself with the nature of the case she is about to assist on? Give specific examples.

4. What is the most important principle of efficient assisting from the scrub nurse? Discuss your answer.

5. Discuss the importance of safe uniform and dress with respect to asepsis as well as explosions.

6. During the course of an operation, a basin of sterile water spills on the instrument table. What steps must be taken to insure that no contamination occurs?

7. Since sterile gloves are worn throughout an operation, why must the hands be rendered surgically clean by preoperative scrubbing?

8. Discuss possible breaks in aseptic technique that may occur during gowning and gloving.

9. Discuss some of the scrub nurse's duties with respect to preparation of sutures and needles.

IMMEDIATE CARE OF THE POSTOPERATIVE PATIENT

10

PURPOSE OF CHAPTER

This chapter is designed to review and explain the over-all nursing care of patients during the first 24 hours after surgery. Pertinent observations and safety factors involved in the care of these patients will be highlighted. Specifics of care necessary for the patient who has had a selected surgical procedure will be found in the last section of each chapter in Part II.

INTRODUCTION

Postoperative management of the patient begins when the incision is closed, the dressing applied, and the patient transported to another area within the operating suite. There are two areas to which the patient may be brought, depending on his over-all condition and the type of surgery that has been performed.

The Recovery Room. The patient coming to this area will stay until he has totally reacted from anesthesia and is awake (from 1 to 2 hours after surgery). His vital signs will stabilize during this period. He will have had a relatively uncomplicated surgical procedure and his immediate postoperative course will be predictably smooth.

The Intensive Care Unit. This patient will have experienced a more complex surgical procedure and, as a result, will require a longer period of time to recover from its effects and for his condition to stabilize. Usually, extraordinary measures will have been taken during the surgical procedure, e.g., being placed on cardiopulmonary by-pass, and requiring constant vigilance and care. His condition may be unstable initially. It may require the use of monitors to continually assess his vital signs. He may need emergency procedures performed at intervals throughout the postoperative period. The surgical and nursing team may also anticipate that this patient's postoperative course may be complicated. Intensive therapy can be administered to him while he remains in this area; the time interval in which such services are available is often crucial and may mean the difference between life and death.

Both units are staffed by knowledgeable and experienced doctors and nurses who genuinely enjoy this type of challenge and have the emotional fortitude and stamina to endure a daily routine of caring for these patients.

For the patient it is quite advantageous to be placed in either unit. It will assure him of constant observation, if his condition so demands. In such specialized areas, physicians and surgeons can be readily called upon to come to the patient's bedside for immediate observation, evaluation, and diagnosis of the current problem. Treatment of unforeseen complications can be managed rapidly and smoothly, thus causing a minimum of anxiety for the patient.

131

Transportation of Patient from Operating Room to Recovery Room

The patient is transferred to the recovery room or intensive care unit following surgery. The anesthesiologist, surgeon, and attendants accompany the patient to the area; the anesthesiologist insures adequate ventilation in transit. The nurse who receives the patient is informed of the patient's condition by the staff anesthesiologist. Immediate orders to be carried out by the staff may be reviewed by the attending doctor.

The head nurse or the nurse who is assigned to the patient must read the *postoperative note.* This note will have the following information on it:
1. The type of surgery performed.
2. The estimated blood loss; fluid replacement.
3. What type of drains are in place, and their total number.
4. Findings at the time of surgery.
5. Complications during surgery.
6. Condition of the patient immediately after surgery.

Recovery Bed and Individual Unit

The patient is admitted to the recovery room or intensive care unit and placed in his own bed or left on a stretcher equipped with side rails. The following basic equipment will be needed at the patient's bedside: a sphygmomanometer and stethoscope, equipment for administering intravenous infusions or transfusion, side rails, suction apparatus, tongue depressors and mouth gag, emesis basin, and mouth wipes. Emergency equipment that should be nearby includes: oxygen, airway, tracheotomy set, dressing tray, and drug tray. The nurse's notes consist of a recovery room sheet or an intensive care sheet, and an intake and output sheet.

Charting on Admission of the Patient

The following details must be observed, measured, reported, or eventually charted by the nurse:
1. The time the patient is received in the recovery room.
2. The level of consciousness.
3. The color of the skin, nail beds, and lips.
4. The presence or absence of peripheral pulses.
5. The condition of the skin.
6. Temperature, pulse, respiration, blood pressure, and neurological data. (If the patient has undergone abdominal aortic by-pass graft surgery, pedal pulses are to be taken.)
7. The amount and type of drainage (if any) on the dressing.
8. The amount and type of intravenous infusion, and the site of the needle or intracatheter being utilized for the infusion.
9. The mode of oxygen administration and the liter flow rate.
10. The presence of an airway, endotracheal tube, or tracheostomy tube.
11. Medications that have been administered in transit.
12. The amount of urine output during the past hour or during the surgical procedure (total quantity).
13. The types of fluids given parenterally during the surgical procedure.
14. Any unusual situations, as in cases where:
a. Precautions against seizure must be taken.
b. The patient has allergies to drugs or other substances (determined from the patient's history).

   c. Cardiac monitoring is necessary because of pre-existing disease problems or an intraoperative event.

   d. Physical abnormalities are present.

   e. Blood reactions occur.

General Postoperative Orders Written by the Doctor

In general, the postoperative orders are concerned with five areas. They are:

1. The patient's vital signs.
2. Intake and output recording — amount *and* frequency.
3. Intravenous fluids to be administered in a specific time interval.
4. Management of any drainage tubes present.
5. Potential crisis situations. The house officer or anesthesiologist should be called when any of the following signs are present:

   a. Blood pressure is below 90–100 (exceptions to the usual acceptable minimum will be noted in specific orders).

   b. The pulse is over 120 beats per minute or below 60.

   c. Temperature is over 101 degrees.

   d. The "due to void" time limit has passed.

   e. Agitation or restlessness is noted.

A list of *common postoperative orders* is presented here for your review:

> Turn the patient; encourage effective coughing, deep breathing, and leg exercises every 2 hours without fail.
>
> Connect drainage tubes to appropriate gravity or suction apparatus.
>
> Allow the patient nothing by mouth until he is awake, at which time sips of water and chips of ice may be permitted; advance intake as tolerated. (The patient with a nasogastric tube is given nothing by mouth.)
>
> Keep an accurate intake and output record.
>
> Record data on hematocrit, complete blood count, and electrolytes the evening of surgery; repeat in the morning if indicated.
>
> Apply elastic stockings or Ace bandages to both legs (optional).
>
> Give medication for pain or restlessness every 3 to 4 hours as necessary.
>
> If the patient has not voided by a designated time, call the doctor.
>
> Follow intravenous therapy orders.
>
> Observe vital signs every 20 minutes until the patient leaves the recovery room; if the patient stays overnight (because his condition is not stable), note the signs once an hour during this time and thereafter.
>
> Apply oropharyngeal suctioning as needed.
>
> Administer oxygen via nasal prongs, catheter, or mask at the specified rate of flow.

IMMEDIATE NURSING CARE

OBSERVING, REPORTING, AND RECORDING

The nurse must be prepared at any time to report to the doctor on the condition of the patient with an *up-to-the-minute summary*. She must communicate the information to the doctor in a clear, concise, and sequential way. Her information must be factual and based on careful observation and monitoring. Moreover, she must be ready to answer the doctor's questions on details of the patient's needs, treatments, and nursing care.

In the early postoperative period, it is the responsibility of the nurse to keep the patient warm, check and record his vital signs, prevent the patient from falling or thrashing about in such a manner as to injure himself, observe and ensure adequate ventilatory exchange, promote and maintain infusions of intravenous fluids, relieve postoperative pain or restlessnes, and be alert to changes in the patient's condition which may indicate the possibility of imminent complications. She must never leave the patient alone until he has recovered from anesthesia and is oriented to his surroundings. She must speak distinctly to the patient and close to his ear in a conversational tone while he is reacting from anesthesia. In addition, the patient may be comforted if the nurse touches his hand or arm while speaking to him during this time.

No matter what type of surgical procedure the patient has undergone, his postoperative care must include the following measures (along with particular treatments described in each chapter of Part II):

1. Providing for privacy as well as personal modesty in the recovery room area.
2. Administering mouth care at least every 2 hours, especially when the patient is receiving nothing by mouth.
3. Applying good back care, which includes massage of the bony prominences at least every 2 hours.
4. Providing for position changes every 1 to 2 hours.
5. Checking for pressure areas on the skin when the patient is moved.
6. Maintenance of proper body alignment in all positions in which the patient is placed in the recovery room bed.
7. Providing adequate and/or additional dressing bulk, especially over drains.
8. Checking the skin around a drain (when practical) to assess its condition.

CARE OF THE PULMONARY SYSTEM

Acute respiratory obstruction and atelectasis constitute the two most significant potential complications affecting the pulmonary system in the first few hours following major surgery. Most of what follows is directed toward maintaining adequate ventilation and respiration in order to prevent atelectasis and pneumonia.

Positioning the Patient

In general, the optimum position for the postoperative patient is on his side with a pillow at his back for support, with the knees slightly flexed and the face turned to the side with the chin extended. This position lessens the danger of aspiration, since any mucous material in the mouth will fall to the side of the oral cavity and drain out. If the patient vomits, his head is turned more to the side, and the head of the bed may be lowered slightly. This tends to prevent aspirations of vomitus into the pulmonary tree. Unless contraindicated, the patient should be placed on his side until the swallowing and gag reflexes return. If the patient is unconscious, it is extremely hazardous to leave him on his back, since his diminished swallowing and gag reflexes may permit him to aspirate mucus or his breathing may be impaired by his tongue obstructing the airway. By placing the patient in a lateral position, the tongue drops to the side of the mouth, allowing air to pass over it and thereby aiding ventilation. Should it be necessary to keep the patient on his back, the danger of aspiration can be lessened by turning the head to one side when he vomits and suctioning the vomitus from the throat as required.

The patient's position should be changed every 2 hours. This is done primarily to ensure adequate ventilation and drainage. The physician will note in his postoperative orders whether the patient can be turned from side to side or whether his movements are to be more restricted. Turning and moving the patient comfortably and safely in the early postoperative period are best accomplished by two or three nurses. When the patient is more alert and responsive, he may help in changing his position when directed by the nurse.

Signs and Symptoms of Anoxia and Anoxemia

Since the nurse is constantly observing the immediate postoperative patient, it behooves her to become familiar with the signs and symptoms of *anoxia.* The patient suffering from oxygen deprivation may manifest:

1. Rapid, shallow breathing.
2. Noisy, snoring, or guttural respirations.
3. Gasping.
4. A fighting response to an oxygen mask on the face.
5. Cyanosis (this may be absent even with severe degrees of anoxia).
6. Rapid, thready pulse.
7. Apprehension.
8. Restlessness and attempts to get into an upright position in bed. The latter is a most important early sign of anoxia.
9. Confusion.

Common causes of upper respiratory tract obstruction are:

1. The tongue falling back into the pharynx while the patient is in the supine position.
2. Secretions (vomitus, thick or copious mucus, saliva) partially or completely blocking the pharynx.
3. Laryngeal spasm — an event which produces an audible "crowing" sound.

When the patient's respiratory tract becomes partially or totally obstructed, the following actions must be taken:

1. Move the patient's lower jaw forward with your hands; push or pull the jaw forward and upward and hold it in this position while you proceed to step 2.
2. Quickly insert an oropharyngeal airway tube; use suction to remove mucus in the pharynx and, if necessary, the trachea.

If the patient's breathing pattern is not corrected, proceed to:

3. Manually respirate the patient through the airway, using oxygen or room air to achieve sufficient rapid ventilation.
4. Call the anesthesia department or the attending physician or surgeon. (This step should be taken by another member of the staff. At least two nurses must be on hand when the patient's breathing problem becomes an emergency.)
5. Bring emergency resuscitative equipment to the bedside. (Again, one of at least two nurses performs this duty.) Prepare to bypass the upper airway by inserting an endotracheal tube or, in special situations, a tracheostomy tube.

Mechanical Respiratory Aids

Under general anesthesia, the muscles of the jaw relax, thereby permitting the tongue to slide back and obstruct the airway. To prevent this, the jaw is grasped and held or supported in a forward position. The complication of obstruction of the airway can also be prevented by the use of several mechanical devices:

Oral Airway. This is a rubber or plastic hollow tube inserted into the oropharyngeal cavity. It prevents the tongue from slipping back into the throat and occluding the airway.

Endotracheal Tube. This respiratory tube is inserted into the trachea by way of the nose or mouth. The size of the tube will depend on the route that is used. Oral tube insertion is called *orotracheal intubation;* nasal tube insertion is called *nasotracheal intubation.* In either case, the tube can be *cuffed* or uncuffed. The cuff is a protective device that prevents the aspiration of secretions from the mouth or gastrointestinal tract; the cuff also serves to keep the tube stationary in the trachea and permits positive pressure respiration.

The endotracheal tube, whether nasal or oral, is effectively designed to prevent respiratory obstruction or aspiration, to allow periodic deep suctioning of tenacious or copious mucus, and to promote adequate ventilation in the unconscious, subconscious, or paralyzed postoperative patient. In general, the main purpose of the endotracheal tube is to *maintain a patent airway.* Such a tube is left in place for 48 to 72 hours (in most cases). The intubated patient may be permitted to breathe humidified atmospheric air or he may have his respiration controlled by a ventilator. When a ventilator or respirator is used, a swivel adapter is attached to the end of the endotracheal tube so that the tube may be connected to a Bird, Emerson, or Monahan respirator. When a patient's breathing is aided by a respirator, the rate and depth of his respirations can be partially or totally controlled by the machine. The respirator can be regulated and set in such a way as to permit the patient himself to trigger the inspiratory phase of the apparatus' cycle (this setting permits what are called "assisted respirations"). Alternatively, the machine may be set to a certain number of respirations per minute and maintain a regulated, timed respiratory cycle (this setting produces what are called "controlled respirations"). Periodic hyperventilation (every 15 minutes) can be accomplished with the machine or by manual technique (the tubing is disconnected from the ventilator and an Ambu bag is used).

Specific concentrations of oxygen (over 60 per cent). compressed air, or room air can be inhaled by the patient or be administered under pressure through the endotracheal tube into the respiratory tract.

Care of the patient with an endotracheal tube should involve the following points:

> Check breath sounds initially and at periodic intervals thereafter on both sides of the chest to assess the quality and depth of respirations after the endotracheal tube has been put in place.
>
> Be certain that the tube does not slip down the trachea, especially when the cuff is deflated. Be equally certain that there is no slippage when an uncuffed tube without a flange at its tip is used.
>
> Use a gauze mouth gag or oral airway even with the orotracheal tube in place so that the patient will not bite down on the tube and occlude its lumen.
>
> Have an Ambu bag at the patient's bedside in case of respirator malfunction. Should there be any malfunction, the patient must be manually respirated until another machine is set up.
>
> Using the Ambu bag, manually induce 10 to 15 breaths of 100 per cent pure oxygen every 15 minutes (hyperventilation).
>
> Suction the endotracheal tube, using sterile technique; suction the mouth with clean technique.
>
> Deflate the cuff of the tube and check the amount of air that is withdrawn; determine whether this amount is adequate or appropriate for the tube's size.
>
> Release the cuff every 2 hours and reinflate it or its alternate cuff so that tracheal trauma and pressure in one area will be minimized.
>
> When the tube cuff is released, and secretions from the mouth fall back down

the trachea, causing the patient to choke, reinflate the cuff, suction the tube, and proceed again with cuff deflation.

Administer mouth care at least every 2 hours.

Tracheotomy. The surgeon may elect to perform a tracheotomy for a number of reasons. The patient may not be ventilating or exchanging gases adequately, or he may require respiratory assistance for over 72 hours. Perhaps the orotracheal or nasotracheal tube causes the patient intolerable discomfort. In some cases, the patient's secretions are excessive, and require frequent, sterile aspiration. Whatever the reason for the surgeon's decision, his procedure in performing the tracheotomy is straightforward, consisting of making an opening in the patient's trachea and inserting a rubber or metal tracheotomy tube. The patient may then breathe humidified atmospheric air or oxygen-enriched air via a Briggs adapter or by means of a mechanical ventilator or respirator attached to the end of the tracheotomy tube (see the preceding discussion of the endotracheal tube).

Suctioning the Patient

As a result of the preoperative administration of sedatives or opiates and the intraoperative effects of anesthesias, the mucous membrane of the patient's respiratory tract is stimulated to produce abundant amounts of mucus. Since the patient's reflexes are depressed and he is generally weak, he may be unable to expectorate respiratory secretions. When air flows through these secretions in the trachea, bronchi, and alveoli, the result is audible as *rales.* The sounds of rales will vary, depending on the amount of secretions present, the distribution of fluid in the lungs and bronchi, and the exact location of fluid in the respiratory tract.

Fine rales will have a crackling, sharp sound, produced in the alveoli.

Medium rales are sounds emanating from secretions in the bronchioles.

Coarse rales are loud, gurgling sounds from secretions in the trachea, bronchi, and smaller bronchi.

The suctioning procedure is only undertaken when a patient's secretions are audible. Suctioning always carries with it a risk in the critically ill patient; prolonged suctioning may lead to sustained anoxia and cardiac arrest. In order to obtain the full cooperation of the conscious patient, the nurse must tell him what to expect and ask that he bear with the discomfort of the procedure for a period of a few seconds. The discomfort should be minimized and compared or contrasted with the danger of the patient developing respiratory obstruction leading to atelectasis, hypoxia, and pneumonia.

Technique of Suctioning

1. Preoxygenate the patient with 100 per cent pure oxygen for 5 minutes before initiating the suction procedure.

2. Instill 2.5 to 5 cc's of normal saline (sterile) into the trachea by way of the endotracheal tube. Alternatively, the saline may be injected directly into the trachea by the doctor (the use of a hypodermic needle is recommended for this method).

3. Use the Ambu bag to respirate the patient for 10 to 15 breaths (optional).

4. Gather the equipment. On hand should be:

a. Sterile #14 French catheter.

b. Sterile saline or water-soluble lubricant.

c. Sterile bowl for saline.

d. Sterile gloves.

e. Oxygen apparatus.

f. Suction apparatus (source of negative pressure).

g. Heated nebulizer attached to oxygen outlet.

5. Hyperextend the patient's neck.

6. Using sterile technique, pass the lubricated catheter (without suction attached to the end) through the nose or mouth (there will be less resistance on the patient's part if the catheter is passed nasally). The catheter should be passed in a gloved hand.

7. Listen at the end of the catheter for audible breath sounds after the catheter is in place in the trachea.

8. Attach the suction source to the end of the French catheter. Suction for *10 seconds only.*

9. Interrupt suction source and disconnect suction tubing from the catheter after completing suctioning (10 seconds).

10. With the catheter still in place in the trachea, hold the heated nebulizer over the end of the catheter so that the patient can again receive room air enriched with oxygen and saturated totally with water vapor.

11. Resume the suctioning procedure, beginning with step 5 (hyperextending the patient's neck).

12. Record the amount, color, odor, and consistency of secretions and report any changes to the house officer or surgeon.

In some institutions, only a certified nurse may perform deep endotracheal suctioning; other establishments will allow the nurse to perform this procedure only if the patient has an orotracheal or a nasotracheal tube in place in the respiratory tract.

Contraindications

The use of deep endotracheal suctioning is restricted in certain cases; it should not be administered to patients with any of the following conditions:

1. Acute status asthmaticus.

2. Upper airway obstruction (caused, for example, by peritonsillar abscess, laryngeal edema, or croup).

3. Bleeding tendencies (as a result of leukemia, hemophilia, nasopharyngeal bleeding, or bleeding esophageal varices).

4. Fractures or abnormalities of the nasal passage.

5. Tracheal stenosis.

6. Acute myocardial infarction.

Hazards

The following complications can occur during and as a result of the act of suctioning:

1. Hypoxia.

2. Cardiac arrhythmias.

3. Cardiac arrest.

4. Respiratory arrest.

5. Bronchospasm.

6. Respiratory mucosal trauma.

7. Aspiration pneumonia.

Use of Oxygen

Oxygen is administered to the patient postoperatively by way of nasal catheter, face mask, or prongs. Whatever the method of administration, it is necessary to deliver humidified oxygen to the patient, because regular oxygen produces excessive drying of the mucous membrane of the respiratory tract. The oxygen equipment and tubing should be checked periodically for its ability to deliver the set liter flow to the patient. A nasal catheter must be changed to the alternate nostril at least every 8 hours; a face mask must be removed for face care every 2 hours. The patient who is receiving oxygen by face mask must have an exact fit of the mask to his facial size and contour.

Respiratory Complications

In the immediate postoperative period, the most common and potentially the most disastrous pulmonary complications are atelectasis and pneumonia. Partial or massive collapse of a lung is heralded by tachycardia, fever, restlessness, and, at times, cyanosis. The basic etiology of this condition is the inspissation of mucus and excess secretions as well as dehydration and a poor cough reflex. These secretions are not adequately handled by the postoperative patient who finds it painful and, at times, impossible to cough adequately in order to clear his pulmonary tree. The preoperative use of atropine as a drying agent partially reduces these secretions but, in the patient with chronic bronchitis and emphysema (such as the heavy smoker), these secretions occur in great abundance postoperatively.

In the vast majority of patients, these mucous inspissations or "plugs" can be cleared by aiding and urging the patient to breathe deeply and cough at frequent time intervals. The pain that the coughing will cause at the surgical site can be reduced with a pillow or blanket applied to the patient's incision when he coughs. The liberal use of analgesic medications for the first 24 hours also will enable the patient to cooperate more effectively. Some patients will require stimulation of their cough centers with a nasal catheter. Intermittent positive pressure machines aid greatly in assisting deep respirations. In the occasional intractable case, bronchoscopy with direct removal of mucous plugs may become necessary.

CARE OF THE CARDIOVASCULAR SYSTEM

The Vital Signs

These physiological indices (pulse, blood pressure, temperature, and respirations) are most important criteria of the status of the patient at any one time. Each must be monitored carefully and frequently by the nurse in the early postoperative period. A brief description of their significance will aid the nurse in understanding the importance of these signs in the care of her patient.

The Pulse. The pulse is the peripheral mirror of the heartbeat. Its characteristics are threefold — rate, rhythm, and volume.

Pulse Rate. The early postoperative patient may be expected to run a pulse slightly above normal (e.g., 100 per minute). Bradycardia (pulse below 60), with no other symptoms or signs, is often due to the anesthetic agents used in the case and, provided the patient is tolerating it well, is of no consequence. Tachycardia (pulse above 110) is distinctly abnormal and calls for an explanation. It may be due to excess blood loss during or following surgery, to a cardiac arrhythmia, to high fever, to atelectasis, to a pneumothorax, or to pain. An occasional patient who is extremely anxious may register a tachycardia of no particular significance. Nevertheless, when the pulse rises to 110 per minute or higher, *it calls for a satisfactory explanation.*

Rhythm. The nurse should describe the rhythm of the pulse beat. Is it totally irregular? Is it regular with an occasional "skipped beat"? Of even greater significance is a previously regular rhythm which suddenly converts to an irregular pattern. Any alteration in the normal pulse rhythm should be called to the physician's attention immediately.

Volume. The pulse volume measures the ejection force of the heart, as well as the volume of blood being circulated in the body. A strong regular pulse is a healthy sign. A feeble pulse, however regular and slow it may be, may signal the onset of hypotension and shock. The nurse should accustom herself to recognizing, through touch, a normal pulse volume and should record any deviations from this norm.

The Blood Pressure. Falls in blood pressure in the early postoperative period may be due to many causes. It is difficult to estimate what constitutes a significantly low blood pressure. Certainly a systolic pressure below 80 mm. Hg (mercury) should be called to the physician's attention. More important than the actual blood pressure level are the changes occurring over several readings. Thus, for example, a patient with a baseline blood pressure of 140 mm. Hg systolic, who begins to show falls in these readings to 130, 120, and 110, may be developing a significant problem; this should be called to the physician's attention long before the pressure reaches 80 systolic.

Respiration. Rapid respirations (tachypnea) as well as shortness of breath (dyspnea) may signify cardiovascular complications in that the patient attempts to compensate for the anoxia of shock by breathing more frequently or more deeply. It is often extremely difficult to distinguish a primary pulmonary complication from a cardiovascular problem on the basis of respirations alone. This will require careful physical examination, electrocardiogram, blood gases study, venous pressures, and a chest x-ray. Whatever the cause, the sudden or gradual development of dyspnea, tachypnea, or both in the early postoperative period may signify the onset of a serious cardiovascular or pulmonary problem.

Respiratory complications can result from the patient's conscious or unconscious movements to constrict or compress his chest when he feels postoperative pain. Do not underestimate the importance of providing the patient with analgesic medication for this pain — when his pain is reduced, he can breathe freely and deeply, thereby circumventing potential respiratory problems.

Body Temperature. Initially, the patient comes to the recovery room with a body temperature ranging from 96 to 99 degrees. He is cold and in need of rewarming; the nurse should cover him with warm blankets and allow his body temperature to reach a normal level again. Thereafter, there is a physiological rise in temperature to about 100 degrees. Of and by itself, it is of no significance. However, any further elevation in temperature may mean the onset of a more serious problem. By far the most common early cause of temperature elevation is atelectasis. The temperature should be taken every 1 to 4 hours for the first 24 hours. Rectal temperature is the most accurate, and should be taken unless there is a specific contraindication (e.g., anal surgery).

Precautions to be Taken when Giving the Initial Dose of a Narcotic

Unless the anesthesiologist has given you an order to administer a narcotic drug to the patient immediately upon his arrival in the recovery room, *the usual procedure* when the patient arrives in the recovery room is to take two sets of vital signs in the first 40 minutes after admission and to administer pain medication soon thereafter. A narcotic drug may still be systemically circulating in the patient when he leaves the operating room. Therefore, if the patient is sleepy, or if he falls asleep immediately after admission to the recovery room, beware of being quick to give a narcotic drug. Pain will be manifested by specific activities or behaviors on the patient's part — crying, moaning, restlessness, or complaining. The nurse should keep these signs in mind as she observes the patient's condition for a reasonable length of time in order to assess his need for pain medication. Narcotics are usually administered any time after the first hour in the recovery room. However, if the patient is awake in the first half hour and is very uncomfortable, he will be medicated for pain if his vital signs are stable.

Prevention of Venous Stasis

The patient may have elastic stockings applied to his legs after surgery. This is a prophylactic measure designed to prevent venous stasis in the legs — a prime factor in the development of thrombophlebitis. The patient's knees should not be kept flexed for any great length of time. This may predispose him to venous stasis by compression on the femoral or popliteal veins. It is important that the nurse check the elastic stockings periodically to make certain that they do not roll below the knee. If this happens, the tight constricting band of the stocking may impede the venous return of blood. Leg exercises, which consist of flexion and extension of the joints of the legs and dorsiflexion of the feet, should be encouraged to promote venous return by muscular contraction.

Cardiovascular Complication

Shock. Shock is basically the inability of the circulatory system to meet the oxygen demands of the body. It is manifested in the patient by:

Apprehension.
Restlessness.
Cold, moist skin.
Cyanotic lips.
Rapid, thready pulse.
Rapid, shallow respirations.
Thirst.
Decreased temperature of the body.
Hypotension.
Decreased urine output.
Decreased central venous pressure.

Causes of Shock

1. Central — the failure of the heart to act as an effective pump. This may be the result of:
a. Coronary occlusion.
b. Congestive heart failure.
c. Cardiac arrest.
2. Peripheral — this occurs as a result of decreased volume of circulating blood being returned to the heart.
a. Hemorrhage:
1) Primary — occurring at the time of surgery.
2) Secondary — occurring the first few hours postoperatively.
b. Severe fluid losses.
c. Neurogenic:
1) Secondary to anesthetic agents.
2) Acute adrenal insufficiency.
3) Septic shock (the result of massive infection).

Treatment of Shock

When the doctor has evaluated the patient's condition and determined the cause of shock, treatment is begun:

1. Patients who suffer from myocardial failure may receive:
a. Cedilanid (rapid-acting intravenous digitalizing drug).
b. A vasoconstrictor, such as norepinephrine.
c. Oxygen.
d. Rotating tourniquets.
e. Aminophylline.
2. Patients who need replacement of blood or fluid volume due to hypovolemia may receive:
a. Whole blood replacement.
b. Plasma replacement.
c. Fluid and electrolyte replacement.

3. Patients who need peripheral vasoconstriction may receive:

a. Vasopressor drugs.

b. Cortisone. When used, this is given in massive doses (e.g., 1 to 2 grams daily intravenously).

Cardiac Arrest. The sudden cessation of heartbeat is an ever-present threat before, during, and after surgery. No form of surgery or anesthesia is immune to the possibility of cardiac arrest. The signs and symptoms are recognized immediately and include:

Loss of consciousness.

Loss of blood pressure.

Loss of pulse beat.

Dilated pupils.

Cold, clammy skin.

Cyanosis of lips and extremities.

Absence of reflexes.

Causes of Cardiac Arrest

1. Hypoxia of the myocardium due to:

a. Respiratory obstruction during induction of anesthesia.

b. Aspiration causing respiratory obstruction and resulting in hypoxia.

c. Inadequate ventilatory exchange of gases.

d. Respiratory acidosis.

e. Severe shock secondary to volume depletion.

2. Drugs:

a. Epinephrine.

b. Digitalis (in toxic doses).

c. Quinidine.

d. Penicillin.

e. Tetanus toxoid or a sulfa drug (producing an anaphylactic reaction).

3. Air embolism.

4. Acute coronary thrombosis (ventricular fibrillation).

5. Asphyxia.

6. Electrocution.

7. Severe electrolyte imbalance, particularly a high serum potassium level.

8. Stimulation of the pharynx.

Treatment of Cardiac Arrest. The patient's chest should be given an initial hard, quick, firm blow with a closed fist at a point on the sternum corresponding to the area over the heart. An Ambu bag should be used to initiate positive pressure breathing; EKG leads are to be placed on the patient and the "cardiac arrest board" positioned underneath him. The "code" or arrest signal is made known to the surgeon or anesthesiologist. External cardiac massage (external manual systole) and pulmonary ventilation are applied together while the defibrillator is readied for delivering the first external electric shock to the heart muscle. External manual systole can be quite effective in maintaining circulation, especially to the brain, provided that the systolic blood pressure is kept at 80 mm Hg. Often, an endotracheal tube is inserted and attached to a respirator so that adequate ventilation can be maintained during the resuscitative efforts. A number of drugs should be available for ready use:

Those injected intracardially:

10 per cent calcium chloride

1:10,000 epinephrine

Those given intravenously:

sodium lactate

sodium bicarbonate

epinephrine
Neo-Synephrine
Levophed
dopamine
lidocaine

These drugs are used during attempts at cardiac conversion with the defibrillator. If the first countershock is not successful, continuous cardiopulmonary resuscitation is continued and the drugs administered again as necessary (determined by evaluation of the EKG pattern and the laboratory analysis of arterial blood gases). *Note:* No one should touch the patient or anything metallic in contact with the patient while the countershock or conversion shock is being administered. Contact with wet spots on the floor (caused by leakage of dripped intravenous solution) must be avoided as well during the resuscitative events.

Resuscitative efforts with external defibrillation are continued until the heartbeat is resumed or effective cardiac action has been restored.

GASTROINTESTINAL CARE

Nausea

If the patient experiences nausea, deep breathing may alleviate the subjective feeling. The doctor may order antiemetic drugs or tranquilizing drugs to be administered; in some cases, a nasogastric tube may be passed into the stomach.

Analgesic drugs such as morphine sulfate and Demerol often produce feelings of nausea, and the nurse may wish to explain this to the patient.

Vomiting

It is most important to turn the patient's head and assist him in expectorating the vomitus into an emesis basin. Preventing the patient from swallowing or aspirating the vomitus may be accomplished by: (1) positioning the patient on his side with his head turned to the same side and (2) applying oral suction.

If the patient has had thoracic or abdominal surgery, it may be helpful to support the wound while he vomits.

Gastrointestinal Tubes

A Levin tube may be inserted at the completion of surgery on the gastrointestinal tract or its accessory organs. When the patient arrives in the recovery room, this tube may be clamped off with a Kelly or Hoffman clamp; intestinal or gastric drainage may be accomplished en route to the recovery room by placing a plastic bag over the unclamped tube. The nurse irrigates the intestinal or gastric tube with normal saline in order to determine the patency of the tube. She also checks to see that the tube (whether intestinal or gastric) is attached to the specific type of suction apparatus designated by the surgeon. In most cases a sump apparatus is used for gastrointestinal drainage because it does not exert continuous suction on the mucosa of the tract. The amount of drainage (as well as the kind of drainage) is observed and measured every 8 to 24 hours, depending on hospital policy or specific postoperative orders. Measurement of the drained gastrointestinal fluid must be accurate, for the figures on drainage are a decisive factor in estimating how much fluid replacement will be necessary to offset fluid loss. If the patient loses a great deal of fluid through gastric or intestinal suction, replacement with an equal amount of electrolyte-balanced isotonic parenteral fluid (similar to the lost fluid) is required. Fluid replacement must be accomplished within 24 to 48 hours if a positive fluid balance is to be maintained.

Fluids by Mouth

Patients who have had general anesthesia usually will not be permitted to have fluids by mouth until they have sufficiently recovered from the effects of anesthesia, are not nauseated, and have not vomited. Ice chips may help diminish the sensation of thirst.

PARENTERAL FLUID ADMINISTRATION

Parenteral fluids given by the intravenous route will be administered at a certain rate over a period of hours. When parenteral fluids are ordered by the doctor, the following information must be included in the original order:
1. The amount in cc's to be infused over a one-hour period.
2. The flow rate of the administration unit (the IV set) — that is, how many drops there are in one cc.

When both of these variables are known, the nurse may compute the flow rate in *drops per minute* by use of the following formula:

$$\frac{\text{Drops per cc (or ml) of given set}}{60 \text{ (minutes in an hour)}} \times \text{total hourly volume} = \text{drops per minute}^*$$

Dangers of Intravenous Fluid Administration

The nurse must be alert to the following complications of intravenous fluid therapy.
Pyrogenic reactions from unsterile equipment.
Pulmonary edema from vascular overload.
Allergic reaction to blood products.
Infiltration of the IV fluid, causing local phlebitis.

Charting of Intravenous Fluids

It is imperative that the nurse chart parenteral fluids administered to the patient at the completion of each bottle. These fluids are totaled on a 8-hour basis, and then a grand total for a 24-hour period is tallied. The nurse may have to know how much fluid the patient has taken or lost on an hourly basis so that she may report this to the doctor.

---

*From A. L. Plumer, *Principles and Practice of Intravenous Therapy* (Boston: Little, Brown, and Company, 1970), p. 68.

TRANSFUSIONS

Blood may be given to the patient postoperatively when his hematocrit level falls or his blood pressure drops to significantly low systolic readings indicating incipient shock as a result of internal or external hemorrhage.

The following factors must be checked by the nurse or the doctor before a transfusion is initiated:

The blood bottle must be checked for type, Rh. factor, and patient's name (some hospitals check a hospital identification number of the recipient with the chart).

Cross-check the patient's chart with the transfusion bottle to determine the correct blood type and Rh. factor of the donor and the recipient.

Check the patient himself for correct identification (some hospitals place identification bracelets on all patients for this purpose).

The nurse should chart the time the transfusion was initiated, any reactions noted, and time of completion of the unit of blood. It is most important for a nurse or doctor to stay with the patient for the administration of the first 50 cc. of blood to evaluate the patient's reaction to the transfusion.

Symptoms of untoward reactions include:

Chills.

Fever.

Urticaria.

Dyspnea.

Orthopnea.

Hemoptysis.

Gurgling sound in the chest (indicative of pulmonary edema).

Pain in the lumbar region or posterior chest.

Hematuria.

If an untoward reaction is observed, the transfusion should be stopped immediately and the doctor notified of the reaction. The blood and equipment used in the transfusion must be returned to the blood bank for analysis. A sample of venous blood is drawn from a site other than that at which blood is being infused and is sent to the blood bank. Usually, a 24-hour urine specimen is collected and the patient is administered Benadryl.

URINARY SYSTEM CONSIDERATIONS

After surgery, the patient will have an 8- to 10-hour period in which he is expected to void. After this time, the doctor may order the patient to be catheterized to prevent distention, distress, and the possibility of urinary tract infection from stasis of urine.

The patient who is distended may have a palpable fullness above the symphysis pubis and may express a desire to void. He may also have a spasmodic type of pain associated with distention of the bladder.

At the completion of some surgical procedures, the surgeon may order a catheter to be inserted to establish continuous urinary drainage and accurate measurement. The catheter is attached to a sterile collecting bag or bottle. The amount is recorded on an 8-hour basis; the grand total is tallied at the end of 24 hours. If the urinary output is to be measured and recorded and the patient does not have a urinary catheter in place, the nurse should collect the urine voided by the patient and note the time it is passed.

Care of a Patient with a Foley or Indwelling Urinary Catheter

1. Anchor the catheter on the patient's inner thigh with tape, permitting freedom of movement without resulting tension on the urethrovesical area of the urinary bladder.

2. Keep the urethral meatus free of accumulated material and secretions, which not only cause discomfort but predispose the patient to urinary tract infection. Cleanse the catheter-meatus junction with sterile water or sterile saline daily, or every eight hours as indicated or as ordered by the physician. In some instances, the physician may order that a Neomycin 1 per cent soaked gauze pledget be applied to the meatus 4 times a day. Alternatively, Neosporin ointment may be applied to the same area every 6 hours. When this ointment is applied, retract the catheter gently away from the urinary meatus, and apply a layer of the ointment directly on the area of the catheter nearest the meatal point.

3. Irrigate the urinary catheter on the doctor's order only; acetic acid 0.25 per cent or another type of antibiotic solution may be ordered. Use 30 cc's per irrigation and note on the intake and output sheet that this procedure has been carried out. Record the precise amount of fluid instilled through the catheter into the bladder.

4. Make certain that at all times the drainage apparatus permits urine to drain by gravity. In this way adequate urine drainage can be ensured whether the patient is in or out of bed.

5. Remove the urinary catheter at least every 5 days, or change it as ordered by the physician.

OTHER CONSIDERATIONS

Pain

When the patient complains of pain postoperatively, it is the responsibility of the nurse to note the location. There are two types of postoperative pain:
1. Incisional pain.
2. Pain in an area other than that of the incision.

Incisional pain is localized to the area of surgery. Pain in any other area should be evaluated in terms of these questions:
1. What is the exact location of the pain?
2. Is the pain intermittent or constant?
3. Is the pain sharp, dull, or colicky?
4. Does the pain radiate to another part of the body?
5. Does the pain occur upon inhalation or exhalation?

When the answers to these questions have been determined, the nurse should record the information for the physician's reference. If it appears to the nurse that the location and the intensity of the pain are abnormal for the surgery that has been performed, she should report this to the physician.

Common Drugs Used to Relieve Postoperative Pain

Morphine.
Demerol.
Methadone.
Dilaudid.
Talwin.

Percodan.

Codeine.

The nurse should note how long it takes the narcotic or analgesic to relieve the patient's pain and whether this pain is relieved adequately. She must note when the drug is given and the prescribed dose administered. Because some medications and anesthetic drugs used at the time of surgery have lingering effects (e.g., Innovar), the dose of the narcotic drug administered postoperatively must be cut in half. In every case, the nurse must be knowledgeable of the drugs that have been administered intraoperatively and the effects these drugs have on the patient in the immediate postoperative period.

Restlessness

The most common causes of restlessness are:

1. Postoperative pain.
2. Tight, constricting dressings.
3. Cerebral anoxia.
4. Urinary retention.
5. Anxiety.
6. Intestinal or gastric distention.
7. The remaining effects of anesthesia (e.g., ketamine).

If the patient is uncomfortable, excited, or agitated from one of these causes, he will move about or thrash in his bed until the condition is rectified. The restless patient may injure himself by hurling his arms or legs or both against the side rails of the bed. He may even attempt to climb out of his bed. The nurse should protect the patient during this period of restlessness. The side rails of the bed should be padded. If necessary, a written restraint order should be obtained from the doctor (e.g., Posey belt). An analgesic or sedative may be administered. If the patient has any drainage tubes in place, the nurse must be on guard lest he pull out these tubes in his agitated state. She should also give these tubes additional slack so no stress is placed on the wound.

DISCHARGE OF THE PATIENT FROM THE RECOVERY AREA

The doctor will evaluate the patient's condition when he has reacted from the anesthesia. The vital signs should be stable, and the patient should be free of complications. A written order may be needed from the doctor; the staff of the clinical area should be notified that the patient is to be transported from the recovery room, and the head nurse on this unit will then see that the patient's room is ready. An escort and a nurse will usually accompany the patient during transfer. Portable stands for intravenous infusions, a portable oxygen tank, and additional side rails may be needed for the transfer. If the patient is to be moved to a new clinical area, the admitting office may have to be notified as well as the head nurse on the new clinical unit. The patient's clothes and valuables must also be transferred to the new room. When the patient is brought to his room, all drainage tubes must be connected to proper apparatus. The nurse who accompanies the patient must discuss the condition of the patient, treatments, and medications with the head nurse so that an individualized nursing care plan can be written and implemented. Any special aspects of nursing care should also be discussed with the head nurse at this time.

In summary, then, there are certain criteria which must be met and certain procedures which must be followed in discharging the patient from the recovery room:

1. The patient must have recovered from the effects of general anesthesia. This usually requires a two-hour stay in the recovery room.

2. The vital signs must have stabilized.

3. There must be no excessive drainage or bleeding from any site or body cavity.

4. The physiological effects of any narcotic medication must have stabilized (this will require about one half hour from the time of administration).

5. The patient must have regained consciousness, and the level of consciousness must be satisfactory.

6. All essential orders must be carried out and completed by the recovery room personnel.

7. Should the situation arise, provisions for attendance by a private duty nurse must be made on the clinical unit where the patient is to be moved.

8. The urine output must be adequate (30 cc's per hour). The amount must be noted and recorded.

9. The staff of the clinical unit to which the patient is to be transferred must be alerted and make the necessary preparations for receiving the patient in his room.

TRANSFER OF THE PATIENT FROM THE RECOVERY ROOM

The following routines should be observed during the transfer procedure:

1. An escort and a nurse must accompany the patient from the recovery room to the new clinical area. One other person may be needed to transfer equipment.

2. Safety measures for all drainage tubes must be observed. In addition, the side rails of the stretcher must be up. The patient should be adequately covered with top bedding.

3. On arrival at the clinical unit, notify the head nurse of the patient's return.

4. Get assistance in moving the patient onto his bed.

5. Put the patient on his side when he is placed in the bed if he is still sleepy; otherwise, place him in an optimum position for comfort.

6. Provide a basin at the bedside and attach a call light to the patient's gown or pillow. The side rails of the bed should be up.

7. The bed must be placed in the lowest position after the patient is transferred into it.

8. Check functioning of tubes, drainage equipment, and suction apparatus.

9. Show the staff nurse on the clinical unit the patient's dressing; explain the type of drainage tubes in place and indicate which of the tubes already in place must be irrigated.

10. The initial set of vital signs are to be taken by the staff nurse on the clinical unit.

11. A verbal report must be given by the recovery room nurse to the staff nurse on the clinical unit. This report should include:

a. A review of all the recovery room records.

b. The condition of the patient during the immediate postoperative period.

12. The recovery room nurse should write a note on the patient's progress record indicating when the patient was transferred to the clinical unit and his condition at that time.

STUDY QUESTIONS

1. What are the specific advantages of the recovery room and the intensive care unit?

2. What are some important observations you as a nurse must make when a patient is brought to the recovery room or intensive care unit? Select a specific patient and list these observations.

3. List some safety precautions for optimum patient care that are employed in the recovery room and intensive care units.

4. What are the hazards involved in transporting a patient from the operating room to the recovery area?

5. What emergency equipment should each recovery room and I.C.U. have? Why is each piece used, and when would it be used?

6. What are the principles underlying the general postoperative orders written by the doctor?

7. List the types of mechanical devices that may be used to assist the patient to breathe.

8. What are some signs and symptoms of respiratory distress and resultant hypoxia that the nurse must anticipate?

9. What are some indications for deep endotracheal suctioning of a patient postoperatively?

10. What principles are employed in the deep endotracheal suctioning procedure?

11. Review and list the nursing care of a patient receiving oxygen therapy by the following modes of administration:
    a. Face mask
    b. Face tent
    c. Nasal catheter
    d. Nasal prongs

12. What variations of the vital signs might occur in the immediate postoperative period and why?

13. Describe the physiological basis of postoperative pain in the postsurgical patient.

Part II

SPECIFIC OPERATIVE PROCEDURES

ABDOMINAL AND PELVIC SURGERY

INTRODUCTION

11

BOUNDARIES, ANATOMY, AND CONTENTS

The abdominopelvic regions are considered together as they form one continuous cavity extending from the respiratory diaphragm to the pelvic diaphragm, and the surgical principles involved in these two areas are fundamentally similar.

The simplest way of understanding the anatomic nature of this region is to look upon it as a large sac (the peritoneum) containing several organs, and supported on the outside by several layers of muscles anteriorly as well as posteriorly.

Surgical entrance into this sac is usually obtained by the anterior approach through one of several standard incisions. While varying from area to area on the abdomen, several distinct layers of tissue must be penetrated during abdominopelvic surgery:

1. Skin
2. Subcutaneous fat
3. Superficial fascia
4. Deep fascia
5. Muscle
6. Fascia
7. Peritoneum

The abdominopelvic cavity contains the following organs and tissues:

The *gastrointestinal tract* and its *appendages,* exclusive of the esophagus and the anus. The gastrointestinal appendages include (moving downward):

1. Liver, gallbladder, pancreas, portal vein
2. Appendix

The spleen and splenic vein.

The *female reproductive* organs:

1. Uterus
2. Ovaries
3. Fallopian tubes or oviducts

SURGICAL APPROACHES

Innumerable incisions have been developed in the history of abdominal surgery all incorporating, with varying degrees of success, certain characteristics of a *well-planned* incision:
1. Ease and speed of entrance into the abdominal cavity
2. Maximum exposure
3. Ease and speed of extension of incision
4. Ease and speed of closure
5. Minimum postoperative discomfort
6. Maximum postoperative wound strength

TYPES OF INCISIONS

Direction

Vertical or "up and down"
Horizontal or transverse
Oblique

Location

Midline
1. Upper abdominal
2. Lower abdominal
Paramedian
1. Upper abdominal
2. Lower abdominal
Subcostal
Suprapubic
Inguinal
Transverse
1. Upper abdominal
2. Lower abdominal

COMMONLY USED INCISIONS, THEIR CHARACTERISTICS AND USES

Kocher's Subcostal Incision

Location and Direction. This is an oblique subcostal incision (right or left) (Fig. 11–1 a).
Characteristics. The incision is begun in the epigastrium and is carried obliquely downward approximately two fingerbreadths below, and parallel to, the costal margin. This incision gives excellent exposure of the upper abdominal contents; it is, however, extended only with difficulty, is executed slowly, and is quite painful postoperatively. The most important aspect of the Kocher subcostal incision is its postoperative strength, there being few instances of wound dehiscence following its use.

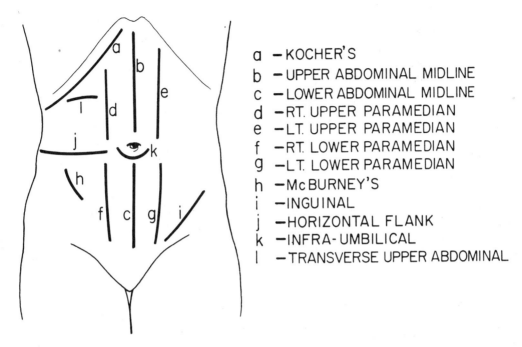

a – KOCHER'S
b – UPPER ABDOMINAL MIDLINE
c – LOWER ABDOMINAL MIDLINE
d – RT. UPPER PARAMEDIAN
e – LT. UPPER PARAMEDIAN
f – RT. LOWER PARAMEDIAN
g – LT. LOWER PARAMEDIAN
h – McBURNEY'S
i – INGUINAL
j – HORIZONTAL FLANK
k – INFRA-UMBILICAL
l – TRANSVERSE UPPER ABDOMINAL

FIGURE 11–1 Commonly used abdominopelvic incisions.

Uses
1. Right Side: gallbladder and biliary tract surgery
2. Left Side: surgery of the spleen

Upper Abdominal Midline Incision

Location and Direction. This is an upper abdominal, vertical incision (Fig. 11–1 b).
Characteristics. The incision is begun in the epigastrium at the level of the xiphoid process and is carried vertically downward to the level of the umbilicus. This incision provides excellent exposure of the upper abdominal contents; it is easily extended, quickly executed and easily closed. It is not considered a strong incision and the incidence of wound dehiscence is high. When your patient has had an upper abdominal incision, watch carefully for signs of dehiscence.

Uses
1. Rapid entry into the abdomen to control a bleeding ulcer
2. Gastrectomy

Lower Abdominal Midline Incision

Location and Direction. This is a lower abdominal, vertical incision (Fig. 11–1 c).
Characteristics. The incision is begun opposite the umbilicus and is extended vertically downward in the midline to the suprapubic region. This incision provides excellent exposure of the pelvic organs including bladder, prostate, uterus, tubes, ovaries, and sigmoid colon. It is easily extended and quickly executed and closed, but lacks the strength of a transverse or paramedian lower abdominal incision.

Uses
1. Hysterectomy
2. Suprapubic prostatectomy
3. Cystostomy
4. Salpingectomy
5. Presacral neurectomy

Paramedian Incision

Location and Direction. This is a vertical incision which is confined to an area approximately two fingerbreadths to the right or left of the midline, and may be in the upper or lower abdomen.

Characteristics. The incision is extended in a vertical direction parallel to and two fingers lateral to the midline. When the rectus muscle is reached, it may be split vertically or retracted laterally. This incision allows excellent exposure of the nearby organs, according to its location. It is slowly executed and closed, but is very easily extended and gives a firm closure. Its *uses* depend on its location.

Uses
1. Right Upper Paramedian (Fig. 11-1 d):
a. Biliary tract surgery
2. Left Upper Paramedian (Fig. 11-1 e):
a. Surgery on the spleen
b. Gastrectomy
c. Vagectomy
d. Repair of hiatus hernia
3. Right Lower Paramedian (Fig. 11-1 f):
a. Appendectomy
b. Small bowel resection
c. Surgery on right adnexae
4. Left Lower Paramedian (Fig. 11-1 g):
a. Sigmoid colon resection
b. Miles' resection
c. Hysterectomy
d. Surgery on left adnexae

McBurney's Incision (Fig. 11-1 h):

Location and Direction. This is an oblique incision over McBurney's point in the right lower quadrant.

Characteristics. The incision is extended obliquely from just below the umbilicus, through McBurney's point upward, toward the right flank. This incision is quickly executed and closed. It allows a firm wound closure but it is difficult to extend and gives poor exposure.

Use. Appendectomy.

Inguinal Incision

Location and Direction. This is an oblique incision in the inguinal region (Fig. 11-1 i).

Characteristics. The incision is extended from the pubic tubercle one fingerbreadth above and parallel to the inguinal crease up to the anterior iliac crest. This incision does not enter the abdomen, but is used for exploration of the inguinal canal.

Uses
1. Repair of inguinal hernia
2. Excision of hydrocele of the cord

Horizontal Flank Incision

Location and Direction. This is a midabdominal incision which extends out into the flank (Fig. 11-1 j).

Characteristics. This incision is begun at the lateral border of the rectus sheath at the level of the umbilicus. It is extended horizontally out to the flank. The underlying muscles are split in the direction of their fibers, and the retroperitoneal space is thereby reached. This incision is rapidly executed and closed, can easily be extended, and provides for a secure wound.

Uses
1. Lumbar sympathectomy
2. Nephrectomy
3. Ureterolithotomy
4. Inferior vena cava ligation

Infraumbilical Incision

The infraumbilical incision is curvilinear. It is located below the umbilicus and is used only for an umbilical hernia repair (Fig. 11-1 k).

SKIN PREPS

Preoperative shaving of the skin and operative cleansing encompass the same area determined by the nature of the surgical procedure.

The area to be prepped must always be considerably wider than the contemplated incision, particularly since further unexpected extension of the incision may be required.

Figure 11-2 and the shaded areas to be prepped are self-explanatory. They will be referred to throughout subsequent chapters of this section.

POSITION

Figure 11-3 is self-explanatory. It will be referred to throughout subsequent chapters of this section.

SPECIAL FEATURES OF ABDOMINOPELVIC SURGERY

Wound Sepsis. The abdominal wall is particularly apt to become infected for reasons not clearly understood. In addition, many cases of abdominal surgery involve opening into the

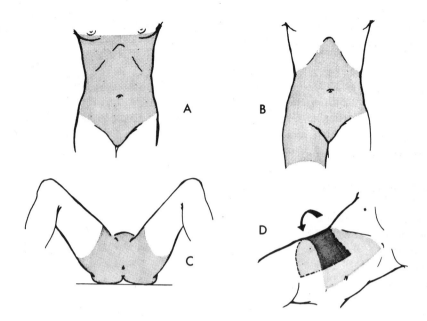

FIGURE 11–2 Skin preps. A. All procedures except as listed under B, C, and D. B. Inguinal hernia. C. Perineal phase of Miles' resection, dilatation and curettage, and cervical biopsy. D. Nephrectomy, lumbar sympathectomy, vena cava ligation, and ureterolithotomy.

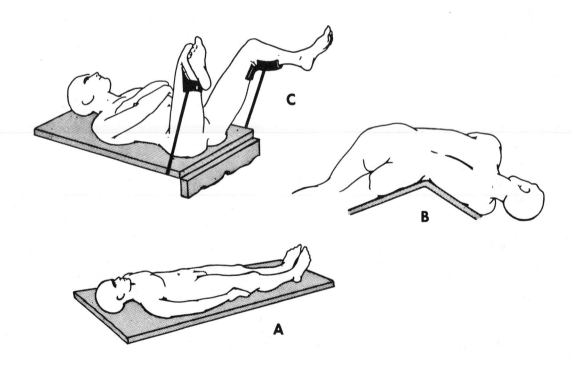

FIGURE 11–3 Positions. A. All procedures except as listed under B and C. B. Nephrectomy, lumbar sympathectomy, vena cava ligation, and ureterolithotomy. C. Perineal phase of Miles' resection, dilatation and curettage, and cervical biopsy.

intestinal tract, which is teeming with pathogenic microorganisms. Consequently, every effort must be made to protect the abdominal incision. These measures include:

Adequate skin shaving and preparation

Proper use of skin towels

Emptying of the bowel and sterilization when intestinal surgery is planned

Fine surgical technique

Exposure. The loops of intestine (34 running feet of bowel packed into this small area) create the problem of difficult surgical exposure. In addition, the many deep abdominal recesses make it difficult to obtain good lighting. Measures to improve abdominal exposure include:

Proper packing off of intestinal loops with laparotomy towels

Proper use of self-retaining and other abdominal retractors

Use of supplementary "spot" lights which must be frequently readjusted by the circulating nurse when requested

Wound Closure. The abdominal incision is subjected postoperatively to many stresses during breathing, straining, and coughing. In no other surgical region is wound dehiscence a more frequent or more serious problem than in abdominopelvic surgery. Measures to prevent wound dehiscence include:

Attention to nutritional deficiencies preoperatively, particularly with reference to vitamin C and total protein levels

Use of a properly planned incision

Meticulous wound closure

Avoidance of postoperative abdominal distention

Immediate Postoperative Management. The general principles of postoperative management, as found in Part I of this manual, are applicable. Certain special features of abdominopelvic surgery are as follows:

Postoperative Ileus. Most major abdominopelvic operations are complicated by a certain degree of postoperative ileus. The patient is therefore allowed nothing by mouth (NPO) until peristalsis returns and flatus is passed. To prevent abdominal distention, a Levin tube is frequently passed through the nose into the stomach and kept in place until peristalsis returns.

Postoperative Atelectasis. The painful *upper abdominal incision* makes it difficult for the patient to respire normally and this situation may result in accumulation of mucus in the lung. If small bronchi are plugged by mucus, atelectasis results and pneumonia ensues. Careful attention to pulmonary care must be given in the early postoperative period.

Urinary Retention. The painful abdominal incision may also limit the patient's ability to void in the early postoperative period. This is why it is important to check output of urine. The surgeon should be notified if bladder distention occurs.

Wound Care. The undrained abdominal cavity represents no problem in the early postoperative period. When drains are used, the dressing may soak through shortly after surgery. This should be called to the surgeon's attention.

12

THE PATIENT
WITH AN
UMBILICAL HERNIA

Operation: Repair of an Umbilical Hernia

TYPICAL HISTORY

A 3-year-old male was born with a small umbilical hernia and has been followed for 2 years. The hernia has shown no signs of closure and, although there have been no episodes suggesting intestinal obstruction, the patient has been hospitalized for repair of the hernia.

PHYSICAL EXAMINATION

The patient is a well-developed, well-nourished, male child with an obvious umbilical hernia, but otherwise in no distress (the child is lying quietly in bed).

Significant Findings

1. There is a protrusion in the region of the umbilicus which stands out prominently, particularly when the child strains and coughs. When he is resting quietly there is no suggestion of an umbilical hernia.

2. On examination of the umbilical area, two fingers are easily admitted into the abdominal cavity through the defect in the abdominal wall.

DIAGNOSTIC STUDIES

There are no pertinent diagnostic studies in the evaluation of an umbilical hernia.

PROBABLE HOSPITAL COURSE

The patient will undergo routine laboratory studies and any special studies in relationship to other problems. There are no particular laboratory or x-ray studies necessary in the evaluation and treatment of an umbilical hernia.

PREPARATION FOR SURGERY

1. *Skin Prep.*   The entire abdomen from the nipple line as far as and including the pubis is cleansed with pHisoHex. (See Introduction.)
2. *Enema.*   Not necessary.
3. *Levin Tube.*   Not necessary.
4. *Blood.*   Not necessary.
5. *Premedications.*   Routine.
6. *Special Medications.*   None.
7. *Operating Room Skin Prep.*   From the nipple line as far as and including the pubis. (See Introduction.)
8. *Position.*   Horizontal supine. (See Introduction.)

PATHOLOGY

Umbilical hernia represents a congenital defect in which there is a failure of closure of the umbilical foramen which was patent during fetal development. This aperture usually allows for the escape of intestines into the yolk sac during embryological development. The intestines return in the early months of development and the fascial wall generally closes.

GENERAL RATIONALE AND SCHEME

Most umbilical herniae close spontaneously within a year or two of birth. They generally present very little danger of intestinal obstruction and, except for the anxiety they cause the parents, are of no concern. There is some disagreement among authorities as to which types of herniae probably will not close. Some authorities feel that if the fascial defect in the abdominal wall permits the insertion of one finger it probably will not close. Others feel that even larger herniae will close spontaneously. At any rate, if in the surgeon's opinion the umbilical hernia is not likely to close spontaneously, operative closure is indicated.

Scheme

1. A supra- or infraumbilical curvilinear incision is made.
2. The hernial sac is excised.
3. The peritoneum and rectus sheath are closed.
4. The skin is closed.

PROCEDURE

1. *Skin Incision.*   A small curvilinear incision is made in the supraumbilical or infraumbilical area in the normal skin found in these areas. In this way, the umbilicus is preserved and there is usually no evidence of scarring following the operation.
2. An opening is made into the peritoneal cavity and the contents of the sac are reduced. Following this step, the excess sac tissue is excised.
3. The peritoneum is closed as a separate layer with interrupted sutures.
4. The anterior rectus sheath is closed transversely in an overlapping fashion.
5. The skin is closed with interrupted sutures.

SURGICAL HAZARD

Injury to Contents within the Sac. Occasionally a loop of small intestine is found within the sac of the umbilical hernia adherent to the sac lining. Careless dissection in this area may result in injury to the small intestine which, if unnoticed, may lead to leakage with generalized peritonitis.

EARLY POSTOPERATIVE MANAGEMENT

The patient is kept in the recovery room until he is sufficiently reactive from the anesthetic. Routine management is discussed in Chapter 4, Part I and should be carefully reviewed at this time. The usual course of the postherniorrhaphy patient is smooth, and one of the few problems to be anticipated is *bleeding through the dressing.* Occasionally a small vessel that has been left unligated may begin to bleed. This can result in loss of blood or formation of a hematoma with consequent infection and disruption of the suture lines. Therefore, if the dressing soaks through, the surgeon should be notified immediately. As for other procedures followed postoperatively, the child is usually given liquids by mouth as soon as he is alert, and he may be discharged the day after surgery.

STUDY QUESTIONS

1. What methods may be used to maintain reduction of an umbilical hernia during the waiting period to determine whether the hernia will close spontaneously?

2. Are there any complications if an umbilical hernia remains unrepaired?

3. The mother of a 6-month-old infant who has a very small umbilical hernia that barely admits the finger, asks your opinion whether or not this hernia should be repaired surgically. How would you handle the mother's question and her anxiety?

4. Can you explain the presence of an umbilical hernia on embryological grounds?

5. What other herniae may be found in an infant? Where are they located? How are they managed?

6. Discuss the surgical steps in the repair of an umbilical hernia.

7. What other organs besides the intestines may be found in an umbilical hernia?

8. What is the usual postoperative course of an infant who has undergone umbilical hernia repair? Discuss specifically: *diet, medication, nursing care,* and *home care.*

THE PATIENT WITH AN INGUINAL HERNIA
13

Operation: Inguinal Herniorrhaphy or Hernioplasty

TYPICAL HISTORY

A 36-year-old male, in excellent health previously, noted the sudden onset of sharp steady pain in the groin while lifting a heavy article. Over the next few days he became aware of a small, slightly tender lump in the right groin which disappeared on his lying down, only to recur when he stood.

PHYSICAL EXAMINATION

The patient is a well-developed, well-nourished male in no acute distress.

Significant Findings

There is a slight bulge in the right groin which increases when the patient coughs or strains.

DIAGNOSTIC STUDIES

There are no x-ray or laboratory studies used to diagnose or confirm a simple, reducible inguinal hernia. The diagnosis is made simply on the basis of the physical examination.

PROBABLE HOSPITAL COURSE

Provided no other associated problems have been discovered during the initial examination of the patient, surgery will be planned within a day or two after admission. Certain conditions may predispose individuals to the development of an inguinal hernia by causing an increase in intra-abdominal pressure (Fig. 13–1). These include:

1. *Chronic Cough.* A chest x-ray may be required to rule out such conditions as carcinoma of the lung.

2. *Straining at Stool.* Sigmoidoscopy and barium enema may be indicated to rule out carcinoma of the rectum.

3. *Ascites.* Liver studies and cardiac studies are indicated to rule out cirrhosis or cardiac failure.

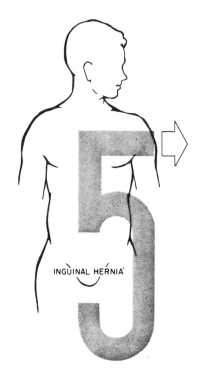

1	STRAINING AT WORK
2	CHRONIC COUGH
3	STRAINING TO VOID
4	STRAINING AT STOOL
5	ASCITES

FIGURE 13–1   The five major predisposing factors in hernia development.

4. *Straining to Void.*   Intravenous pyelography, postvoiding residuals, and cystoscopy may be indicated to rule out prostatic obstruction.

5. *Straining at Work.*

PREPARATION FOR SURGERY

In addition to the general measures outlined in Part I, the particular approach to the hernia patient is as follows:

1. Complete history and physical examination.

2. *Psychological and Legal Aspects.*   The male patient undergoing an inguinal hernia repair is often somewhat concerned over loss of sexual potency or "manhood." If such concern be expressed by the patient, the nurse should reassure him on this point. Occasionally, a large, recurrent hernia may require castration on the involved side in order to effect a radical cure of the hernia. Should this be anticipated by the surgeon, special consent forms should be signed by the patient.

3. *Skin Prep.*   The entire abdomen from the costal margins as far as and including the pubis and the upper thigh on the involved side is cleanly shaven on the ward. (See Introduction.)

4. *Enema.*   A soapsuds or Fleet enema should be given either the evening before or the day of surgery, as the patient will find it most uncomfortable to attempt to move his bowels the day following surgery.

5. *Levin Tube.*   Unnecessary.

6. *Blood.*   Unnecessary.

7. *Premedications.*   Same as for appendectomy.

8. Patient should be encouraged to void preoperatively.

9. *Operating Room Skin Prep.* The entire abdomen, pubic area, and upper thigh on the involved side are thoroughly washed with pHisoHex and rinsed; then they are painted with tincture of Zephiran. (See Introduction.)

10. *Position.* Horizontal supine. (See Introduction.)

PATHOLOGY

A hernia represents any protrusion of organs into a space they would not occupy normally. There are two types of inguinal herniae:

Indirect (congenital). This represents a herniation of a segment of peritoneum (the sac) through the internal abdominal ring and down the inguinal canal; sometimes the herniation continues into the scrotum. It may be accompanied by a segment of intestine.

Direct. This represents a herniation of a segment of peritoneum through a weakness in the abdominal wall in the inguinal region. The herniation does not pass through the internal abdominal ring. The significance of the distinction is as follows:

1. Fundamentally, an *indirect hernia* is a congenital defect in which a sac of peritoneum is found in the inguinal canal. Repair is usually simple and the recurrence rate low.

2. A *direct hernia* usually occurs in older men and represents an acquired weakness of the lower abdominal wall. Such a weakness is particularly apt to follow chronic increases in intraabdominal pressure. Consequently, this type of hernia must alert the surgeon to the possible presence of one of the five causes of increased abdominal pressure already discussed. Also, the recurrence rate following repair is usually higher than in indirect herniae.

GENERAL RATIONALE AND SCHEME

A hernia is progressive and tends to become larger with time. Generally, the larger the hernia is, the more difficult it is to repair. The great danger with a hernia is the possibility of a loop of bowel becoming strangulated within the narrow confines of the inguinal ring and canal, resulting in *intestinal strangulation* and gangrene of the bowel.

Scheme

1. The inguinal canal is opened.
2. The peritoneal sac is located and excised as close to its exit from the abdomen as possible.
3. The weakness in the abdominal musculature is strengthened with sutures.

PROCEDURE

1. *Skin Incision.* Oblique, one finger above and parallel to inguinal ligament from pubic tubercle to anterior iliac spine (Fig. 11–1, p. 155).

2. *Deepening Incision.* Superficial fascia is incised until aponeurosis of external oblique muscle is reached. This is incised, exposing the inguinal canal. A self-retaining retractor may now be requested by the surgeon.

3. *Exploring for Sac.* The sac is usually adherent to cord structures and is carefully sought in the inguinal canal. In the case of *indirect hernia,* a finger-like projection of peritoneum is found and followed to internal abdominal ring. In the case of *direct hernia,* a bulge will be seen in the floor of the inguinal canal but there will be no discrete peritoneal sac.

4. *Ligation of Sac* (indirect hernia only). The sac is usually opened, then ligated at the level of the internal abdominal ring; the excess tissue is then excised.

5. *Repair ·of Abdominal Wall.* The conjoined tendon is then sutured to the inguinal ligament. (The variations in the types of repairs are too numerous to mention.)

6. *Closure.* The external oblique aponeurosis is closed, the wound is irrigated, and the superficial fascia and skin are closed.

SURGICAL HAZARDS

1. *Damage to Spermatic Cord.* Severance of the cord can occur during dissection of the hernial sac. If severance is unilateral, it will not cause sterility, if bilateral, permanent sterility will occur.

2. *Damage to Blood Supply of Testis.* This can also occur during dissection of the hernial sac and may lead to infarction of the testis.

3. Rarely, damage to the nearby femoral artery or vein can occur.

EARLY POSTOPERATIVE MANAGEMENT

The patient is brought to the recovery room and kept there until sufficiently reactive from the anesthetic. (See Part I for routine management.) The usual course of the posthernioplasty patient is smooth, and among the few problems to be anticipated are:

1. *Acute Urinary Retention.* This is prone to occur as the patient finds it most uncomfortable to void spontaneously. He should be catheterized if his bladder is painfully distended. He may stand to void as soon as he has recovered from anesthesia.

2. *Scrotal Hematoma.* Though uncommon, slow bleeding may result in massive accumulation of blood in the scrotum which may lead to scrotal infection and require prolonged hospitalization. The scrotal area should be examined frequently and any signs of swelling reported to the surgeon immediately.

3. *Care of the Wound.* Unless bleeding has occurred, care of the wound in the recovery room is minimal, and the dressing may be removed the day after surgery. If bleeding occurs, the dressing should not be reinforced until the surgeon has been informed.

4. The patient may resume his usual diet as soon as he is alert. He may ambulate within 12 to 24 hours after surgery and is usually discharged in 3 to 4 days.

STUDY QUESTIONS

1. What are the different types of inguinal herniae? Are they all repaired in the same way?

2. What is the difference between a strangulated hernia and an incarcerated one?

3. What is a femoral hernia? Describe its repair.

4. What abdominal organs may be found within the sac of an inguinal hernia?

5. Can you visualize the internal abdominal ring? Ask the surgeon to demonstrate this as well as the hernia sac during a surgical procedure.

6. What cord structures are found in the male? In the female?

7. What is the conjoined tendon? Ask the surgeon to demonstrate it.

8. What methods may be used to encourage voiding after herniorrhaphy?

9. Are there any hazards associated with catheterizing a patient? What are they? How are they prevented?

10. Are there any hazards attributable to severe distention of the urinary bladder?

11. Why is a strangulated hernia dangerous?

12. Should a small asymptomatic hernia be repaired?

13. How does intestinal obstruction result from an inguinal hernia?

14. Are all incarcerated herniae surgical emergencies?

15. What nonoperative measures may, at times, accomplish reduction of an incarcerated hernia?

16. Make a list of pre- and postoperative activities the nurse should carry out in caring for the patient who is to have a herniorrhaphy.

17. What are the potential psychological effects of castration in the male? How should these fears be managed?

14

THE PATIENT
WITH AN
INCISIONAL HERNIA

Operation: Repair of Incisional Hernia

TYPICAL HISTORY

A 55-year-old obese female underwent cholecystectomy 8 years ago. Following surgery, she noted a lump in her incision which persisted to the current admission. From time to time there is mild, dull, aching pain in the region of this lump which disappears when the patient lies down. She has been keeping the lump reduced with a girdle for several years, but now enters for repair of this incisional hernia.

PHYSICAL EXAMINATION

The patient is a well-developed, obese female in no acute distress.

Significant Findings

1. There is a very loose, redundant abdominal wall.
2. There is a large protruding hernial mass in the upper region of a vertical incision.
3. Many loops of intestine can be palpated through this mass.

LABORATORY DATA

There are no pertinent laboratory data associated with an incisional hernia. A barium enema may be done which may reveal loops of colon within the incisional hernia.

PROBABLE HOSPITAL COURSE

Following routine studies, as well as a barium enema, the patient will be ready for operative repair of the incisional hernia. There are no specific studies that need be done for such a case. Consequently, the patient will probably be operated on within a day or two of her hospitalization unless some problem is uncovered during the routine studies. If chronic cough, secondary to chronic pulmonary disease, is present, a few days may be set aside for pulmonary therapy. This will diminish the cough and aid in the patient's postoperative course.

PREPARATION FOR SURGERY

1. *Levin Tube.*   Not usually necessary unless there is significant intestinal distention.
2. *Blood.*   The patient is typed and cross-matched for one to two units of whole blood as a good deal of blood may be lost during surgery.
3. *Skin Prep.*   The abdominal wall is prepped from the nipples as far as and including the pubis. (See Introduction.)
4. *Enema.*   A cleansing enema is given the night prior to surgery or the morning of surgery.
5. *Premedications.*   Routine.
6. *Special Medications.*   None.
7. *Operating Room Skin Prep.*   (See Introduction.)
8. *Position.*   Horizontal supine. (See Introduction.)

PATHOLOGY

An incisional hernia usually occurs when the fascia of the abdominal wall is disrupted or weakened postoperatively. The peritoneum protrudes through this fascial opening and projects in all directions over the abdominal wall, creating several finger-like projections of peritoneum that contain segments of bowel. If the fascial ring or weakness through which the peritoneum originally protruded is sufficiently small, and if the fascial wall is of good consistency otherwise, a very firm permanent repair can be obtained. At times, the entire fascial wall is perforated with areas of weakness and thinness — so-called *fenestrated fascia.* In these cases, repair if often unsuccessful and a synthetic, such as Dacron or wire mesh, may be used to reinforce the repair.

GENERAL RATIONALE AND SCHEME

An incisional hernia very often creates an uncomfortable and unsightly mass. If feasible, the hernia should be reduced and abdominal wall repair should be carried out.

Scheme

1. The old scar is excised.
2. The skin and subcutaneous tissue are reflected laterally in all directions, care being taken to prevent injury to loops of intestine.
3. The peritoneal sac is opened and the intestine is reduced.
4. The peritoneum is then closed firmly, following which the several layers of fascia are repaired over the peritoneal closure.

PROCEDURE

1. *Skin Incision.*   As a rule, this follows the line of the old incision. The entire original scar is excised, care being taken not to penetrate too deeply, as loops of intestine may be injured easily.
2. *Draping Skin.*   This is important, particularly since inadvertent injury to the intestine may result in contamination of the incision.
3. The entire projection of peritoneum and intestine over the fascia is dissected free from surrounding tissue before the peritoneal cavity is opened.

4. The peritoneum is opened and several loops of intestine are usually visualized immediately. These may be adherent to the inner wall of the peritoneal sac, and must be carefully dissected free from the peritoneum and reduced into the adbominal cavity.

5. The peritoneum is carefully and firmly approximated in the midline, and any redundant tissue that might remain is excised.

6. The fascial edge is carefully approximated. This may be done in several fashions. Some surgeons merely approximate the fascial edges, whereas others create a double-layer closure by folding the fascial edges one over the other — the so-called Mayo repair.

7. Large drainage tubes are left in place over the fascial closure to afford adequate drainage of serum and blood that will accumulate postoperatively. Penrose drains or suction catheters may be used for this purpose (Fig. 14–1).

8. The skin is carefully approximated as a final layer, following which a heavy compression dressing is applied.

SURGICAL HAZARDS

The most important hazard in repair of incisional hernia is the possibility of inadvertently injuring loops of intestine while making the skin incision and dissection. This is avoided by performing very careful dissection of tissue prior to reducing the bowel into the abdominal cavity.

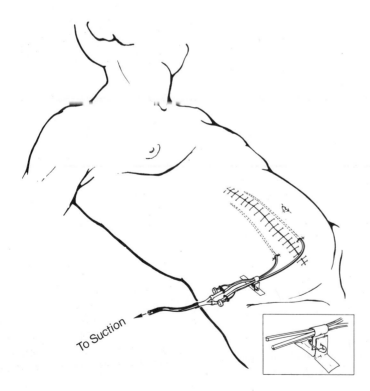

To Suction

FIGURE 14–1 Suction catheters for large incisional hernia. They are well secured to the skin and are not kinked.

EARLY POSTOPERATIVE MANAGEMENT

1. *Levin Tube.* Routine management.

2. If suction catheters are used, these are connected to low suction. They should be observed carefully, as kinking of the catheters results in obstruction and poor functioning of the catheter. The catheters usually are removed 3 to 4 days after surgery.

3. To avoid abdominal distention, the patient's diet is limited to light liquids until she passes flatus.

4. The patient may be ambulated within 12 to 24 hours after surgery. Some surgeons use abdominal binders when ambulating their patients; others feel the binders are of no value.

5. *Wound Care.* In spite of the use of drains or suction catheters, the extensive dissection of skin flaps that accompanies repair of an incisional hernia predisposes to seroma and hematoma formation, the forerunners of wound infection. Frequent inspection and palpation of the incision by the nurse may detect the early signs of fluid collection. Any fluid collection that is found will be aspirated and cultured by the surgeon. If treatment is indicated, the appropriate soaks and antibiotics will be applied.

STUDY QUESTIONS

1. What are some of the complications of an incisional hernia?

2. What are some of the predisposing factors which lead to the formation of an incisional hernia?

3. Be able to describe the Mayo type of incisional hernia repair to your class.

4. Discuss the nursing management of wound suction catheters.

5. Describe the surgical steps involved in the repair of an incisional hernia.

6. What is the relationship, if any, of a previous incisional infection to the development of an incisional hernia?

7. Review and plan the postoperative nursing care of a patient who has had a repair of an incisional hernia.

8. What learning needs might the patient have to help him cope with his home care?

9. How should you assess the wound in an effort to detect early sepsis following incisional hernia repair?

15

THE PATIENT WITH
HEPATOMEGALY
AND JAUNDICE

Operation: Laparoscopy

TYPICAL HISTORY

A 67-year-old female with a history of heavy alcoholic intake of many years' duration enters the hospital for evaluation of an enlarged liver and slight scleral icterus. She has noticed recent anorexia and increasing abdominal distention; she has also noted that she tires very easily.

PHYSICAL EXAMINATION

The patient is a well-developed, chronically ill-appearing female, in no particular distress.

Significant Findings

1. Scleral and cutaneous icterus.
2. The abdomen is distended and the liver edge is palpable about four fingers below the right costal margin.
3. The patient demonstrates palmar erythema, cutaneous "spiders," and loss of axillary hair.

DIAGNOSTIC STUDIES

1. Liver function tests show a slightly elevated bilirubin, moderately elevated alkaline phosphatase, decreased albumin, abnormal prothrombin time, and elevated transaminase.
2. A liver scan shows diffuse filling defects consistent with cirrhosis, with a large filling defect in the right lobe suspicious for malignancy.

PROBABLE HOSPITAL COURSE

Hepatomegaly and jaundice are always serious but not always easily evaluated. The jaundice precludes a Graham-Cole series, yet it is vital that extrahepatic obstructive disease be excluded, as this could be treated surgically.

The possible malignant process seen on the liver scan must be evaluated further as well. Percutaneous liver biopsy with a needle could help to establish the diagnosis of cirrhosis or hepatitis, but often this procedure is hazardous. A blind liver biopsy with a needle could fail to

172

"hit" the lesion and lead to a false sense of security. The laparoscope, on the other hand, permits selective biopsies and complete visualization of the liver, without submitting the patient to a major operation. It is quite safe in experienced hands and is gaining in popularity. The surgeon will attempt to correct the prothrombin time before performing laparoscopy.

PREPARATION FOR SURGERY

1. An effort is made to correct the prothrombin time with intravenous vitamin K.
2. *Skin Prep.* The entire abdomen from the costal margins as far as and including the pubis is cleanly shaven while the patient is on the ward.
3. *Enema.* Not necessary.
4. *Blood.* One unit of whole blood is prepared.
5. *Premedications.* Routine.
6. *Special Medications.* None.
7. *Operating Room Skin Prep.* The entire abdomen from the costal margins as far as and including the pubis should be prepped according to the hospital routine.
8. *Position.* Horizontal supine.

PATHOLOGY

Any pathological findings will of course depend on the exact organ being evaluated with the laparoscope. In the case of liver disease, one usually expects to find an enlarged, swollen organ which may show diffuse parenchymal changes consistent with cirrhosis, hepatitis, or metastatic nodules from some primary source. Occasionally a hepatoma forms in the course of chronic cirrhosis of many years' duration.

GENERAL RATIONALE AND SCHEME

Hepatomegaly and jaundice may be due to many causes, some correctable with surgery. The clinician, faced with the problem of jaundice, must rule out these correctable causes. The work-up is very difficult and frequently requires some kind of biopsy to obtain liver tissue.

Scheme

1. A small incision is made in the abdomen.
2. A pneumoperitoneum is created.
3. The laparoscope is inserted and an entire abdominal examination carried out.
4. Liver biopsies may be taken if necessary.

PROCEDURE

1. *Skin Incision.* This is usually a 2 cm incision made at an appropriate spot depending on the organ or organs which the surgeon wishes to evaluate.
2. A verres needle is inserted into the abdomen and connected to tubing which delivers carbon dioxide and oxygen at about 2 liters per minute.

3. After the pneumoperitoneum has been established, the verres needle is removed, a large trochar is inserted through the same incision, and the laparoscope is inserted through the trochar.

4. A general inspection of the entire abdominal cavity is now carried out. Organs that can easily be visualized through the laparoscope include (1) the liver and gallbladder, (2) the anterior surface of the stomach, (3) the spleen, (4) the large and small bowel, (5) the appendix, and (6) the ovaries, tubes and uterus.

5. If any pathology is noted, especially in the liver, a separate incision is made, biopsy forceps are inserted and, under direct examination through the laparoscope, biopsies are taken.

6. The biopsy sites will bleed and must be cauterized. This is usually done with the tip of the biopsy instrument (Fig. 15–1).

7. The laparoscope is withdrawn, the pneumoperitoneum is deflated, and the skin incisions are closed with 4–0 silk sutures. Band-Aids may be used over the incisions.

SURGICAL HAZARDS

1. The verres needle or trochar could perforate a loop of intestine. This is rare but particularly apt to happen if there are adhesions from previous surgery.

2. The carbon-dioxide/oxygen gas could cause an embolism if the needle is inadvertently inserted into an intra-abdominal vein.

3. Persistent bleeding from a biopsy site may occur.

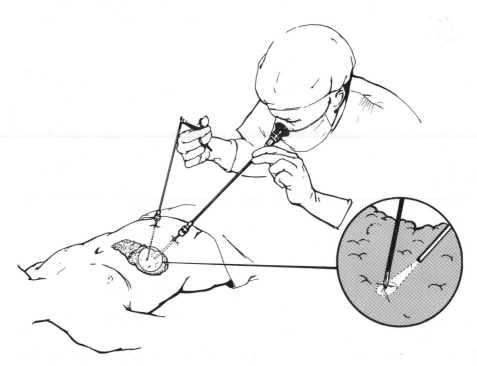

FIGURE 15–1 Laparoscopy with biopsy of cirrhotic liver under direct visualization.

EARLY POSTOPERATIVE MANAGEMENT

1. The patient is awake at the conclusion of the procedure. She may complain of moderate abdominal discomfort and some shoulder pain.

2. Diet can be resumed immediately and the patient can be ambulated as soon as the effects of anesthesia have passed.

3. The vital signs should be checked for the first 24 hours in view of the slight possibility of continued bleeding.

4. Severe or persistent abdominal pain is a sign that a complication, such as perforation of the intestine, has occurred. If pain is unusually severe and not relieved with minimal narcotics, the physician should be notified.

STUDY QUESTIONS

1. Name five uses for the laparoscope.

2. Compare the advantages and disadvantages of closed needle biopsy of the liver, open liver biopsy, and translaparoscopic biopsy.

3. Why does the surgeon establish a pneumoperitoneum before inserting the laparoscope?

4. What causes shoulder pain after laparoscopy?

5. Discuss the differential diagnosis of jaundice; list and describe the clinical procedures available for evaluating a patient with jaundice.

6. List 10 "liver function tests" and state for each the significance of any abnormal results.

7. What intra-abdominal organs cannot be evaluated with the laparoscope?

8. Obtain a laparoscope from the operating room and demonstrate its parts to your class.

16

Operation: Cholecystectomy

TYPICAL HISTORY

A 46-year-old obese mother of four children has noted increasing intolerance to fatty or fried foods. Following ingestion of these foods, she develops belching, nausea, flatulence, and occasional episodes of right upper quadrant pain. Her past history has been otherwise unremarkable and she denies any other significant gastrointestinal symptoms.

PHYSICAL EXAMINATION

The patient is a well-developed, somewhat obese female in no acute distress.

Significant Findings

1. There is no evidence of scleral or cutaneous icterus.
2. The abdomen is obese.
3. The liver is not felt.
4. There is some mild tenderness in the region of the gallbladder.
5. Rectal examination reveals normal-colored stool.

DIAGNOSTIC STUDIES

1. *Alkaline Phosphatase.* Normal.
2. *Bilirubin.* Normal.
3. *Graham-Cole Test.* Confirmation of the diagnosis of cholelithiasis (stones in the gallbladder) rests upon this test.

A radiopaque dye, in the form of tablets, is administered orally the evening prior to the tests; the patient is then fasted until the test is performed. The dye is absorbed from the gastrointestinal tract, passes into the liver, and is then excreted into the gastrointestinal tract and *stored in the gallbladder.* Several x-rays are then taken of the gallbladder, which can be visualized because it has stored the dye. Stones contained within the gallbladder are visualized as *radiolucent areas* since they displace the radiopaque dye.

The absence of visualization of the gallbladder *may* point to gallbladder dysfunction, as it may be assumed that a gallbladder which fails to store the dye is diseased. However, should the patient have vomited the tablets soon after ingestion, a false assumption of a diseased gallbladder may be made. It is important, therefore, that the nurse ascertain whether or not the patient has retained the tablets.

PROBABLE HOSPITAL COURSE

Provided no other associated problems have been discovered during the initial examination and routine studies, surgery will be planned 2 to 3 days after admission, as soon as the diagnosis has been confirmed.

PREPARATION FOR SURGERY

In addition to the general measures outlined in Part I, the particular approach in cholecystectomy is as follows:

1. Complete history and physical examination.

2. *Skin Prep.* The entire abdomen from the costal margins as far as and including the pubis is cleanly shaven on the ward. (See Introduction.)

3. *Enema.* A soapsuds or Fleet enema is given the evening prior to surgery.

4. *Levin Tube.* Some surgeons prefer to have their patients intubated prior to surgery, usually in the morning. Others do not use a Levin tube routinely for cholecystectomy. The preoperative orders should specify the surgeon's desire in this regard.

5. *Blood.* It is wise to type and cross-match for at least one unit of whole blood for cholecystectomy. This, again, is highly variable, and the surgeon should request whether or not he wishes blood to be available and in what quantity.

6. *Premedications.* Same as for appendectomy.

7. *Special Medications.* None.

8. The patient should be encouraged to void preoperatively.

9. *Operating Room Skin Prep.* The entire abdomen from the costal margins as far as and including the pubis should be prepped according to the hospital routine. (See Introduction.)

10. *Position.* Horizontal supine. (See Introduction.)

PATHOLOGY

The chronically inflamed gallbladder is usually thick-walled, is often scarred, and may show residual edema or inflammation from a recent acute attack. There may also be local adhesions indicative of prior acute inflammation. The gallbladder usually contains one or more stones.

GENERAL RATIONALE AND SCHEME

A chronically inflamed gallbladder, particularly if it contains stones, is a source of recurrent gastrointestinal distress, and should be removed on that account alone. In addition, there is the ever-present danger of an acute attack of cholecystitis occurring as well as the danger of a stone lodging in the common duct and causing obstructive jaundice. This latter complication of gallbladder disease is very serious and can be fatal.

Scheme

1. The gallbladder is exposed through a subcostal or paramedian incision.
2. The cystic duct and cystic artery are exposed, ligated, and divided.
3. The peritoneal covering of the gallbladder is incised and the diseased organ removed.

Note: If only cholecystectomy is planned, a general laparotomy kit is all that is required. Should a common duct exploration be anticipated, however, common duct probes, dilators of the sphincter of Oddi, and irrigating equipment will be required.

The circulating or scrub nurse should try to learn whether common duct exploration is anticipated some time before surgery is begun so that all necessary instruments will be available. In addition, some surgeons will desire to do *cholangiography* in the operating room (see Chapter 18). This will require that the x-ray department be notified well in advance and that a cassette be placed on the operating table prior to surgery.

PROCEDURE

1. *Skin Incision.*   A right subcostal incision or a right upper paramedian incision is the most frequently used in cholecystectomy. (See Introduction.)

2. *Deepening Incision.*   The superficial fascia and fat are incised below the skin. A good deal of bleeding may occur, and will require control with ligatures at this point. The anterior fascia overlying the rectus muscle is incised. In the case of the subcostal incision, the rectus muscle is divided transversely. For the paramedian incision, the rectus muscle is either split vertically or retracted to the right.

3. *Opening Peritoneum.*   This is done very cautiously to avoid injuring underlying structures, such as the liver, the stomach, or the transverse colon.

4. *Draping Wounds.*   This is done according to the surgeon's instructions.

5. *Exploration.*   A general exploration of the abdomen is carried out. Any associated disease is noted. The common duct is carefully palpated. If it appears to be enlarged or if a stone is felt within it, the surgeon will inform the nurse that a common duct exploration is to be carried out.

6. *Identification of Cystic Duct and Artery.*   It is extremely important that absolute identification of the cystic duct and artery be made prior to clamping or ligating of any structures. When this has been accomplished, the surgeon will proceed with the next step. Identification may take but a few minutes or may occupy 20 to 30 minutes, as it requires meticulous dissection of the local anatomy.

7. *Ligation and Division of Duct and Artery.*   The cystic duct is ligated with catgut suture close to its junction with the common duct, and the cystic artery is ligated with silk or catgut (Fig. 16–1).

8. *Incision of Peritoneal Cuff over Gallbladder.*   The gallbladder is contained within a fold of peritoneum of variable thickness. The surgeon incises this cuff, leaving a sufficient edge for reapproximation after removal of the gallbladder. A good deal of bleeding may occur at this stage of the procedure, and the nurse should anticipate the need for hemostats. The gallbladder is shelled out of its bed in the liver and handed to the nurse.

9. *Closure of Peritoneal Cuff.*   A running catgut suture is used to close the remaining peritoneal cuff. This acts as a hemostatic mechanism, controlling oozing of blood from the gallbladder bed.

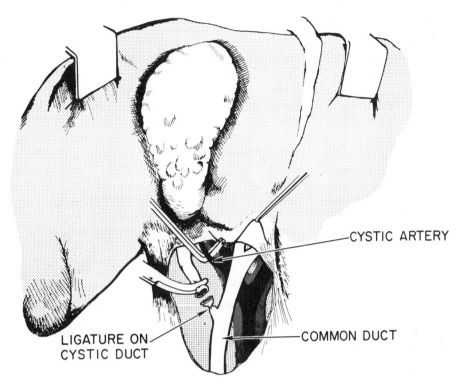

FIGURE 16–1 Procedure for cholecystectomy. The surgeon has ligated and divided the cystic duct. He is in the process of ligating the cystic artery.

10. *Drainage.* A large Penrose drain is then inserted into the foramen of Winslow. It will be brought out through the wound or through a separate stab wound, according to the surgeon's preference.

11. *Closure of Wound.* Routine.

SURGICAL HAZARDS

1. *Injury to Common Duct.* This can be a tragic complication of gallbladder surgery, particularly if it is not recognized. Partial severance of the common duct may lead to an unusual amount of bile drainage postoperatively and this should alert the nurse to the possibility of duct injury. Ligation of the common duct will lead to postoperative jaundice, which may occur several days following surgery.

2. *Operative Hemorrhage.* This may be caused by accidental division of the cystic or hepatic artery. Attempts to blindly clamp a vigorously bleeding vessel are the most common cause of injury to the common duct or hepatic artery.

3. *Accidental Ligation of Hepatic Artery.* Improper identification of the cystic artery may lead to this complication. It is often fatal because it may lead to necrosis of the right lobe of the liver.

EARLY POSTOPERATIVE MANAGEMENT

The patient is kept in the recovery room until he is sufficiently reactive from the anesthetic.

1. *Pain Medication.* Upper abdominal incisions can be extremely painful, and may require as much as 100 mg. of Demerol or 10 to 15 mg. of morphine for relief.

2. *Levin Tube.* If present, this should be connected immediately to an intermittent suction apparatus. Every 2 to 4 hours saline should be instilled into the tube and aspirated. Failure to obtain fluid on aspiration usually indicates that the tube is incorrectly positioned. The situation should be corrected or the tube will not function properly.

3. *Pulmonary Complications.* Upper abdominal incisions lead to splinting of the diaphragm on the affected side, which can cause atelectasis and pneumonia. In spite of the discomfort he will feel, the patient must be urged to breathe deeply and to cough frequently in order to prevent such complications.

4. *Dressing.* This may require frequent changes due to drainage of bile and blood around and through the Penrose drain. The first dressing change should be done by the surgeon.

5. *Shock.* Rarely, the ligature on the cystic artery may be dislodged. Hemorrhage is rapid, leading to hypotension and shock. Any significant change in the vital signs or the appearance of excessive bloody drainage on the dressing should be noted and reported to the surgeon immediately.

6. The Levin tube is usually removed 1 or 2 days after surgery, depending on the amount of serous and bilious drainage noted. Diet is advanced from liquids to solids over a 2 to 3 day period, and convalescence is usually very smooth. The patient may be ambulated the day after surgery. The drain is removed 5 or 6 days after surgery, and discharge from the hospital may be anticipated 1 or 2 days after that.

STUDY QUESTIONS

1. Define cholelithiasis and choledocholithiasis.

2. Trace the migration of bile from the liver to the duodenum.

3. What factors predispose to gallbladder disease?

4. Do you think chronic cholecystitis would respond to antibiotics?

5. A 67-year-old female is admitted to the hospital with jaundice. List five causes of this condition. Which of these causes is treated surgically?

6. Be prepared to discuss in class the construction, function, and management of a Levin tube. What are some of the complications attending prolonged use of a Levin tube? What is the nursing care of a patient on Levin tube drainage?

7. On the evening following cholecystectomy, the nurse notes the appearance of a completely soaked dressing containing bile and blood. What are some of the causes of this condition? What should the nurse do in its management?

8. Make a list of preoperative and postoperative activities the nurse should carry out in caring for the patient undergoing cholecystectomy.

9. Discuss the Graham-Cole test. What dyes are used and how are they administered? What type of gastrointestinal preparation should precede a Graham-Cole test?

10. What are the nursing implications inherent in patient preparation for this test?

11. What are the benefits of early ambulation following cholecystectomy?

12. Diagram the cystic duct, the common duct, and the cystic artery and be prepared to discuss this anatomy in class.

13. Why does the surgeon use a Penrose drain following cholecystectomy? What problems may result if this drain is accidentally pulled out during a dressing change?

THE PATIENT WITH ACUTE CHOLECYSTITIS   17

Operation: Cholecystostomy (Drainage of Inflamed Gallbladder)

TYPICAL HISTORY

A 52-year-old obese female, mother of six children, enters the hospital with acute right upper quadrant pain radiating below the right costal margin and into the back. The pain is severe and steady, and is associated with nausea and vomiting. Past history reveals intolerance to fried and fatty foods.

PHYSICAL EXAMINATION

The examination reveals a well-developed, obese female, lying quietly in bed in acute abdominal distress.

Significant Findings

1. Temperature is 101°F.
2. Pulse is 110 per minute.

3. Skin is warm and flushed.
4. Abdomen is obese.
5. The patient experiences acute tenderness in the right upper quadrant.
6. There is a globular tender mass palpable just below the right costal margin.

DIAGNOSTIC STUDIES

1. WBC is 21,000 per cu. mm.: polymorphonuclear cells, 87 per cent; lymphocytes, 6 per cent; and band forms, 7 per cent.
2. Hematocrit level is 39 per cent.
3. Flat and upright abdominal x-rays reveal the presence of a globular mass in the right upper quadrant.

PROBABLE HOSPITAL COURSE

The patient is suffering from acute cholecystitis, with evidence of hydrops of the gallbladder. There are three schools of thought as to the proper treatment, and her hospital course will depend largely on what mode of therapy is favored by her surgeon:

1. *Immediate Emergency Surgery.* Some surgeons believe that acute cholecystitis, once diagnosed, constitutes an urgent case for surgery, similar to a case of acute appendicitis. The main danger in waiting, it is argued, is the fear of perforation of the gallbladder which might lead to bile peritonitis and death. According to this school of thought, then, the patient is prepped and taken to the operating room shortly after admission.

2. *Delayed Emergency Surgery.* A second group of surgeons also believe that acute cholecystitis represents a serious affliction warranting emergency surgery. However, it is felt by this group that the fluid and electrolyte imbalances, as well as the patient's state of shock, demand a 24- to 36-hour period of treatment prior to surgery. The patient will be given intravenous fluids and antibiotics and will be operated upon a day or two after admission.

3. *Elective Surgery.* A third group of surgeons is not as impressed with the danger of perforation of an acutely inflamed gallbladder, arguing that the distorted anatomy which results from acute cholecystitis increases the hazards of injury to vital structures. Accordingly, the patient is treated with I.V. fluids and antibiotics for several days and then discharged when improved. Several weeks later, she will be readmitted for elective cholecystectomy.

PREPARATION FOR SURGERY

Assuming that emergency surgery is planned, the routine preparation for cholecystectomy is carried out, as outlined in the preceding chapter. As with any emergency procedure, the psychological preparation of the patient is vital. Intravenous fluids, including water and saline, will probably be ordered prior to surgery, and the surgeon may also order intravenous antibiotics, depending on the amount of sepsis he judges to be present.

PATHOLOGY

The gallbladder may show varying degrees of acute inflammation:
1. *Hydrops.* A large, swollen, bile-filled gallbladder.

2. *Acute cholecystitis* with edema, thickening and inflammation of the walls, as well as varying degrees of patchy necrosis due to thrombosis of vessels.

3. *Gangrenous cholecystitis* with advanced areas of necrosis and slough.

4. *Perforation.*   There is leakage of bile from the gallbladder into the abdominal cavity.

GENERAL RATIONALE AND SCHEME

The acutely inflamed gallbladder should be removed: it will never function properly again, it represents a source of recurrent sepsis, and it also presents the hazard of rupture. In the vast majority of cases, cholecystectomy is carried out and the operative scheme is similar to that described in the preceding chapter. If age and the general condition of the patient contraindicate a lengthy procedure, or if the anatomic distortion has created formidable technical hazards, a cholecystostomy may be undertaken. This is described below.

Scheme

1. The surgeon opens the abdomen.

2. He inserts a suction trochar into the fundus of the gallbladder to decompress it (Fig. 17–1).

3. He then widens the aperture created by the trochar and removes all stones contained within the diseased gallbladder.

4. Lastly, a large drainage tube is left in the gallbladder for postoperative drainage.

PROCEDURE

1. *Opening Abdomen.*   Similar to steps 1 to 5 in preceding chapter.

2. *Pursestring Suture in Fundus of Gallbladder.*   Using a heavy silk or chromic catgut suture swaged on a noncutting needle.

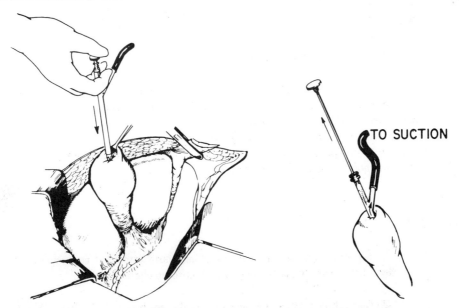

TO SUCTION

FIGURE 17–1 Trochar decompression of the gallbladder. Note the structure of the suction trochar.

3. *Trochar decompression of gallbladder* (Fig. 17–1).
4. *Culture of any fluid or bile escaping.*
5. *Aperture* in fundus of gallbladder enlarged.
6. *Stones removed* with spoons or stone forceps.
7. *Catheter drainage* of gallbladder, using large (e.g., No. 20) Foley or mushroom catheter.
8. *Reinforcing pursestring suture* used to further secure tube in the gallbladder fundus.
9. *Suturing Fundus of Gallbladder to Abdominal Wall.* This is done to avoid leakage of bile into the abdominal cavity.
10. *Catheter* is brought out through a separate stab wound or through the incision.
11. *In addition a Penrose drain* is used to drain the gallbladder bed.
12. *Catheter is secured* to skin of the abdominal wall.
13. *Routine Wound Closure.*

SURGICAL HAZARDS

Contamination of wound and peritoneal cavity may occur from spillage of infected bile into the peritoneal cavity during decompression.

POSTOPERATIVE MANAGEMENT

Mangement of patients following cholecystostomy and cholecystectomy is similar except for the tube used in cholecystostomy. It should be secured to the dressing and abdominal binder, and observed frequently. Should the patient inadvertently remove this tube, fatal bile peritonitis may result. The tube is placed on dependent drainage unless suction is specifically ordered by the surgeon. It should not be aspirated or irrigated unless this is requested by the surgeon. The bile drainage through the tube must be *measured and recorded separately* under a column headed "cholecystostomy tube drainage." The color and consistency of the fluid should be recorded in the nurse's notes.

Summary of Postoperative Management of Cholecystostomy Tube

1. Check security of tube attachment to dressing frequently. If the patient is restless, she should be restrained to prevent her from accidentally pulling out the tube.
2. Connect tube to *dependent drainage.*
3. Do not irrigate or aspirate tube unless ordered to do so.
4. Record output in separate column headed "cholecystostomy tube drainage."
5. Record color and consistency of drainage in nurse's notes.

STUDY QUESTIONS

1. List the signs and symptoms of an acute attack of cholecystitis. How do they differ from those associated with chronic cholecystitis?

2. Can cholecystitis be treated with antibiotics? Discuss the "medical management" of this condition.

3. List the preoperative nursing care in preparing a patient for a cholecystectomy.

4. What *special* instruments must the scrub nurse have available for the cholecystostomy procedure?

5. Describe the function and management of a cholecystostomy tube. Emphasize the nurse's role.

6. On the evening following cholecystostomy, the nurse finds the patient delirious and thrashing about in bed. What are the dangers involved with specific reference to the cholecystostomy tube? What measures should the nurse take to minimize these dangers?

7. On this same evening the nurse notes that *no drainage* has occurred for 6 to 8 hours from the cholecystostomy tube. She chooses to irrigate the tube in the hope of dislodging a plug of mucus. Discuss this form of management in class.

8. A patient recovering from cholecystostomy asks you whether more surgery will be needed in the future. How would you handle this question?

9. Why must cholecystectomy be done several weeks or months following cholecystostomy?

10. What are the particular learning needs of the patient during his home care phase of convalescence?

THE PATIENT WITH OBSTRUCTIVE JAUNDICE

18

Operation: Choledochotomy (Opening and Exploring the Common Bile Duct)

TYPICAL HISTORY

A 61-year-old male, with a long history of belching and intolerance to fatty foods, noted the onset of jaundice 2 weeks prior to admission. This was accompanied by moderate epigastric and right upper quadrant pains and production of clay-colored stools and dark urine. He denies heavy alcohol intake or exposure to known hepatotoxins.

PHYSICAL EXAMINATION

The patient is a well-developed, jaundiced male, complaining of epigastric pain.

Significant Findings

1. Jaundice is noted.
2. The liver and gallbladder are not felt, but there is tenderness over the gallbladder.
3. The stool is clay-colored.
4. There are none of the stigmata associated with cirrhosis.

DIAGNOSTIC STUDIES

1. WBC is 11,000 per cu. mm.
2. Hematocrit value is 37 per cent.
3. Urine is positive for bile.
4. Blood chemistries:
a. Total bilirubin is 23.
b. Direct bilirubin is 18.
c. Alkaline phosphatase is 16.
d. Cephalin flocculation is 1 plus.
e. Serum transaminase is 30.
5. X-ray of the abdomen is negative.
6. Liver scan is normal.

PROBABLE HOSPITAL COURSE

The jaundiced patient represents a difficult diagnostic problem at times. The jaundice may be "medical," in which case surgery is of no value and may even lead to serious morbidity or death. Conditions causing "medical" jaundice include:
a. Cirrhosis.
b. Hepatitis.
c. Hepatic necrosis.
d. Hemolytic anemia.
The important causes of "surgical" jaundice include:
a. Stones in the common bile duct.
b. Tumor of the bile ducts or ampulla of Vater.
c. Tumor of the head of the pancreas.
The surgeon often consults with an internist, and both evaluate the patient in the hope of arriving at an accurate preoperative diagnosis. The history and physical examination, as well as a battery of "liver function" tests, aid in the diagnosis. In addition, at times, a *needle biopsy* of the liver may be done. The tissue obtained is submitted to the pathologist, who may be able to arrive at the cause of the jaundiced state. The studies may require as little as 3 to 4 days or as much as 2 to 3 weeks. Should a diagnosis of "surgical" jaundice finally evolve, surgery will be undertaken.

PREPARATION FOR SURGERY

The jaundiced patient often suffers from the effects of a damaged liver. The resulting chemical abnormalities must be adjusted to provide values *as nearly normal as possible* prior to surgery. Some of the preparatory steps, then, include the following:

1. *Anemia,* when present, is corrected with transfusions of *packed red cells* and whole blood.

2. *Hypoproteinemia,* particularly low albumin levels, is corrected with blood transfusions and with infusions of serum albumin.

3. *Low prothrombin time,* which could lead to serious hemorrhagic tendencies, is corrected with parenteral administration of vitamin K.

4. *Electrolyte deficiencies,* particularly low serum sodium, are corrected with administration of appropriate fluids.

5. *Low liver stores of glycogen* are corrected with a high carbohydrate intake.

When all chemical deficiencies have been corrected, the routine prep for cholecystectomy is carried out and surgery undertaken.

PATHOLOGY

1. The gallbladder may be chronically inflamed, contracted, and filled with stones. One would then expect to find *stones* obstructing the common bile duct as well.

2. The gallbladder may show surprisingly little inflammation, may be extremely distended, and may contain no stones. In this case, a more likely cause for the common duct obstruction and resulting jaundice will be a tumor, either of the bile duct or in the head of the pancreas.

3. In each case, one would expect to find a swollen, congested, and darkly bile-stained liver secondary to the obstruction of the bile outflow.

GENERAL RATIONALE AND SCHEME

Obstructive jaundice must be relieved, as the liver injury is progressive and ultimately fatal.

Scheme

1. The surgeon opens the common duct.

2. If stones are found, these are removed and the obstruction is relieved.

3. The surgeon then drains the common duct temporarily with a t-tube and removes the gallbladder in the usual manner.

4. If a tumor is discovered, the surgeon must decide whether it is resectable or not. Most such tumors are not resectable, and the only surgery possible is to perform a by-pass procedure which will temporarily relieve the jaundice and its distressing symptoms.

PROCEDURE

(It is assumed that stones are found to be the cause of jaundice.)

1. *Opening Abdomen.* See Chapters 16 and 17.

2. *Exploration and Evaluation:*

a. Surgeon palpates gallbladder for stones.

b. Surgeon visualizes and palpates common duct for dilation and stones.

c. He inspects liver for possible metastases.

d. He palpates pancreas for possible tumor.

3. *Opening Common Bile Duct:*

a. Two sutures are placed in common duct to serve as stabilizers when duct is opened.

b. A long-handled knife with a small blade is used to cut a small vertical incision in the common duct. Suction should be available, as a large amount of bile may flow out under considerable pressure.

4. *Probing and Exploring Duct.* A malleable probe and stone-retrieving forceps are used to remove any stones that may be present in the common duct.

5. *Dilating Ampulla of Vater.* After the obstructing stones are removed, Bake's dilators are used to dilate the ampulla of Vater, which usually is inflamed or spastic, owing to the presence of ductal stones.

6. *Irrigation of Duct.* Small French catheters are inserted proximally and distally in the common duct and sterile saline irrigations are carried out to insure that no small stones or bits of debris are left behind.

7. *Insertion of T-tube.* In order to insure complete decompression of the liver, a temporary t-tube is sutured into the common duct, the long arm of which is brought out through the incision or through a separate stab wound (Fig. 18–1).

8. *Cholangiography.* As a final check for retained ductal stones, the surgeon may choose to inject 15 to 20 cc. of radiopaque dye through the t-tube before closing the abdomen. The x-ray report is immediately made available to the surgeon. If further stones are visualized, he will reopen the common duct and remove these stones.

9. *Penrose Drains.* As in cholecystectomy.

10. *Routine Wound Closure.*

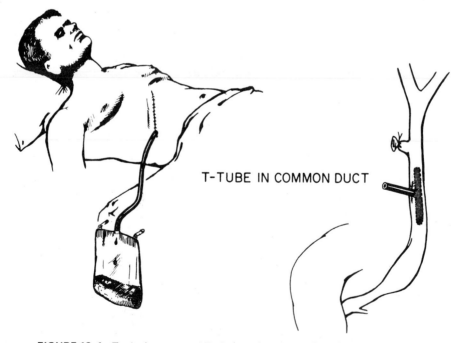

T-TUBE IN COMMON DUCT

FIGURE 18–1   T-tube in common bile duct, and postoperative bile drainage system.

SURGICAL HAZARDS

1. Same as for cholecystectomy, *plus*:
2. Possibility of overlooking a stone in common duct.
3. Perforation of common duct with dilator.

EARLY POSTOPERATIVE MANAGEMENT

1. Same as for cholecystectomy, *plus*:
2. Management of t-tube (Fig. 18–1);
a. Secure to dressing and check this frequently.
b. Connect tube to *dependent drainage.*
c. Do not irrigate or aspirate tube unless specifically ordered to do so.
d. Record output in separate column headed "t-tube drainage."
e. Note color and consistency of drainage in nurse's notes.

STUDY QUESTIONS

1. List 10 causes of jaundice. Which are treated surgically? Which medically?

2. Why is a gallbladder x-ray (Graham-Cole series) *not ordered* in the jaundiced patient?

3. What psychological problems would you anticipate in the severely jaundiced patient? Discuss in class how you would cope with these problems.

4. Make a list of "liver function tests" from any standard surgical or laboratory textbook. In this list, describe:
   a. The nature of the test.
   b. Rationale for this in the diagnosis of jaundice.
   c. The preparation of the patient for this test (emphasizing the nurse's role).

5. Describe to your class the rationale of a needle biopsy of the liver. What equipment is needed? What is the nurse's role in preparing the patient for this test? What information could be gained from a laparoscopy?

6. How does hemolytic anemia cause jaundice?

7. What are the dietary modifications needed by the jaundiced patient?

8. List and describe the features and function of all surgical instruments used to explore the common bile duct.

9. A patient, 1 day following common duct exploration, inadvertently pulls out his t-tube. What are the possible ill effects of this accident? What would you, as the nurse caring for this patient, do?

10. Describe the structure and function of a t-tube to your class. How should the nurse *chart* the bile output from a t-tube? What is the importance of charting t-tube output?

11. Define Courvoisier's law. Explain its significance in the jaundiced patient.

12. What is a t-tube cholangiogram? How and why is it done?

13. What serious postoperative complications might ensue after this procedure?

14. What are the nursing implications and observations necessary in helping to *prevent* or to quickly *detect* these complications?

19 THE PATIENT WITH INOPERABLE CANCER OF THE PANCREAS

Operation: Cholecystojejunostomy

TYPICAL HISTORY

A 60-year-old male enters the hospital complaining of yellow skin and dark-colored urine of about 6 weeks' duration. The patient began noticing rather vague, dull, epigastric and mid-back pain about 3 months ago. He thought he had an ulcer and treated himself with antacids and aspirins. He became concerned because of rapid, unexplained weight loss, anorexia, and "loss of energy and ambition." His friends first noted the jaundice, and this finding prompted him to seek medical attention. The jaundice has been deepening, the urine has become "dark like coffee," and his stools have taken on a clay-colored appearance. The pain has worsened, and has remained steady and dull. It is felt mostly in the epigastrium.

PHYSICAL EXAMINATION

The patient is a well-developed, thin, chronically ill-appearing male who is deeply jaundiced and complains of continuous, dull epigastric pain.

Significant Findings

1. The skin and sclerae are deeply jaundiced.
2. The facies shows all the signs of chronic wasting disease.
3. The stool is paste-like and clay-colored.
4. The urine is dark and has a strong, foul odor.

DIAGNOSTIC STUDIES

1. *Alkaline phosphatase.*   Markedly elevated.
2. *Bilirubin.*   Markedly elevated.
3. *Upper gastrointestinal series.*   This may be normal or may reveal a widening of the duodenal loop consistent with an enlarged mass in the head of the pancreas.
4. *X-rays of the gallbladder.*   These are not ordered in most cases, because the jaundice precludes visualization of the biliary tree in the usual manner. *Percutaneous transhepatic cholangiography* is sometimes performed and may be of value.
5. *Pancreatic scan.*   The scan is rarely of any value, particularly in detecting small tumors of the pancreas.
6. *Pancreatic arteriography.*   In experienced hands, this test sometimes displays a "tumor blush" in the pancreas. Most surgeons have not yet found this test to be of real value.

PROBABLE HOSPITAL COURSE

The deeply jaundiced patient with steady abdominal pain, weight loss, and anorexia is assumed to be harboring a tumor in the pancreas or extrahepatic biliary tree until otherwise is proven on exploratory laparotomy. A careful search is made by whatever diagnostic tests are thought fruitful and are indicated by the surgeon. Evidence of distant metastases (e.g., to a supraclavicular lymph node) may preclude surgery and therefore must be sought out before the laparotomy. Widespread liver metastases or long-term biliary obstruction can damage the liver and increase the risk of surgery. This organ must, therefore, be carefully evaluated before proceeding with surgery.

PREPARATION FOR SURGERY

1. Complete history and physical examination, with particular emphasis on searching for metastatic disease and evaluating the functional reserve of the liver.
2. Vitamin K must be given if the prothrombin time is prolonged.
3. *Skin Prep.*   The entire abdomen from the costal margins as far as and including the pubis is cleanly shaven while the patient is on the ward.
4. *Levin Tube.*   This may be inserted before surgery or after general anesthesia has been completed.
5. *Blood.*   Eight to ten units of blood are typed and cross-matched.
6. *Premedications.*   Standard for any general anesthetic.
7. *Special Medications.*   Vitamin K.
8. *Operation Room Skin Prep.*   The entire abdomen from the costal margins as far as and including the pubis should be prepped according to the hospital routine.
9. *Position.*   Horizontal supine.
10. *Foley Catheter.*   This is inserted preoperatively because of the possibility of a long, radical cancer operation.

PATHOLOGY

Cancer of the pancreas may demonstrate many anatomical variations, and treatment is based on the findings at the time of surgery.
1. *Cancer of the ampullary region.*   This type of tumor may be only pea-sized and completely limited to the outlet of the pancreas into the duodenum. Such a tumor produces early

jaundice because of the obstruction it forms in the common bile duct. The lesion may be amenable to pancreatectomy, with a fair chance of cure.

2. *Cancer of the head or body of the pancreas.* Often the tumor is localized to the head or body of the pancreas (more rarely, it appears in the tail). These lesions cause later jaundice and are usually much more advanced and less apt to be cured than ampullary lesions.

3. *Cancer of the pancreas with widespread metastases.* Often, by the time laparotomy is performed, the tumor has (a) invaded regional lymph nodes around the pancreas, (b) fixed itself to vital structures such as the superior mesenteric artery, or (c) spread to the liver. In any of these cases, radical extirpative surgery is not feasible, and the surgeon can only palliate the condition (by means of a by-pass procedure). The tumor may also have caused narrowing of the duodenum, threatening pyloric obstruction. This may require a by-passing gastrojejunostomy as well as a by-passing cholecystojejunostomy.

GENERAL RATIONALE AND SCHEME

Obstructive jaundice, regardless of its cause, leads inexorably to progressive liver failure and death. The obstruction may be due to biliary calculi or to malignancy; the cause ultimately must be determined by exploratory laparotomy.

Scheme

1. The abdomen is opened and a careful evaluation of the liver, extrahepatic biliary tree, and pancreas is carried out.

2. If a curable form of malignancy is discovered, the surgeon will proceed with a radical pancreaticoduodenectomy. More often, the disease will be found in an advanced, unresectable form, and a simple by-pass will be carried out between the biliary tree and the intestines to overcome the obstructive jaundice.

PROCEDURE

1. *Skin Incision.* A right subcostal or a right upper paramedian incision is the most frequently used in biliary and pancreatic procedures.

2. *Deepening Incision.* Same as for cholecystectomy.

3. *Opening Peritoneum.* Same as for cholecystectomy.

4. *Draping Wounds.* Draping is carried out according to the surgeon's instructions. Since the biliary tree and the intestinal tract contain contaminant organisms, the chances of a wound infection are increased. Efforts should be made to protect the entire thickness of the wound edges, as can be achieved with the use of a "ring drape."

5. *Exploration.* A general exploration of the abdomen is carried out first. Then the liver is carefully evaluated for signs of metastatic disease. Often, the gallbladder is markedly dilated when the common bile duct is obstructed by malignant disease. The common duct will be carefully palpated for gallstones, as will be the entire head, body, and tail of the pancreas for tumors.

6. *Determining the Type and Extent of Tumor.* Assuming that the surgeon has excluded gallstones as a cause of the obstruction and has noted a tumor in the head of the pancreas, he must now carry out a careful evaluation to determine whether the tumor can be removed. If there is evidence of metastatic disease in the liver or in the lymph nodes within the portal area, no cure is possible, and surgery will be abandoned. If the tumor is localized to the head of the pancreas but

has invaded the superior mesenteric artery or the aorta, the resection will probably be abandoned because a cure is most unlikely and the mortality from resection formidable. Under any of these conditions, the surgeon *will* elect to by-pass the obstruction in the biliary tree by anastomosing the gallbladder or the common bile duct to some segment of the gastrointestinal tract.

7. *Decompression of gallbladder.*   A trochar is inserted into the fundus of the gallbladder to decompress it.

8. *Identifying the Jejunum.*   The ligament of Treitz is used to identify the jejunum. A loop of jejunum is brought up over or through the transverse mesocolon for anastomosis with the gallbladder.

9. *The Anastomosis.*   The gallbladder fundus and the side wall of the jejunum are approximated with interrupted seromuscular sutures, usually 3–0 silk. The jejunum and the fundus of the gallbladder are opened and any brisk bleeders ligated with fine catgut. A through-and-through running 3–0 catgut suture is then used to join the gallbladder to the jejunum. Finally, a second layer of interrupted 3–0 silk sutures is used to join the anterior seromuscular surfaces to complete the anastomosis (Fig. 19–1).

10. *Drainage.*   Because of the fear of bile leakage from the anastomosis as well as from the liver bed, a small Penrose drain is placed in the foramen of Winslow and brought out through a stab incision.

11. *Closure of Wound.*   Routine.

SURGICAL HAZARDS

1. *Defective Anastomosis.*   A water-tight seal of the anastomosis is necessary to prevent fatal postoperative leakage. Defective anastomoses may be due to (a) tension on the suture line, (b) poor blood supply, or (c) failure to invert the entire mucosa.

2. *Injury to the Pancreas.*   Any rough handling of the pancreas can injure this friable organ and lead to serious postoperative pancreatitis.

3. *Excess Hemorrhage.*   Hypoprothrombinemia, a result of defective liver function, can lead to serious hemorrhage during surgery. This may be minimized by the appropriate use of vitamin K.

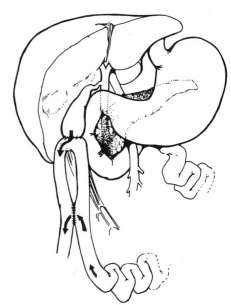

FIGURE 19–1 A completed cholecystojejunostomy. *Question:* Why is a side-to-side enteroenterostomy also depicted here?

POSTOPERATIVE MANAGEMENT

The patient is kept in the recovery room until he is sufficiently reactive from the anesthetic.

1. *Levin Tube.* This is managed exactly as it is for cholecystectomy.

2. *Dressings.* Dressings may require frequent changes, owing to drainage of bile and blood around the Penrose drain. The first dressing change should be performed by the surgeon. After 2 or 3 days, drainage should be minimal. Any drainage occurring after that time, particularly if more than a scant amount, suggests leakage from the anastomosis until otherwise is proven.

3. The patient is ambulated the day after surgery. Diet is rapidly advanced over a 3 or 4 day period, depending on the return of normal peristaltic activity. The patient may be ready for discharge on the seventh day after surgery. He may still be jaundiced at this early date, as it will take 2 to 3 weeks for the yellow pigment to be cleared from the subcutaneous tissues. The surgeon may check the patient's bilirubin and alkaline phosphatase in the early postoperative period. These are often early indicators of the efficacy of the by-pass procedure.

STUDY QUESTIONS

1. Describe all the signs of *chronic wasting disease.*

2. What is *percutaneous transhepatic cholangiography*? Describe the procedure, indications for its use, and its hazards.

3. What liver tests suggest obstructive jaundice? Nonobstructive jaundice?

4. Why does liver disease predispose to bleeding tendencies? How is the disease discovered by the surgeon and what can be done about it?

5. What and where is the ampulla of Vater?

6. Can a person survive following *total pancreatectomy*? If so, what supportive therapy would he need?

7. What is a ring drape? What theoretical advantages does it have over a plastic stick-on skin drape?

8. Three days after a cholecystojejunostomy for carcinoma of the head of the pancreas, the patient develops rather severe abdominal and mid-dorsal back pain, a rapid pulse, dehydrated mucous membranes, and oliguria. His hematocrit has risen to 56; the white blood cell count is 23,000; amylase 2000 units. Over the next 2 hours, the pain worsens, the pulse becomes more rapid, and the patient goes into shock.
    a. What is the most likely single cause of this syndrome?
    b. What is the patient's immediate need?
    c. What bedside diagnostic procedures might the surgeon institute to further evaluate the state of shock and to monitor the efficacy of his treatment?

d. Select the one central venous pressure which you think is most likely to be registered before treatment is instituted:
    (1) 2 cm of water
    (2) 10 cm of water
    (3) 20 cm of water
Explain in detail to your class your choice.

9. Following appropriate therapy for 3 hours, the patient described in question 8 demonstrates a hematocrit of 46, excellent urine output, a normal blood pressure, and a strong, slow pulse. Select the one central venous pressure likely to be registered at this time:
    (1) 2 cm of water
    (2) 10 cm of water
    (3) 20 cm of water
Explain in detail to your class your choice.

THE PATIENT WITH OPERABLE CANCER OF THE PANCREAS

20

Operation: Radical Pancreaticoduodenectomy

TYPICAL HISTORY

A 56-year-old patient enters the hospital complaining of dull, persistent epigastric distress and some vague back pains of about 6 weeks' duration. This has been accompanied by anorexia, easy fatigue, and a 6-pound weight loss. In the past week, he noted dark urine and a yellow color to his sclerae.

PHYSICAL EXAMINATION

The patient is a well-developed, thin, well-nourished male with a slight yellow tinge to his sclerae and skin. He is complaining of vague epigastric distress and back pains.

Significant Findings

1. The skin and sclerae are slightly jaundiced.
2. The urine is bile-tinged.
3. There is slight tenderness on palpation of the abdomen, but no masses are palpable.

DIAGNOSTIC STUDIES

1. *Alkaline phosphatase.*   Moderately elevated.
2. *Bilirubin.*   Moderately elevated.
3. *Upper gastrointestinal series.*   Normal.
4. *Pancreatic scan.*   Normal.
5. *Pancreatic arteriogram.*   Normal.

PROBABLE HOSPITAL COURSE

When obstructive jaundice, as manifested by an elevated bilirubin and alkaline phosphatase, is associated with weight loss, epigastric distress, and anorexia in a 56-year-old patient, the probable cause is either calculous disease of the biliary tree or a malignancy involving the pancreas or extrahepatic biliary system. In spite of the normal x-rays and scans, an exploratory laparotomy is mandatory.

PREPARATION FOR SURGERY

The patient is prepared in the same fashion as in cholecystojejunostomy (see previous chapter).

PATHOLOGY

Operable cancer of the pancreas involves either a lesion of the ampulla of Vater or a lesion localized to the head of the pancreas with no regional metastases and no involvement of the superior mesenteric artery. Either lesion will require an extensive resection for cure and, consequently, every effort will be made to define the limits of the tumor before proceeding with the operation.

GENERAL RATIONALE AND SCHEME

1. The abdomen is opened and a careful evaluation of the liver, extrahepatic biliary tree, and pancreas is carried out.
2. A resectable lesion of the ampulla of Vater or of the head of the pancreas will require pancreatectomy and duodenectomy if a complete extirpation of the lesion is to be effected.

PROCEDURE

Steps 1 to 6.   The preliminary steps are the same as for cholecystojejunostomy. (See preceding chapter.)

7. Once a decision is made to continue with the procedure, the surgeon should notify the anesthesiologist and the operating room supervisor. The procedure may take from 5 to 6 hours and will require multiple blood transfusions. The blood lab should be apprised of the decision to proceed with the operation.

8. The procedure followed in a pancreaticoduodenectomy is one of the most extensive of all abdominal procedures. In many ways, the intricacy and complexity of the surgery exclude it from detailed discussion in a text such as this. Consequently, important *general* principles will be outlined here, and further study in specialized surgical texts is recommended.

9. Early in the course of a pancreaticoduodenectomy, the dilated common bile duct is dissected and isolated with a Penrose drain to prevent injury to this structure.

10. The duodenum and head of the pancreas are mobilized, and multiple vessels joining the pancreas to the mesenteric vessels are carefully ligated and divided.

11. Because the distal half of the stomach is to be included in the specimen, a hemigastrectomy is carried out. Postoperative hyperacidity can be a frequent occurrence, though, and some surgeons routinely perform a bilateral vagotomy as part of the procedure.

12. After the specimen has been removed (including the duodenum, the spleen, half or more of the pancreas, and the distal half of the stomach), the jejunum is sutured to the pancreas and stomach, and the common bile duct is sutured into the side wall of the jejunum, often over a rubber stent.

13. A number of Penrose drains are placed in the abdomen, particularly in the area of the pancreaticojejunostomy, in anticipation of anastomotic leaks.

14. *Closure of Wound.* Routine.

SURGICAL HAZARDS

1. *Shock.* Radical pancreaticoduodenectomy carries with it one of the highest risks of shock in general surgery. Next to septic shock secondary to multiple organ trauma, few procedures equal radical pancreatectomy in terms of overwhelming hemodynamic, cardiopulmonary, and renal alterations within the body. All of the cardiac, respiratory, renal, and metabolic problems frequently attending the shock state may manifest themselves during or after this procedure, and the "stress" state may last several days under the best of circumstances.

2. *Defective Anastomoses.* There are at least three anastomoses carried out in the course of the surgical procedure. Leakage can result in fatal pancreatitis or bile peritonitis.

3. *Massive Hemorrhage.* The pancreatic blood supply is closely associated with the celiac and mesenteric vessels, which are often quite inaccessible. Major and sudden hemorrhage can occur at any time during or after the operation.

POSTOPERATIVE MANAGEMENT

The patient undergoing radical pancreaticoduodenectomy should be kept in the intensive care unit for several days because of the likelihood that shock will result from the surgery. The patient often will require assisted respirations for 2 or 3 days. General principles of management include the following.

Cardiorespiratory Monitoring

1. Continuous cardiac monitoring.
2. Assisted or controlled ventilation.
3. Frequent electrocardiograms.
4. Frequent monitoring of arterial blood gases.
5. Monitoring of central venous pressure or pulmonary wedge pressure.

Renal Monitoring

1. Hourly urine output.
2. Daily creatinine.
3. Daily serum and urine electrolytes.
4. Plasma and urine osmolality daily.
5. Careful checking of daily fluid intake and output.
6. Daily weighing of patient.

Metabolic Care

Hyperalimentation may be started soon after surgery.

Wound and Catheter Care

1. Dressings should be changed daily; the wound area should be checked for any leakage of intestinal contents and for any signs of excoriation of the skin.
2. A careful check should be made to ensure that all catheters are secured to the dressings. Among the catheters may be:
   a. A tube gastrostomy.
   b. A tube choledochojejunostomy.
   c. Various sump catheters used to collect drainage from anastomoses.

STUDY QUESTIONS

1. What is the value of measuring pulmonary arterial pressures?

2. What is acute tubular necrosis? List some of its causes. Why is it apt to occur after a pancreaticoduodenectomy?

3. What is the value of measuring urine and plasma osmolality?

4. How could you monitor the patient to detect the early development of acute postoperative pancreatitis?

5. Shortly after a pancreaticoduodenectomy in which major blood loss had been offset by replacement, the surgeon's order calls for Ringer's lactate to be given at 150 cc per hour. You observe that the urine output is scant and that the CVP reading is 19 cm of water. What is the best course of action?
   a. Continue present management, because the patient's vital signs are stable, he is alert, color is good, and he seems to be doing quite well.
   b. Speed up the infusion of Ringer's lactate, because the oliguria needs to be treated in order to prevent renal failure.
   c. Inform the surgeon of the situation, with the expectation that he will order a reduction in the rate of intravenous fluid infusion or request that a diuretic be administered.

6. Continue with the situation presented in question 5; assume that you chose to inform the surgeon and that he ordered an intravenous diuretic in massive dosages. When the diuretic is administered, the oliguria persists, and the CVP still reads 19 to 20 cm. What are some of the possible explanations for this situation? What complications may soon ensue? What observations should you be making? What treatment(s) might the surgeon order? These problems should be discussed in your class and different students assigned the tasks of looking up information on the various aspects of these problems.

THE PATIENT WITH A LACERATED LIVER   21

Operation: Repair of A Lacerated Liver

TYPICAL HISTORY

A 25-year-old male was admitted through the emergency room following an injury sustained in a motorcycle accident. Witnesses state that the man was thrown from the motorcycle and that he injured his upper abdominal wall against the handlebars of his motorcycle.

PHYSICAL EXAMINATION

A well-developed male is admitted complaining of right upper abdominal pain and right shoulder pain.

Significant Findings

1. Pallor is noted, particularly around the lips.
2. Hypotension is noted (90/50).
3. Pulse is 110 per minute.
4. There is tenderness in the upper abdomen, particularly on the right side.
5. Some rigidity of the right rectus muscle is found.
6. There is tenderness over the right tenth and eleventh ribs.
7. Bowel sounds are diminished or absent.
8. Bruises are seen across the upper abdomen.

DIAGNOSTIC STUDIES

1. WBC is 27,000 per cu. mm.
2. Hematocrit level is 34 per cent.

3. Chest x-rays show fractured ribs 10 and 11 on right.
4. Flat and upright x-rays of the abdomen are negative.

PROBABLE HOSPITAL COURSE

1. The history and physical findings are very suggestive of hemorrhagic shock secondary to a lacerated liver. No time can be wasted in preparing this patient for immediate surgery.

2. If the diagnosis is not clear-cut, a period of observation will be instituted. The points to watch for during this period of observation are similar to those for a ruptured spleen. If there is serious doubt about the diagnosis of lacerated liver, a laparoscopic examination can be invaluable.

PREPARATION FOR SURGERY

1. A Levin tube is inserted preoperatively.
2. The abdomen is prepped from the nipple line as far as and including the pubis. (See Introduction.)
3. Type and cross-match six to eight units of blood.
4. A large intravenous needle or, preferably, intracatheter is inserted on the ward.
5. Enema is not necessary.
6. Routine premedications.
7. No special medications.
8. *Operating Room Skin Prep.* From nipples as far as and including pubis. (See Introduction.)
9. *Position.* Horizontal supine. (See Introduction.)

PATHOLOGY

1. Often, a small laceration in the capsule of the right lobe of the liver is found surrounded by a small hematoma and with adjacent liver contusion.

2. At the other extreme, a markedly lacerated and avulsed liver, particularly involving the right lobe, may be found with a good deal of free blood in the peritoneal cavity.

GENERAL RATIONALE AND SCHEME

The liver is an extremely friable and difficult organ to repair. In most cases, debridement of necrotic tissue is done, followed by repair of the laceration. In severe lacerations, a right or left hepatic lobectomy may be required.

Scheme

1. Blood clots and destroyed liver tissue are removed.
2. A large hot saline pack is placed over the bleeding liver surface until the plan for hemostasis is determined.
3. The lacerated liver is closed with appropriate suture material.
4. Thorough irrigation of all blood clots, particularly above the liver and below the diaphragm and in the pelvis, is accomplished.

5. Drainage is established.
6. The abdomen is closed.

PROCEDURE

1. *Opening the Abdomen.*   A right upper abdominal vertical incision is the most commonly used. (See Introduction.) The diagnosis of intraperitoneal hemorrhage is usually confirmed immediately when blood rushes forth as the peritoneum is opened. Occasionally, bleeding has ceased and a large hematoma is found over the region of the lacerated liver.

2. *Exploration.*   The source of the bleeding is confirmed. Further exploration for other trauma is deferred until the injured liver is repaired and bleeding controlled. Following this, the entire abdominal cavity and all its organs are carefully examined for signs of other injury.

3. A hot saline pack is placed over the bleeding surface of the liver preparatory to suturing of the laceration.

4. Large chromic sutures are placed through the liver tissue and tied carefully in an attempt to control the bleeding from the liver surface. Often, the tissue is quite friable and will not hold sutures. In this case, either Surgicel or Gelfoam, or some other hemostatic substance, is placed in the crevice of the laceration and sutures are loosely tied to approximate the tissue against this hemostatic substance.

5. The best needle for suturing a lacerated liver is a large curved noncutting needle with a blunt tip.

6. After bleeding is controlled, a general exploration is carried out, with particular attention paid to the bile ducts, the duodenum, and the pancreas.

7. When it is determined that no other trauma exists, all remaining blood and clots are removed from the suprahepatic regions as well as the pelvis.

8. The area of repair is again inspected to be certain that no further hemorrhage is occurring.

9. Large Penrose drains are placed in the region of the laceration and brought out through the incision or through drain sites placed near the incision. Some surgeons advocate routine decompression of the common bile duct with a t-tube after significant liver trauma (Fig. 21–1). The precise rationale for this procedure has not yet been well established. However, hemobilia can

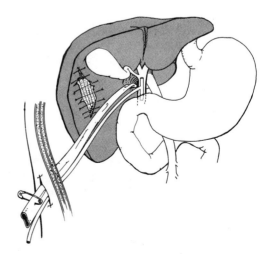

FIGURE 21–1 Repair of a lacerated liver. Note the use of a Penrose drain and a t-tube.

certainly be diagnosed earlier with a t-tube in place, and the tube permits postoperative x-ray evaluation of the extrahepatic biliary tree should this be necessary.

10. The abdominal wound is closed in the usual manner.

SURGICAL HAZARDS

1. *Failure to Control Massive Hemorrhage.*   Death may intervene due to the massive blood loss from severely traumatized liver tissue in spite of all attempts to reach and control the bleeding areas.

2. *Injury to Nearby Organs.*   Because of the massive bleeding and large blood clots found in the region of the liver bed, there is a distinct hazard of injury to the common duct and associated structures in the portal bed.

3. *Overlooking Other Injuries.*   There is the danger of assuming that only one organ has been injured, once the major source of hemorrhage has been controlled. A thorough investigation must be carried out before the operation is completed.

EARLY POSTOPERATIVE MANAGEMENT

1. A Levin tube is placed on low suction.

2. Careful monitoring of vital signs must be carried out, because of the possibility of underreplacement of lost blood or continued bleeding.

3. Pulmonary complications, particularly right lower lobe pneumonia, are prone to occur due to splinting of the diaphragm on the involved side. Coughing, deep breathing, and turning must be urged frequently.

4. *Care of the Dressing.*   The dressing will often soak through with blood and bile because of the large drains which have been placed at the site of trauma. Should this happen, the surgeon should be called immediately and a fresh dressing applied.

5. The t-tube, if used, is placed on dependent drainage and is secured to the dressing. The amount of bile drainage is noted every eight hours.

STUDY QUESTIONS

1. Why is the right lobe of the liver more prone to injury than the left lobe?

2. Describe the mechanism of action of Surgicel and Gelfoam as hemostatic agents.

3. What type of suture material and needle are optimum for the surgical repair of a liver laceration?

4. In a patient who is being observed for possible intraperitoneal hemorrhage following an abdominal injury, describe the nurse's role in the careful observation of this patient.

5. What are some of the signs to look for which might indicate the presence of continued intraperitoneal hemorrhage?

6. What is the significance of excessive thirst in a patient being observed for possible intraperitoneal hemorrhage?

7. Review and be able to discuss the comprehensive nursing care of a patient who has had liver surgery.

8. What is the significance of continued postoperative bile leakage onto the dressing of a patient who has suffered a liver laceration?

9. What is the significance of deepening jaundice postoperatively in this patient?

THE PATIENT WITH A PERFORATED DUODENAL ULCER

22

Operation: Closure of A Perforated Ulcer

TYPICAL HISTORY

A 42-year-old male, with a 4-year history of epigastric pains suggesting the presence of a duodenal ulcer, was awakened from sleep with acute, severe epigastric pain. The pain rapidly worsened and became generalized throughout the abdomen. He also complained of dyspnea and right shoulder pain.

PHYSICAL EXAMINATION

The patient is a well-developed, thin male in agonizing abdominal pain.

Significant Findings

1. There are grunting respirations.
2. Pulse is 110 per minute.
3. The abdomen is boardlike.
4. There is diffuse abdominal tenderness.
5. There is no audible peristalsis.

DIAGNOSTIC STUDIES

1. WBC is 14,000 per cu. mm.
2. Amylase is normal.

3. X-ray of abdomen indicates presence of air under the diaphragm, consistent with perforation somewhere in the gastrointestinal tract.

4. ECG is normal, except for a rapid rate.

5. Urine is negative.

PROBABLE HOSPITAL COURSE

1. If the diagnosis is certain, the patient is prepared for immediate surgery. Each hour of delay results in increased morbidity and mortality.

2. If there is doubt about the diagnosis, time must be spent in ruling out other causes of severe, sudden epigastric pain. The differential diagnosis includes:

Acute Pancreatitis.   Some of the points to be considered in this diagnosis are:

1. Lack of air under the diaphragm.
2. Highly elevated amylase level.
3. History of heavy alcohol intake, gallbladder disease, or recent abdominal trauma.

Coronary Thrombosis

1. ECG may demonstrate infarction, although this may not appear for 2 to 3 days.
2. Usually no abdominal rigidity.

Ruptured Esophagus

1. Air usually visible in mediastinum by chest x-ray.
2. Greater degree of pulmonary distress.
3. Less abdominal rigidity.

Acute Cholecystitis

1. Tenderness often localized to right upper quadrant.
2. Less abdominal rigidity.
3. History of much less abrupt onset.

Acute Ureteral Colic

1. Less abdominal tenderness.
2. Pain usually in flank, radiating into groin.
3. Often, microscopic hematuria.

Ruptured Aortic Aneurysm

1. Shock more prominent.
2. Pulsatile mass usually felt.

Once the diagnosis of perforated ulcer has been made, the patient is prepared for surgery.

PREPARATION FOR SURGERY

1. *Levin Tube.*   This should be inserted on the ward, as gastric aspiration should be started at once.

2. The patient should be kept in semi-Fowler's position to prevent the leaking gastric contents from gravitating toward the subdiaphragmatic space.

3. If the patient appears to be dehydrated or toxic, a saline infusion should be started soon after admission.

4. *Prep.*   From the nipple line as far as and including the pubis. (See Introduction.)

5. *Blood.*   One unit of blood should be typed and cross-matched.

6. *Enema.*   Not necessary.

7. *Premedications.*   Routine.

8. *Special Medications.*   None.

9. *Psychological Preparation.* As with any emergency operation.
10. *Operating Room Skin Prep.* (See Introduction.)
11. *Position.* Horizontal supine. (See Introduction.)

PATHOLOGY

1. *Location.* The acute perforated ulcer is usually found in the superior portion of the duodenum on its anterior surface (Fig. 22-1).
2. *Size.* It may vary from 1 mm. to 2 cm.
3. *Reaction.* There is often a purulent edematous process surrounding the ragged perforation in the duodenum. Gastric contents may be seen freely flowing from the perforation, or a small tag of omentum may have sealed the perforation.
Chemical or bacterial peritonitis will be found in association with the perforation.

GENERAL RATIONALE AND SCHEME

Continual leakage of gastric contents from a perforated ulcer usually causes death. The surgeon must close off the source of peritoneal contamination caused by the duodenal perforation. If the perforation is recent (within 6 hours), there will be little bacterial peritonitis, and the surgeon may elect to perform emergency gastrectomy and vagotomy. Usually he will be content with plication of the perforated ulcer, often a safer option in light of potential infection.

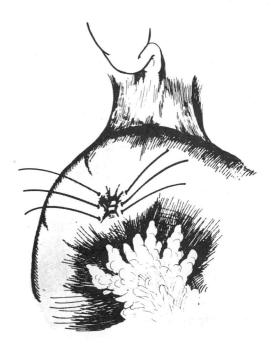

FIGURE 22-1 Through-and-through sutures being used to close a perforated ulcer in the superior portion of the duodenum.

Scheme

1. Abdomen is opened and explored and the diagnosis confirmed.

2. Through-and-through sutures are used to close the perforation, which is then reinforced with adjacent omentum.

3. Peritoneal exudate is aspirated.

4. The abdomen is closed after considerable irrigation with normal saline.

PROCEDURE

1. *Skin Incision.* A vertical midline epigastric or upper right paramedian incision is made. (See Introduction.)

2. *Draping Skin.* Bacterial contamination from a perforated ulcer can result in wound sepsis. Consequently, the edges of the incision must be protected. A "ring drape" is very effective here, as it protects the full thickness of the wound edges.

3. *Opening Abdomen.* Air may be heard escaping as the peritoneum is incised. If free fluid escapes, this should be aspirated and cultured.

4. *Exploration.* This is done cautiously to avoid destroying any natural barriers that may have been set up to ward off generalized contamination.

5. *The perforation* may be handled in one of two ways:

a. Through-and-through simple sutures are used to close the perforation (Fig. 22–1).

b. A pursestring suture may be used at times.

6. *The closed perforation* is further reinforced by suturing a tag of omentum over the perforated area.

7. The abdominal cavity is aspirated to remove all free fluid.

8. *Drains.* Some surgeons prefer to drain the subdiaphragmatic spaces to prevent the development of a subdiaphragmatic abscess. Other surgeons close the abdomen without drainage.

9. *Closure.* Routine.

SURGICAL HAZARDS

Failure to obtain a watertight closure of the perforation may lead to continuing leakage postoperatively, with death ensuing from peritonitis.

EARLY POSTOPERATIVE COURSE

1. *Levin Tube.* Routine management.

2. *Semi-Fowler's Position.* To avoid subdiaphragmatic collection of septic fluid.

3. *Pulmonary Function.* Deep breathing and coughing must be urged to prevent development of atelectasis and pneumonia.

4. Intravenous therapy with supplemental antibiotics.

5. Convalescence is usually smooth. The Levin tube is removed the second or third day after surgery, as soon as bowel sounds are audible. Diet is advanced from liquids to bland solids over a 3 to 6 day period, and often the patient is discharged 7 to 10 days after surgery.

6. Late temperature elevations occurring 5 to 8 days after surgery usually suggest subdiaphragmatic, pelvic, or wound sepsis, and efforts will be made to localize the infection.

STUDY QUESTIONS

1. Why does a patient with a perforated ulcer usually have difficulty in breathing?

2. What is meant by a "boardlike abdomen"?

3. Discuss the meaning of the serum amylase test. Name three illnesses which may result in highly elevated amylases.

4. What is the importance of the semi-Fowler's position in the patient with a perforated ulcer?

5. Why is an electrocardiogram important in the evaluation of a patient in whom a perforated ulcer is suspected?

6. What is pneumoperitoneum? What is its significance? Is it always present on x-rays of patients with perforated ulcers? What other illnesses may cause pneumoperitoneum?

7. What is the treatment of acute pancreatitis?

8. List the important nursing procedures to be carried out *preoperatively* for a patient awaiting surgery on a perforated ulcer.

9. Describe the essential steps in the surgical closure of a perforated ulcer. Why is the abdomen irrigated with saline after closure of the ulcer?

10. Describe the comprehensive nursing care of a postoperative patient who has had a closure of a perforated ulcer.

11. What steps must the nurse take to insure *continuous efficient* functioning of the Levin tube both pre- and postoperatively? Why is this tube very important in this illness?

12. Discuss an emergency gastrectomy or emergency vagotomy plus pyloroplasty as the treatment for a perforated duodenal ulcer.

Operation: Gastroenterostomy

TYPICAL HISTORY

A 70-year-old male has had recurrent attacks of epigastric pain and vomiting for several months. A previous upper gastrointestinal series revealed the presence of a deformed duodenal bulb secondary to a chronic duodenal ulcer. For the preceding 5 days, the patient has had recurrent attacks of vomiting, and is unable to retain solids or liquids.

PHYSICAL EXAMINATION

A well-developed but emaciated and dehydrated male is admitted complaining of epigastric distress.

Significant Findings

1. Emaciation, loss of skin turgor, and dehydration of mucous membranes are noted.
2. There is slight epigastric tenderness.
3. The stomach is distended on percussion over the left upper quadrant.

DIAGNOSTIC STUDIES

1. Flat and upright x-rays of the abdomen may reveal the presence of a dilated and distended stomach. If a swallow of barium is given, this will show complete obstruction at the pylorus of the stomach, and no barium will flow into the small intestine.
2. Electrolyte studies will reveal signs of dehydration, as well as alkalosis due to loss of gastric acid. The serum $[K]^+$ values may be low because of chronic vomiting.
3. Serum albumin may be diminished as a result of chronic malnutrition.

PROBABLE HOSPITAL COURSE

A large Levin tube is passed into the stomach and connected to low suction. Intravenous fluids are given to replace the lost fluids and electrolytes. Because of the chronicity of the patient's ulcer disease, it is highly unlikely that the obstruction will subside and, consequently, preparations are made for surgery as soon as his condition is acceptable.

PREPARATION FOR SURGERY

The patient who has been ill with obstruction of the pylorus for several days usually reveals significant electrolyte and fluid derangements. These must be corrected prior to surgery. The following matters must be treated:

1. The *blood level* is tested and adjusted so that the patient is brought to surgery with hemoglobin and hematocrit levels as close to normal as is feasible.

2. The *electrolytes* are checked carefully and any tendency toward development of *alkalosis* and *hypokalemia* is corrected with appropriate electrolyte solutions.

3. A patient with long-term ulcer disease and obstruction is often *malnourished* and his *protein* balance is low. Consequently, his protein balance must be brought to normal and this often requires the use of packed red cells, whole blood, and serum albumin.

4. *Skin Prep.* The entire abdomen from the costal margins as far as and including the pubis is cleanly shaven while the patient is on the ward. (See Introduction.)

5. *Enema.* A soapsuds or Fleet enema should be given the evening before or on the day of surgery.

6. *Blood.* Two to three units of whole blood are typed and cross-matched and kept available for the patient.

7. *Premedications.* Same as for appendectomy.

8. *Special medications.* None.

9. *Operating Room Skin Prep.* The entire abdomen from the costal margins as far as and including the pubis should be prepped according to the hospital routine. (See Introduction.)

10. *Position.* Horizontal supine. (See Introduction.)

PATHOLOGY

A chronic active duodenal ulcer causes surrounding inflammation and edema of the duodenal mucosa. If this continues, the narrow pyloric canal becomes stenosed and finally obstructed. Often, there is a large mass in the region of the pyloric canal due to localized perforation of the ulcer into the surrounding pancreatic or paraduodenal tissue. If this obstruction has developed over a long period of time, the stomach will be thick-walled and distended as a result of its attempt to overcome the obstruction. The stomach may be extremely large and contain a large amount of gastric sections (Fig. 23–1).

GENERAL RATIONALE AND SCHEME

In the elderly and chronically ill patient, often all that can or need be done is to by-pass the area of obstruction in the pyloric canal. In so doing, the gastric secretions are allowed to pass from the stomach into the jejunum, thereby avoiding the obstructed area. In the absence of any further secretions that would bathe the ulcer, it may subside and no further trouble may occur. Hyperacidity is not usually a problem in the elderly; therefore vagotomy and gastrectomy are not always necessary.

Scheme

1. The stomach and pyloric area are exposed through a left paramedian muscle retracting incision or a vertical midline incision.

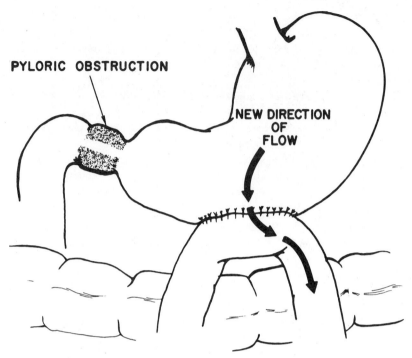

FIGURE 23-1 Gastroenterostomy for pyloric obstruction.

   2. The jejunum is brought up to the posterior wall of the stomach near the antrum of the stomach in the vicinity of the pyloric obstruction.
   3. An anastomosis is created between the stomach and the jejunum in this area (Fig. 23–1).

PROCEDURE

   1. A left paramedian muscle retracting or a vertical midline incision is made in the usual fashion. (See Introduction.)
   2. The abdomen is opened and general exploration is carried out. Carcinoma of the stomach must be ruled out.
   3. Wound towels are applied in the usual fashion.
   4. The ligament of Treitz, which suspends the first part of the jejunum, is used as a landmark to identify the jejunum.
   5. *The first part of the jejunum* is brought up and approximated to the posterior antral area of the stomach.
   6. The first posterior row of sutures to create the anastomosis consists of interrupted silk sutures between the serosa of the stomach and the serosa of the jejunum. This is usually 2–0 or 3–0 suture material.
   7. The stomach and jejunum are opened, bleeding vessels being clamped and ligated.
   8. The stomach is then usually aspirated with a sump suction device.
   9. The internal mucosal sutures usually consist of running absorbable suture material such as 2–0 or 3–0 chromic catgut.
   10. The anterior outer row of suture material again consists of interrupted 2–0 or 3–0 silk suture.

11. *Testing the Anastomosis.* The surgeon then palpates the anastomotic area to determine whether a good opening has been created between the stomach and jejunum. He will proceed to check the function and placement of the Levin tube; he may fashion a tube gastrostomy to substitute for a Levin tube.

12. *Closure of Wound.*

SURGICAL HAZARDS

1. *Uncontrollable Hemorrhage.* An obstructing, inflammatory mass in the head of the pancreas in the first part of the duodenum often produces highly vascular tissue in this area. There is an increased tendency to bleed because of this vascularity and care must be taken to avoid excessive hemorrhage with possible trauma resulting from an attempt to control this hemorrhage.

2. *Spillage of Gastric Contents.* During the incision into the stomach, a good deal of fluid which had not been aspirated by the Levin tube may spill out into the surrounding tissue. This fluid often contains innumerable microorganisms because it has stagnated in the obstructed stomach. Consequently, every effort must be made to drape the area and to use properly functioning suction equipment so as to avoid contamination of the peritoneal cavity.

EARLY POSTOPERATIVE MANAGEMENT

1. The Levin tube is connected to low suction and managed as described in preceding chapters.

2. If the patient has had a significant fluid and electrolyte problem preoperatively, it is wise to insert a Foley catheter into his bladder and monitor the urine output every 2 to 3 hours.

3. Pulmonary complications are quite prone to occur because of the upper abdominal incision. The patient must be urged to breathe deeply and to cough frequently in order to prevent atelectasis and pneumonia.

4. *Care of the Wound.* The incision usually does not drain and it is not usually drained by the surgeon. Consequently, the wound should require no particular immediate care in the recovery room.

5. In most cases the Levin tube is removed in 2 to 3 days if drainage is minimal. Diet is advanced rapidly over 3 to 5 days to soft foods.

6. Generally the patient is discharged 7 to 10 days after surgery.

STUDY QUESTIONS

1. Describe some electrolyte problems that are usually associated with chronic total pyloric obstruction.

2. Would you expect bilious drainage to be seen in the Levin tube preoperatively in a patient with total pyloric obstruction? Explain your answer.

3. What are the signs and symptoms of pyloric obstruction?

4. What clinical problems can occur in a patient suffering from severe hypokalemia (low potassium level)?

5. List three complications of duodenal ulcer in addition to pyloric obstruction.

6. Is there any form of therapy for total pyloric obstruction besides surgery?

7. Of what importance is the ligament of Treitz to the surgeon? Where is it located?

8. On the evening following gastroenterostomy, a moderate amount of bright red blood is found passing through the Levin tube. Discuss how the nurse should manage this problem.

9. Describe all the factors present in the elderly, debilitated, dehydrated male who was discussed in this chapter which might predispose him to develop *atelectasis* and *pneumonia* postoperatively. How would these factors be incorporated by the nurse in her postoperative nursing care plan?

10. Outline a nursing care plan for a patient who has had gastroenterostomy. Consider:
   a. The preoperative phase
   b. The postoperative phase
   c. Scientific principles underlying nursing actions

11. Following gastroenterostomy in which a tube gastrostomy has been inserted, the patient becomes restless. What major complication of his restlessness can occur, and how would you prevent it?

12. Describe the care of a tube gastrostomy. What are its advantages over a Levin tube? Its disadvantages?

24 THE PATIENT WITH A SEVERE DUODENAL ULCER

Operation: Subtotal Gastrectomy

TYPICAL HISTORY

A 46-year-old businessman has been disabled with recurrent epigastric pains for several years. He has a duodenal ulcer which was demonstrated by a previous upper gastrointestinal series. Repeated exacerbations of severe pain have necessitated hospitalization on several occasions over the past 6 years; during a previous admission the patient had severe gastrointestinal bleeding which required transfusion of five units of blood. The current admission was preceded by steady epigastric pain and recurrent episodes of vomiting of 3 weeks' duration.

PHYSICAL EXAMINATION

A well-developed, thin, apprehensive male, appearing to be somewhat older than his stated age, is admitted with the complaint of gnawing, steady epigastric distress.

Significant Findings

1. Epigastric tenderness is noted.
2. Pallor and signs of recent and chronic weight loss are evident.
3. The patient's countenance is anxious and tense.

DIAGNOSTIC STUDIES

1. WBC is 12,000 per cu. mm.
2. Hematocrit level is 37 per cent.
3. Amylase level is normal.
4. Gastric analysis indicates the presence of over 40 units of free hydrochloric acid.
5. There is a trace of occult blood in the stool.
6. Upper gastrointestinal series indicates marked deformity of the duodenal bulb, with an active ulcer crater.

PROBABLE HOSPITAL COURSE

1. The surgeon will wish to confirm the presence of a duodenal ulcer and to determine, as far as possible, the amount of scarring, destruction, or deformity of the duodenum that has resulted from the ulcer. An upper gastrointestinal series will be done. For this examination, the patient is fasted from midnight on the evening prior to the test. On the following day, he is given a glassful of *barium,* which is radiopaque; following this the stomach and duodenum will be outlined by x-ray.

2. A *gastric analysis* may also be ordered on the fasting stomach. A Levin tube is inserted into the stomach, and a specimen of the stomach contents is aspirated for analysis of free and total acid. Then a subcutaneous injection of histamine is given which will stimulate further acid secretion by the stomach. Forty-five minutes after histamine injection, a second gastric specimen is obtained. The nurse should label the first specimen "fasting" and the second specimen "following histamine." The subject of gastric analysis is very complex. Some surgeons prefer a 12 hour overnight collection of gastric juice followed by serial collections after histamine stimulation. For further information on this subject, the student is referred to gastroenterology texts.

3. On the basis of history, x-ray, study, and gastric analysis, the surgeon must decide whether surgery is indicated. If so, the patient will be prepared for surgery within a day or two following the studies just mentioned.

PREPARATION FOR SURGERY

In addition to routine preparations as for any laparotomy, the following steps are necessary:

1. *Psychological Preparation.* The patient with an ulcer is notoriously an extremely apprehensive patient. He may be overly anxious but, more often, he hides his anxiety under the

façade of docility. The nurse must learn to recognize this docile, introverted patient as one who deeply *worries within* and attempt to allay his fears. Often the patient about to undergo gastrectomy fears he will become a nutritional cripple, losing the *"digestive function"* of his stomach. It may be explained to him that the remaining portion of stomach will soon "stretch" and have full digestive power.

    2. *Type and cross-match* four units of whole blood.

    3. *Levin tube,* No. 18, to be inserted on morning of surgery.

    4. Correction of any anemia or electrolyte deficiencies that might exist.

    5. Correction of hypoproteinemia if this exists.

    6. Abdominal prep from nipple line as far as and including pubis. (See Introduction.)

    7. Fleet enema.

    8. Routine medications.

    9. No special medications.

    10. *Operating Room Skin Prep.* (See Introduction.)

    11. *Position.* Horizontal supine. (See Introduction.)

PATHOLOGY

    1. The early ulcer may show some scarring and deformity of the first part of the duodenum. There is often inflammation and edema around the ulcer which is indicative of previous episodes of acute ulcer disease.

    2. The advanced chronic ulcer may show:

a. Severe scarring and deformity of the duodenum.

b. Partial to total obstruction of the outlet of the stomach.

c. Perforation into the pancreas with inflammation and edema of the pancreas.

GENERAL RATIONALE AND SCHEME

    The advanced, chronically inflamed ulcer is often intractable to medical therapy, and surgery is mandatory. By removing a large segment of stomach, the surgeon hopes to overcome its ulcerogenic potential; the *acid produced by the stomach* is said to cause and aggravate an ulcer. It is not always necessary that the ulcer itself be removed. Indeed, although 70 per cent gastrectomy, as demonstrated here, is a time-honored and very acceptable way to cure ulcer disease, it is rapidly losing favor in the judgment of many surgeons. There is a conservative trend today that strongly recommends *lesser* operative procedures such as (1) vagotomy plus pyloroplasty, (2) vagotomy plus antrectomy, or (3) vagotomy plus hemigastrectomy. These approaches seem at least as effective as subtotal gastrectomy in the control of ulcer disease and appear to produce far fewer gastrointestinal problems.

Scheme

    1. Division of the blood supply to the segment of stomach to be removed.

    2. Transection below the pylorus.

    3. Closure of the transected duodenum.

    4. Transection of the proximal segment of stomach.

    5. Anastomosis of the jejunum with the remaining segment of stomach.

PROCEDURE

1. *Opening Abdomen.*   A left upper abdominal or a midline vertical incision may be used. (See Introduction.)

2. *Exploration.*   The extent of ulcer disease is noted, and a judgment is made as to the safety of the procedure. If gastrectomy is judged to be too hazardous, vagectomy and gastroenterostomy may be elected.

3. *Division of Blood Supply.*   Basically, there are four major sources of blood supply to the stomach. These are classified as follows (Fig. 24–1):

   a. *Right Gastroepiploic.*   These vessels run along the junction of the omentum and stomach from the duodenum toward the spleen.

   b. *Left Gastroepiploic.*   These vessels also run along the junction of the omentum and stomach from the spleen toward the duodenum, meeting the right gastroepiploic vessels. These two sets of vessels are clamped, divided, and ligated along the greater curvature of the stomach.

   c. *Right Gastric Artery.*   On the superior surface of the duodenum.

   d. *Left Gastric Artery.*   Near the esophagogastric junction.

4. *Division of Duodenum.*   After the blood supply to the stomach has been secured, the duodenum is divided just below the pylorus. If possible, the duodenum is divided below the ulcer, although this is not absolutely necessary (Fig. 24–2).

5. *Closure of Duodenum.*   This is usually closed with two layers of suture, one of catgut and one of silk. A third reinforcing silk layer may also be used. Leakage from a poorly closed duodenum may cause death. If there is any doubt about the security of the duodenal closure, a catheter may be inserted into the duodenum for postoperative decompression.

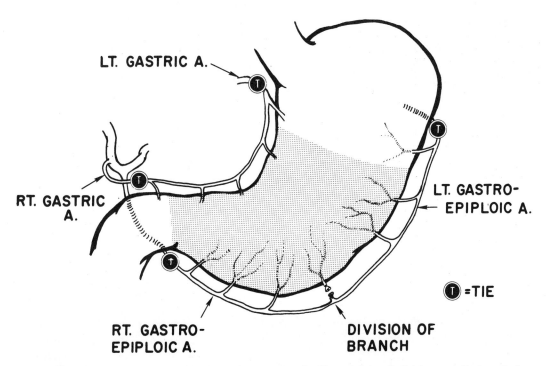

FIGURE 24–1 Gastrectomy. Blood supply to stomach. Note points of division and ligature during gastrectomy.

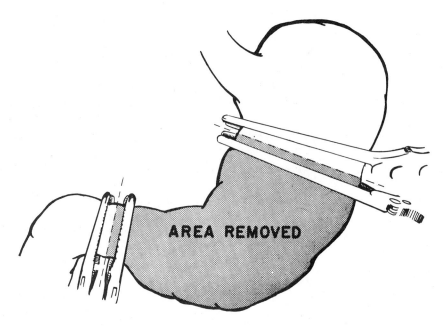

FIGURE 24–2   Clamps on duodenum and stomach prior to excision.

6. *Division of Stomach.*   The surgeon estimates the amount of stomach he wishes to excise (usually 60 to 70 per cent). A clamp is placed across the stomach and the organ is resected (Fig. 24–2).

7. *Gastrojejunostomy.*   The surgeon locates the jejunum and joins it to the remaining segment of stomach, thereby creating a new channel for food. This anastomosis usually requires two layers of suture, one inner and one outer; chromic catgut is used for the inner layer and silk for the outer one.

8. *Closure of Abdomen.*   Routine.

SURGICAL HAZARDS

1. *Excessive Blood Loss.*   Major vessels, particularly those near the duodenum, may be accidentally injured with consequent excessive blood loss.

2. *Injury to Common or Pancreatic Ducts.*   These ducts are often involved in the extensive inflammation caused by a duodenal ulcer. Careless surgical technique in the region of the duodenum may result in injury to these ducts.

3. *Injury to Middle Colic Artery.*   This artery supplies blood to the transverse colon. It passes below the stomach and is quite near the greater omentum. It may be damaged or ligated, thereby causing gangrene of the transverse colon.

EARLY POSTOPERATIVE MANAGEMENT

1. *Management of the Levin Tube.*   This should be connected to low suction in the recovery room. Bleeding from the gastrojejunostomy anastomosis is quite common, so that some bright red blood may be seen in the Levin tube. Persistent or excessive blood loss should be noted and reported to the surgeon. It is important that the Levin tube be irrigated every 2 to 3 hours so as to avoid plugging caused by mucus and blood clots.

2. *Careful Observation of Vital Signs.* Gastrectomy is a lengthy and physiologically shocking procedure to the patient. It is not unusual for two to three units of blood to be lost during this procedure. In addition, continued blood loss may occur postoperatively. The nurse should therefore expect a certain degree of hypotension and tachycardia in the postgastrectomy patient (e.g., blood pressure, 100/60; pulse, 110). A *progressive deterioration* in the blood pressure and pulse, however, should alert the nurse to the development of further difficulties such as continued blood loss, coronary thrombosis, or acute pancreatitis. Consequently, close observation of vital signs is mandatory. Deterioration should be reported to the surgeon at once.

3. *Care of the Wound.* There should be little to no drainage from the wound unless the surgeon has left a drain in place.

4. *Pulmonary Care.* As with any *lengthy upper abdominal* operation, atelectasis and pneumonia are very prone to occur because of splinting of the diaphragm due to the painful incision. Aggressive postoperative pulmonary care should be given (coughing, deep breathing, inhalation therapy as ordered and frequent change of position).

5. If gastrectomy is the only surgery that has been performed, the Levin tube is in many cases removed the day after the operation, and the patient started on water or clear liquids by mouth. Diet is rapidly advanced over the next 4 to 5 days, and the patient is usually ready for discharge 7 to 10 days after surgery.

6. If gastrectomy has been combined with vagotomy, prolonged gastric atony secondary to the paralyzing effect of vagotomy on the smooth muscle of the stomach may occur. The surgeon usually will leave the Levin tube in place and on suction until he is certain that normal gastric function has resumed. This may require 4 to 5 days or longer. Failure to recognize gastric atony may result in a progressive dilatation of the stomach and fatal aspiration. If the Levin tube or the gastrostomy tube has been clamped and the patient has begun to receive liquids, any suspicion of gastric distention should lead to unclamping of the tube to test for residual fluid or gas under pressure. If either is noted, the surgeon should be informed and the tube left on suction until further instructions are given.

CONTROVERSIAL ASPECTS OF ULCER SURGERY

The evolution of ulcer surgery has passed through several distinct stages, and the last word on such surgery has not been heard. The subject is of historical interest, and the student is referred to standard books on ulcer surgery for a detailed description of past and present procedures.

Subtotal gastrectomy, in which 70 to 80 per cent of the stomach is removed, was the standard procedure in this country for many decades and is the method described and illustrated in this chapter. The procedure is very effective in curing ulcer disease but carries with it an unacceptable incidence of long-term metabolic and nutritional defects. With the development of vagotomy and the proof that vagotomy in combination with a lesser gastric resection (30 to 50 per cent) could create anacidity in the remaining stomach pouch, more radical resections lost their popularity in this country and are now being abandoned. The lesser resections, in combination with vagotomy, afford the same high cure rate for ulcer disease as the radical surgery, and with far less devastating effects on nutrition and metabolism.

In an effort to reduce the mortality rate from ulcer surgery, some surgeons have turned to an operation that combines vagotomy with a drainage procedure such as pyloroplasty or gastrojejunostomy. The gastric antrum is resected (50 per cent) in an effort to remove the source of *gastrin,* a stimulant to the production of acid from the body of the stomach. The drainage procedures *do not remove* the antrum but allegedly prevent it from secreting gastrin by preventing antral distention, which is a stimulus to gastrin release. While the mortality rate is slightly reduced by drainage procedures, the recurrence rate for ulcer disease is distinctly increased. There is, therefore, a persistent controversy between the "resectionists" and the "non-resectionists" as to which procedure is ideal for definitive ulcer disease. It may turn out that both types of procedures are valid under different circumstances and that individual tailoring of the procedures to fit these circumstances will offer the best care for each patient.

STUDY QUESTIONS

1. List four indications for surgery for a duodenal ulcer.

2. Describe the technique and rationale of gastric analysis. What is the nurse's role in this test?

3. List some causes of anxiety in the patient about to undergo gastrectomy. How would you manage them?

4. Is there a typical "psychological make-up" of the ulcer patient? Defend your answer with references and examples.

5. Describe some of the factors that predispose a patient to peptic ulcer. Do you think *chronic worrying* is significant in the development of duodenal ulcer? Justify your answer.

6. What place does vagotomy have in the surgical treatment of duodenal ulcer?

7. What is a von Petz gastrectomy clamp? Describe its structure and function to your class, preferably demonstrating its use by obtaining one from the O.R. supervisor.

8. What is a Payr clamp?

9. Why is closure of the duodenum such an important part of gastric surgery?

10. The patient lapses into profound shock 12 hours after gastrectomy. List all possible causes of this episode. Describe all the clinical and laboratory studies which the surgeon may use to arrive at the cause of shock. What role does the nurse play in aiding the surgeon? What patient needs must be attended to? What are the inherent nursing responsibilities?

11. A restless postgastrectomy patient pulls out his Levin Tube. The nurse promptly reinserts the tube. Discuss this action in class.

12. What is the difference between a Billroth I and a Billroth II gastrectomy? Diagram your answer for class.

13. If the patient is forbidden fluids by mouth while on gastric drainage, what nursing measures may be performed to maintain comfort?

14. Outline a 24-hour nursing care plan for the patient who has undergone a subtotal gastrectomy.

15. Discuss the long-term nutritional and metabolic deficiencies resulting from a subtotal gastrectomy.

THE PATIENT WITH
A RUPTURED SPLEEN

25

Operation: Splenectomy

TYPICAL HISTORY

An 18-year-old boy was admitted through the emergency room following an injury sustained in a football game. The exact details of the accident are not clear to the boy, but he believes that he was struck in the upper abdomen by an opposing player's knee. He is complaining of upper abdominal pain and states that he has vomited twice since the injury.

PHYSICAL EXAMINATION

The patient is a well-developed male complaining of upper abdominal and *left shoulder pain.*

Significant Findings

1. Pallor is noted, particularly around the lips.
2. There is hypotension (90/50).
3. The pulse is rapid and thready — 110 beats per minute.
4. There is tenderness in the upper abdomen, particularly on the left side.
5. Rigidity of the left rectus muscle is noted.
6. There is tenderness over the tenth and eleventh ribs.
7. Bowel sounds are diminished to absent.

DIAGNOSTIC STUDIES

1. WBC is 21,000 per cu. mm.
2. Hematocrit level is 37 per cent.
3. Chest x-ray indicates fracture of tenth and eleventh ribs on left side.
4. Flat and upright x-rays of abdomen are negative.

PROBABLE HOSPITAL COURSE

1. The history and physical findings in this case are classic for impending hemorrhagic shock due to a ruptured spleen. *No time can be wasted* in preparing this patient for immediate surgery.

219

2. The history and physical findings are not always as clear-cut as in this case. Quite frequently, the only abnormal finding is slight tenderness over the spleen. The patient will then be observed until a ruptured viscus is entirely ruled out. The points to watch for are:

   a. A falling hematocrit level. This should be tested every 6 to 8 hours initially, then once or twice daily.
   b. Increasing pallor, restlessness, and syncope.
   c. Instability of vital signs.
   d. Increasing abdominal pain or abdominal distention.
   e. Special diagnostic studies may be ordered when there is a slight suspicion of ruptured spleen but not enough evidence to warrant immediate surgery. These studies include:
      (1) splenic scan (Fig. 25–1)
      (2) celiac angiogram
      (3) laparoscopy

PREPARATION FOR SURGERY

1. Levin tube inserted preoperatively.
2. Abdomen prepped from nipple line as far as and including pubis. (See Introduction.)
3. Type and cross-match for four to six units of blood.
4. Large-bore I.V. or, preferably, intracatheter inserted on ward.
5. Enema not necessary.
6. Routine premedications.
7. No special medications.
8. *Operating Room Skin Prep.* From nipples as far as and including pubis. (See Introduction.)
9. *Position.* Horizontal supine. (See Introduction.)

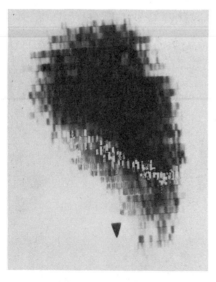 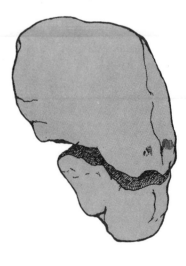

FIGURE 25–1 A ruptured spleen, shown on scan and in a schematic illustration.

PATHOLOGY

The spleen may show all degrees of injury:

1. A *subcapsular hematoma,* due to contusion of the spleen. There may be no free blood in the peritoneal cavity. This hematoma will continue to enlarge, finally rupturing through the capsule, when bleeding becomes profuse.

2. A *lacerated spleen,* which may involve large segments of the spleen or only a tip.

3. *Widespread destruction of the spleen,* which may appear as a large, friable organ filled with fresh and old blood clots. The peritoneal cavity may contain one to several pints of blood.

GENERAL RATIONALE AND SCHEME

The spleen is too friable an organ to be safely repaired following minor trauma. In all instances, it is safer to remove the spleen than to risk delayed bleeding from a sutured area. The *operative scheme* consists of six steps.

1. Exploration through a left upper abdominal vertical incision. (See Introduction.)
2. Delivery of spleen into the wound.
3. Ligation of splenic vein and artery.
4. Excision of spleen.
5. Thorough irrigation of all blood clots.
6. Closure of abdomen.

PROCEDURE

1. *Opening Abdomen.* A left upper abdominal vertical incision is the most commonly used. Diagnosis of intraperitoneal hemorrhage is usually immediately confirmed when blood gushes forth as soon as the peritoneum is opened. (See Introduction.)

2. *Exploration.* The source of bleeding is confirmed. Further exploration for other trauma is deferred until the injured spleen is removed and bleeding controlled.

3. The spleen is delivered into the wound by *rotating* it out of its bed in the left upper quadrant. A large, warm, moist abdominal pack may be placed in the splenic bed.

4. The hilum of the spleen contains the major veins and arteries of the spleen. These are located and *individually* clamped, divided, and ligated with heavy suture. Major bleeding from the spleen is now controlled and the remaining steps can be done slowly and with greater caution.

5. The spleen is easily excised by dividing its mesenteric attachments to *diaphragm, kidney,* and *stomach.*

6. The splenic bed and left subdiaphragmatic area are thoroughly irrigated with warm saline to remove all fluid and blood.

7. Re-exploration of stomach, pancreas, kidney, and intestines is carried out to assure that no other injuries have occurred.

8. The abdominal wound is closed in the usual manner. Many surgeons will place a drain in the left subdiaphragmatic space and bring it out through a stab wound. The drain is intended to prevent collection of blood under the diaphragm and to pick up any drainage from a possible unrecognized injury to the tail of the pancreas.

SURGICAL HAZARDS

1. *Failure to Control Massive Hemorrhage.* Death may be caused by massive blood loss from the splenic artery in spite of all attempts to reach and control the bleeding vessel.

2. *Injury to Nearby Organs.* Surgery for massive bleeding is often necessarily hasty and done with poor visualization due to the uncontrolled bleeding. Nearby structures, *particularly the pancreas,* are prone to injury.

3. *Overlooking Other Injuries.* There is danger of assuming that only one organ has been injured once the major source of hemorrhage has been controlled. A thorough investigation must be carried out before the operation is completed.

EARLY POSTOPERATIVE MANAGEMENT

1. Levin tube connected to low suction. Managed as described in preceding chapters.

2. *Careful Monitoring of Vital Signs.* Under-replacement of lost blood or continued bleeding is the most common cause of postoperative hypotension following surgery for abdominal trauma.

3. *Pulmonary complications,* particularly a left lower lobe pneumonia, are prone to occur due to splinting of diaphragm on involved side. Coughing, deep breathing, and turning must be urged frequently.

4. *Wound Care.* Usually negligible, as wound is often not drained.

5. It is most important in this, as well as in other injuries — particularly those incurred in automobile accidents — to be on constant alert for further complications that may become evident one or more days after the accident. Some of the common problems to anticipate are:

 a. *Pulmonary Contusion* ("wet lung"): This can develop insidiously after any crushing injury of the chest wall. There may be no external signs of chest wall contusion. Unexplained restlessness may indicate early anoxia and impending respiratory failure. The use of sedatives and analgesics can be disastrous here, for further obtunding of the patient's condition can lead to respiratory arrest. Frequent chest x-rays and monitoring of arterial blood gases can indicate serious pulmonary complications, which must *always* be suspected.

 b. *Cerebral Injury:* The vagaries of subdural hematoma, cerebral hemorrhage, and cerebral edema are well known. Careful neurological examination, with particular attention to the level of consciousness, is mandatory if there is the remotest possibility of central nervous system injury.

 c. *Cardiac Contusion:* Any arrhythmia, unexplained hypotension, or shock should suggest cardiac contusion with or without pericardial tamponade. If any significant chest injury is suspected, a continuous monitoring of cardiac function should be instituted, along with careful monitoring of the central venous pressure.

 d. *Occult Injury to Extremities:* Most musculoskeletal injuries that have initially spared the circulation take low priority in the critically injured patient, and may not receive due attention. A fractured long bone, undiagnosed and left unsplinted, can ultimately lead to serious nerve or blood vessel damage. You should carry out careful and frequent evaluations of the upper and lower extremities in order to detect signs of fractures or dislocations.

STUDY QUESTIONS

1. Do you think the patient described in this chapter would have benefited from *diagnostic paracentesis*? From laparoscopy?

2. If the surgeon had chosen to perform a *paracentesis,* what instruments and other equipment would you anticipate he would have needed? What is the nurse's role in aiding the surgeon?

3. Explain why the patient described demonstrated signs of shock shortly after the injury to his spleen *in spite* of a hematocrit value of 37 per cent.

4. What is the signficance of an elevated WBC in ruptured spleen?

5. The abdominal x-ray in this case was negative. What x-ray signs might have been present that would suggest splenic injury? What is the role of celiac angiography in the diagnosis of a ruptured spleen?

6. A 20-year-old male is admitted for observation following blunt trauma to his abdomen. He is under observation by his surgeon to determine whether his spleen has been ruptured. Eight hours after admission he complains to the nurse *of left shoulder pain.* She reassures him that the shoulder might have been sprained in the injury and attempts to ease the pain with use of a hot water bottle. Would you have followed this course of action? Explain.

7. What is so-called *delayed rupture* of the spleen?

8. Discuss the anatomic relationships between the pancreas and the spleen in terms of possible injury to the pancreas during splenectomy.

9. Why is pneumonia a possible complication of splenectomy? What nursing measures should the nurse carry out in an attempt to prevent this complication?

10. What are the indications for administering blood postoperatively in a patient who has undergone splenectomy? What nursing observations might you make that would indicate that the patient would have need of this therapy?

11. Discuss the types of blood reactions that might follow multiple transfusions, touching on signs and symptoms and the nurse's role in management of these reactions. What is the procedure *in your hospital* when a patient has a transfusion reaction?

12. Acute pancreatitis may follow splenectomy. What are the signs and symptoms of this condition? How is acute pancreatitis managed?

Operation: Ileotransverse Colostomy

TYPICAL HISTORY

For several years, a 30-year-old female has had recurrent episodes of lower abdominal pain, periumbilical cramps, and diarrhea alternating with constipation. Recently, she has noted the onset of severe right lower quadrant pain, which is steady and is associated with severe periumbilical cramps, fever, and chills. She has also vomited on several occasions.

PHYSICAL EXAMINATION

The patient is a thin, pale, and poorly nourished female in acute abdominal distress.

Significant Findings

1. Pallor and malnutrition are noted.
2. The patient is dehydrated.
3. Some abdominal distention is evident. Hyperperistaltic and high-pitched rushes can be heard with the stethoscope.
4. There is tenderness and rebound tenderness in the right lower quadrant, with some muscle guarding.

DIAGNOSTIC STUDIES

1. Flat and upright abdominal x-rays reveal distention of loops of small intestine with fluid levels.
2. WBC is 25,000, with a marked shift to the left.
3. Hematocrit is 34 per cent.
4. Sedimentation rate is 40 mm. in 1 hour.
5. Serum albumin is low, serum $[K]^+$ levels are low, and the patient is anemic.

PROBABLE HOSPITAL COURSE

The patient's chronic history as well as her present findings are suggestive of regional ileitis, although acute appendicitis is difficult to rule out prior to surgery. Following x-rays of the abdomen and laboratory studies, the patient will be explored as an emergency procedure. If her fluid balance is in a precarious state, 12 to 15 hours may be required to restore hydration and blood volume prior to surgery. As a rule of thumb, a patient with a pulse rate of greater than 140 per minute is usually too serious a risk for immediate surgery.

PREPARATION FOR SURGERY

1. A Levin tube or long intestinal tube is inserted according to the surgeon's preference.
2. A large-bore intravenous needle or intracatheter should be inserted for I.V. fluid therapy.
3. The patient is typed and cross-matched for two units of blood if regional ileitis is suspected.
4. Skin prep from nipples as far as and including the pubis. (See Introduction.)
5. *Enema.* A Fleet enema may be given.
6. *Premedications.* Routine.
7. *Special Medications.* None.
8. *Operating Room Prep.* From nipples as far as and including the pubis. (See Introduction.)
9. *Position.* Horizontal supine. (See Introduction.)

PATHOLOGY

A wide variety of pathological findings is likely to be found in the presence of regional ileitis.
1. Segmental regional ileitis, localized to the terminal ileum, may present as a boggy, indurated, swollen mass near the cecum, with proximal distention of the small intestine, which will be filled with fluid and gas.
2. There may be multiple perforations of the ileum, with fistulae either to surrounding organs or to the skin. If perforation has occurred, multiple abscesses may be found in the pelvis or free pus may be found.
3. There may be "skip" areas of enteritis, involving any part of the gastrointestinal tract.

GENERAL RATIONALE AND SCHEME

Resection of the grossly inflamed and partially obstructing small bowel affords the best chance of eliminating the mechanically obstructing segment of bowel. In addition, resection of the diseased segment ameliorates the toxic effects of ileitis and usually results in significant nutritional, hematological, and metabolic improvement.

Scheme

1. The abdomen is opened in the usual fasion through a right lower paramedian incision.
2. The diseased segment of small bowel (and in many cases the right colon) is resected, and an ileotransverse colostomy is carried out (Fig. 26–1).

PROCEDURE

1. *Skin Incision.* The commonly used incision is a right paramedian muscle retracting incision. (See Introduction.)

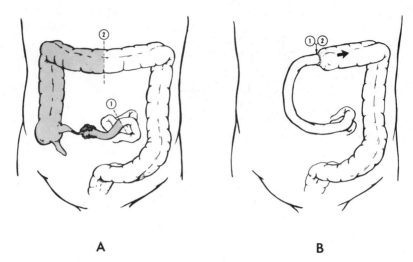

A   B

FIGURE 26-1 *A.* Resection of diseased ileum and right colon for obstructing regional ileitis. *B.* End-to-end ileotransverse colostomy.

2. *Draping the Skin.* This is important, as inadvertent spillage of small intestinal contents may occur during the anastomosis.

3. The abdomen is opened and the diagnosis of regional ileitis and small bowel obstruction is confirmed.

4. If the terminal ileum is diseased, it will be removed along with the right colon.

5. The lateral mesenteric attachment of the right colon is divided. The surgeon must take care to identify and preserve the right ureter during this procedure.

6. The ascending and transverse mesocolon are serially clamped, divided, and ligated. Heavy ligatures are used for this aspect of the surgery.

7. Clamps are placed on the ileum and mid-transverse colon at the point of resection. The intestine is then amputated and the remaining ends brought into approximation for end-to-end anastomosis.

8. A two-layer anastomosis is fashioned, and the rent in the mesentery is closed.

9. The abdomen is closed in the usual manner.

SURGICAL HAZARDS

1. The right ureter is often close to the diseased bowel and may be incorporated in an inflammatory mass in this area. It is easily injured during the process of dissecting the small intestine.

2. The diseased small intestine sometimes is easily ruptured during the course of mobilizing surrounding tissues. Such a rupture will result in immediate massive contamination of the peritoneal cavity.

EARLY POSTOPERATIVE COURSE

1. *Levin Tube.* Routine management.

2. Intravenous fluid therapy is particularly important, as the patient is often dehydrated owing to the tremendous loss of fluid into the small intestine. Consequently, a careful charting of urine

output via a Foley catheter, as well as intravenous intake, must be started upon the patient's arrival in the recovery room.

3. *Vital Signs.* The patient suffering from regional ileitis often is in a precarious state with regard to blood volume and fluid and electrolyte balance. Consequently, the trauma of surgery may initiate stressful mechanisms, resulting in early postoperative hypotension. Vital signs are watched every 15 to 20 minutes during the period in the recovery room.

4. *Care of the Wound.* Drains are not usually required in the operation. Consequently, the wound should be dry and require no immediate care in the recovery room.

5. Postoperative sepsis is a threat because of spillage of intestinal contents during emergency surgery in an already debilitated patient.

STUDY QUESTIONS

1. What synonyms are there for regional ileitis?

2. Can you list some of the proposed theories as to the etiology of this disease?

3. Are all cases of regional ileitis treated surgically? If not, what is the medical therapy for this disease?

4. How would you allay the fears of a patient with regional ileitis preoperatively?

5. A great many articles have been written about emotional support. What does this mean to you as a nurse and how does it affect your patient care?

6. What is the difference between an end-to-end and an end-to-side ileotransverse colostomy? Can you diagram these operations for your class?

7. Describe the surgical steps involved in an end-to-end ileotransverse colostomy to your class.

8. Describe the most important aspects of postoperative nursing care of a patient undergoing ileotransverse colostomy. (Pay particular attention to the possible fluid and electrolyte problems and how they are to be handled.)

9. What hematologic and metabolic derangements are likely to be found in severe, chronic regional enteritis? How might these derangements affect the patient's postoperative course?

10. Discuss regional ileitis with respect to:
    a. Areas of bowel involved.
    b. Lymph node involvement.
    c. Problem of fistulae.
    d. Course of disease.
    e. Signs and symptoms.
    f. "String sign."
    g. Modes of therapy.
    h. Indications for surgery.

27

THE PATIENT WITH
A SMALL BOWEL
PERFORATION

Operation: Small Bowel Resection

TYPICAL HISTORY

A 30-year-old male in excellent health was involved in an automobile accident. He states that his abdomen was thrust against the steering wheel and he now complains of severe, steady, periumbilical abdominal pain. There is no past history of gastrointestinal symptoms.

PHYSICAL EXAMINATION

The patient is a well-developed male experiencing acute abdominal pain.

Significant Findings

1. There is marked pallor and sweating.
2. Blood pressure is 80/60, pulse is 120 and regular.
3. There is guarding of the entire abdomen; bowel sounds are absent; no masses are felt.
4. There is some ecchymosis in the periumbilical region.
5. The remainder of the physical examination is unremarkable.

DIAGNOSTIC STUDIES

1. WBC is 18,000, with a shift to the left.
2. The hematocrit value is 37 per cent.
3. The urinalysis is normal.
4. Chest x-ray demonstrates a small amount of air under both diaphragms.

PROBABLE HOSPITAL COURSE

The patient has suffered acute, blunt trauma to his abdomen. The presence of air under his diaphragm suggests that a hollow viscus has been ruptured, and he will be taken to the operating room as soon as his general condition permits.

228

PREPARATION FOR SURGERY

1. A Levin tube is inserted and connected to low suction.
2. The patient is typed and cross-matched for four to five units of whole blood.
3. The abdomen is prepped from the nipple line as far as and including the pubis. (See Introduction.)
4. An enema is not given.
5. *Premedications.* Routine.
6. *Special Medications.* None.
7. *Operating Room Skin Prep.* The entire abdomen from the nipple line as far as and including the pubis should be prepped according to the hospital routine. (See Introduction.)
8. *Position.* Horizontal supine. (See Introduction.)

PATHOLOGY

The abdomen is opened through an incision chosen by the surgeon on the basis of the probable type of trauma. In the present case, periumbilical pain and the presence of air under the diaphragm suggest that the small bowel may have been injured. Therefore, the surgeon chooses an incision which he feels will be adequate for the entire area of pathology. The abdomen is opened through this incision, which may be a right or left midabdominal vertical incision. Skin towels are applied in the usual fashion. The entire abdomen is explored, and, in this particular case, the small bowel and the mid-ileum show an area of contusion and ecchymosis in the wall of the bowel, with two areas of perforation of the bowel wall.

GENERAL RATIONALE AND SCHEME

The continuity of the gastrointestinal tract obviously must be restored to prevent generalized peritonitis and death. If the area of contusion around the perforated areas of bowel is extensive, the surgeon will elect to do a resection of the bowel rather than attempt to close the small perforation. On the other hand, if these small perforations are not surrounded by unhealthy tissue, the surgeon may elect merely to close the perforations.

Scheme

1. Large rubber-shod clamps are placed distal and proximal to the area of resection to prevent gastrointestinal contents from spilling out through the resected area of bowel.
2. Allin clamps and Ochsner clamps are placed proximal and distal to the perforated area.
3. The perforated bowel is resected and an end-to-end anastomosis created.
4. The mesentery is approximated with running catgut stitches.
5. Drains may or may not be used.
6. The abdomen is closed in the usual fashion.

PROCEDURE

1. *Skin Incision.* A great variety of incisions may be used, depending on the surgeon's preference and his estimate of the area and type of pathologic conditions. Some type of vertical incision is preferred.

2. *Opening Peritoneum.* This is done very cautiously to avoid injuring any underlying structures, particularly the small bowel. The wound edges should be covered with skin drapes to avoid contamination if bowel resection is indicated.

3. *Exploration.* A complete exploration of every viscus contained in the abdomen must be meticulously carried out to be certain multiple injuries to viscera are not present. This is particularly true of the small bowel. The entire small bowel must be carefully examined for other perforations near those which are obvious.

4. Once it has been determined that the injury is limited to perforations of the small bowel, the surgeon must determine whether these perforations can be closed primarily or a resection of bowel is indicated.

5. If resection of the bowel is indicated, the surgeon will milk the gastrointestinal contents from the injured area of bowel and place large rubber-shod clamps proximal and distal to the area of injury to prevent gastrointestinal contents from spilling into the line of anastomosis.

6. Small Allin and Ochsner clamps are used to clamp the bowel proximal and distal to the area of injury. The bowel is divided between these sets of clamps (Fig. 27–1).

7. The antimesenteric borders of both proximal and distal bowel are approximated, and a posterior seromuscular suture of interrupted 3–0 silk suture is used as a first layer. The Allin clamps are removed, care being taken to avoid spillage of bowel contents by using suction and draping of the abdominal contents. A through-and-through suture of 3–0 chromic catgut is used on the posterior wall as a running interlocking stitch. This is converted on the anterior wall to a Connell stitch which inverts the mucosa. The second anterior seromuscular layer again consists of interrupted 3–0 silk sutures.

8. The surgeon now tests the patency of the anastomosis to be certain that the lumen of the anastomosis admits at least one finger.

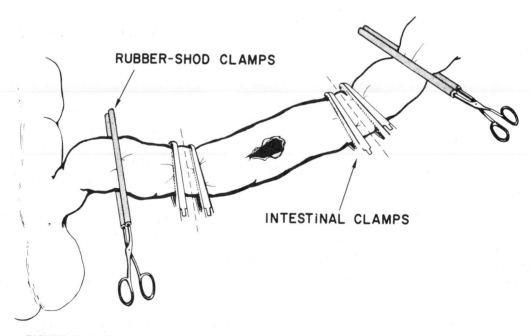

RUBBER-SHOD CLAMPS

INTESTINAL CLAMPS

FIGURE 27–1 Clamps on small bowel prior to resection. Note outer rubber-shod clamps which prevent soilage at time of anastomosis.

9. The mesenteric aperture is now closed with a running 3–0 chromic catgut suture to prevent herniation of the bowel through the rent in the mesentery.

10. The rubber-shod clamps are removed.

11. The abdomen is closed in the usual fashion after liberal irrigation with body-warm saline or Ringer's lactate solution.

SURGICAL HAZARDS

1. *Failure to Recognize Associated Injuries.* This is, by far, the most serious and frequent surgical hazard, and it is avoided by meticulous and thorough investigation of all abdominal viscera.

2. *Contamination of Wound and Peritoneal Cavity.* Failure to apply rubber-shod clamps and to drape the abdominal contents in the wound may result in massive contamination from an unprepared small bowel which can result in serious postoperative sepsis.

3. *Severe Uncontrolled Hemorrhage.* Large vessels contained within the mesentery of the small bowel may have been avulsed or injured by the accident and uncontrolled hemorrhage may occur. Consequently, four to five pints of blood should be available before this type of surgery is contemplated.

EARLY POSTOPERATIVE MANAGEMENT

The patient is returned to the recovery room until sufficiently reactive from the anesthetic.

1. *Levin Tube.* If present, this should be connected immediately to intermittent suction apparatus and cared for in the usual fashion.

2. *Pulmonary Complications.* Associated and unrecognized chest trauma caused by the abdomen's being thrust against the steering wheel may result in accumulation of large amounts of postoperative secretions. These should be carefully watched for and the surgeon notified if the patient has any pulmonary difficulty. If there are any signs of restlessness, anoxia, or pulmonary distress, daily chest x-rays and frequent blood gas analyses should be instituted in order to detect pulmonary contusion.

3. *Management of the Wound.* Unless drains are used, the dressings should remain dry. If blood or fluid soaks through the dressing, the surgeon should be notified.

4. *Postoperative Shock.* The vital signs must be carefully monitored as unrecognized associated injuries may result in massive intra-abdominal bleeding which will manifest itself as postoperative shock.

STUDY QUESTIONS

1. What is the significance of air under the diaphragm in the evaluation of abdominal trauma?

2. List several common chest and abdominal injuries which may result when the driver of a car is crushed against the steering wheel.

3. Describe the structure and function of rubber-shod clamps. In what other areas of surgery might they be used?

4. Describe to your class the steps in a small bowel resection.

5. What are the nutritional implications of a small bowel resection?

6. Why is the frequency of postoperative wound sepsis greater in intestinal surgery performed following trauma than it is in elective intestinal surgery?

7. What is the difference in structure between an Ochsner clamp and an Allin clamp? How does this difference in structure affect the use of each clamp in intestinal surgery?

8. What *complications* might be anticipated by the nurse in caring for a patient who has had surgery on the small bowel?

9. On the first day after small bowel resection for traumatic perforation that occurred in an automobile accident, the patient has become restless, somewhat confused, and dyspneic. His pulse has risen to 110; hematocrit is stable at 40; there is no change in blood pressure. What is the most likely cause of this clinical picture, and what tests should be used to evaluate the patient further?

28

THE PATIENT WITH SMALL BOWEL OBSTRUCTION

Operation: Lysis of Adhesions

TYPICAL HISTORY

A 65-year-old male enters the hospital with a three-day history of colic-like abdominal pains, abdominal distention, vomiting, and inability to move his bowels. He has enjoyed excellent health for 25 years, and his only past medical history was an appendectomy for a ruptured appendix 25 years ago.

PHYSICAL EXAMINATION

The patient is a well-developed, acutely ill male in severe distress with abdominal distention.

Significant Findings

1. Dehydration, with dry mucous membranes and loss of tissue turgor, is present.
2. There is a fecalent odor to the breath.

3. The abdomen is markedly distended, and hypertympany is evident on abdominal percussion.

4. Occasional high-pitched bowel sounds are audible.

5. There is no gas in the rectal ampulla on rectal exam.

DIAGNOSTIC STUDIES

1. Hematocrit is 56 per cent.
2. Urine shows a specific gravity of 1.028.
3. Electrolytes reveal low sodium and chloride levels.
4. Plain film of the abdomen reveals distended and fluid-filled loops of small intestine.

PROBABLE HOSPITAL COURSE

This patient demonstrates rather severe dehydration secondary to vomiting and fluid collection in his small bowel. The obstruction may be due to many causes but is likely related to adhesions resulting from his ruptured appendix 25 years ago. As long as there are no signs of *strangulating obstruction,* surgery is best postponed until bowel decompression is underway and the patient's fluid and electrolyte imbalances have been at least partially corrected. The elevated hematocrit and the specific gravity for the urine reflect rather marked dehydration, and surgery would be very dangerous at this stage. The patient is admitted to an intensive care unit for monitoring during this phase of his illness. A Foley catheter is inserted in order to measure hourly urine output. A central venous pressure line is inserted to make it possible to check for any fluid overload during the period of rehydration. Intravenous fluids are started and should include colloids and some form of saline infusion. Frequent hematocrits and determinations of the specific gravity and hourly output of the urine, together with CVP readings, will accurately reflect any improvement in hydration.

A long intestinal tube is inserted into the stomach and, under fluoroscopic guide, is passed through the pylorus in an effort to decompress the small bowel. Both the state of hydration and the progress in decompression will determine the timing of surgery. Ideally, this should be within 24 to 36 hours after admission, although careful clinical judgment must be used in each case to determine the safest period for each patient.

PREPARATION FOR SURGERY

1. The patient is cross-matched for 3 to 4 units of blood.
2. The abdomen is prepped from the nipple line to and including the pubis.
3. An enema is not necessary.
4. *Premedications.* Routine.
5. *Special Medications.* None.
6. *Operating Room Skin Prep.* The entire abdomen from the nipple line as far as and including the pubis should be prepped according to the hospital routine.
7. *Position.* Horizontal supine.

PATHOLOGY

Markedly distended loops of small bowel will usually be found on opening the abdomen, because even under the best of circumstances the long intestinal tube will probably not have completely decompressed the bowel. Multiple adhesions may be visible, and the point of bowel obstruction will be marked by a rather sharp transition between dilated, edematous, thickened bowel and the more distal thin-walled, soft, non-obstructed bowel. At the point of obstruction, one will usually find a band of adhesions which, in knife-like fashion, has pinned down and obstructed the bowel.

GENERAL RATIONALE AND SCHEME

The abdomen is opened and multiple adhesions are divided. The search is made for the point of obstruction; when it is found, lysis of the adhesions will in most cases release the obstruction and effect a cure. The abdomen is closed in the routine fashion.

Scheme

1. The abdomen is opened in the usual fashion. The choice of incision depends on the suspicion of the surgeon as to the location of the point of obstruction.
2. Adhesions are carefully dissected (the surgeon must take care not to injure any encased loops of small intestine).
3. The bowel is examined for any signs of strangulation. If strangulation is present, a small bowel resection will be required.
4. Once the obstruction has been released, the remainder of the bowel is carefully examined for any other points of obstruction.
5. If the bowel is too distended for a safe closure, a small opening is made in the bowel, and a tube (e.g., a Foley catheter) is used to evacuate retained fluid and gases. The small opening in the bowel is closed with catgut and silk sutures.
6. Drains are usually unnecessary.
7. The abdomen is closed in the usual fashion.

SURGICAL HAZARDS

1. Failure to recognize strangulated bowel. This will result in postoperative peritonitis and death.
2. Damage to bowel during dissection of adhesions.

POSTOPERATIVE MANAGEMENT

The patient is kept in the recovery room until he is sufficiently reactive from his anesthetic. He should then be returned to the intensive care unit for careful management of his fluid and electrolyte balance, which will need to be monitored for a short period of time after surgery.

1. The long intestinal tube is connected to intermittent suction. To encourage further descent into the intestines, the tube should be suspended loosely above the patient's head and *not taped* to his nose.
2. The Foley catheter is connected to dependent drainage, and careful hourly urine measurements are continued. The surgeon may wish to order evaluations of the specific gravity of the urine every 12 to 24 hours to check the patient's state of hydration. If the urine output falls to

less than 30 to 40 cc's per hour, the surgeon should be notified (unless he has left other specific orders regarding the output).

3. The CVP line should be checked for proper functioning, and frequent readings should be taken and recorded. The surgeon will often establish a range of low and high readings and will wish to be notified of any that fall outside the range.

4. If the obstruction has been relieved, the postoperative course should be uneventful. As peristalsis resumes, the abdomen will deflate; the long tube can then be removed and fluids started by mouth. As soon as the fluid and electrolyte abnormalities have been corrected, use of the CVP line, the Foley catheter, and intravenous fluids is discontinued, and the patient is discharged from the intensive care unit.

5. The sutures are removed in 7 to 10 days, at which time the patient may be discharged from the hospital.

STUDY QUESTIONS

1. List some important signs and symptoms of severe dehydration.

2. What are some of the signs of *strangulating obstruction?*

3. Why is surgery dangerous in the face of severe dehydration and abdominal distention from intestinal obstruction?

4. Discuss the function of a long intestinal tube. What factors are involved in the nursing management of such a tube?

5. Discuss the use of colloids and crystalloids in the management of fluid and electrolyte problems.

6. How would you determine that a CVP line is malfunctioning? What are some of the causes of a malfunctioning CVP line? What are the dangers of an unrecognized malfunction in a CVP line?

7. Why is the hematocrit such a valuable laboratory aid in the monitoring of the dehydrated patient? Do you think measurement of the serum potassium level would be a useful way to monitor the dehydrated patient under therapy?

8. Discuss urine and serum osmolality as aids in the management of the dehydrated patient.

Operation: Appendectomy

TYPICAL HISTORY

A 20-year-old male, in previous excellent health, noted the gradual onset of dull epigastric pain followed by anorexia, nausea, and one episode of vomiting. Within 4 to 5 hours, the pain had settled in the right lower quadrant where it became steady, sharp, and moderately severe. The patient denies any history of recent upper respiratory infections. He has had no dysuria, frequency, or hematuria.

PHYSICAL EXAMINATION

The patient is a well-developed, well-nourished male, lying quietly in bed, with his right leg flexed at the hip and knee, and in moderate abdominal distress. He is pale and appears to be somewhat anxious.

Significant Findings

1. There is acute point tenderness in the right lower quadrant over *McBurney's point.* (Fig. 29–1). In the typical case of acute appendicitis, the patient is able to point with one finger to the exact site of maximal tenderness. This "point tenderness" is a very important diagnostic sign.

2. There is some *spasm* of the right rectus muscle and a moderate degree of *rebound tenderness* on the right side. Any process causing localized peritonitis is liable to induce guarding or spasm of the overlying abdominal muscle. This is a reflex protective mechanism.

3. Rectal examination discloses tenderness on the right side. This sign is particularly apt to be present when the inflamed appendix is lying low in the pelvis near the rectum.

4. The pulse and blood pressure are normal.

5. The oral temperature is 99°F. Typically, an acute appendicitis causes very little rise in temperature unless rupture with generalized peritonitis has supervened.

DIAGNOSTIC STUDIES

1. WBC 12,000: polymorphonuclear leukocytes, 86 per cent; lymphocytes, 10 per cent; band forms, 4 per cent.

2. Urinalysis is normal.

3. Hematocrit level is 42 per cent.

4. Hemoglobin is 13 gm. per 100 ml.

5. Chest x-ray is normal.

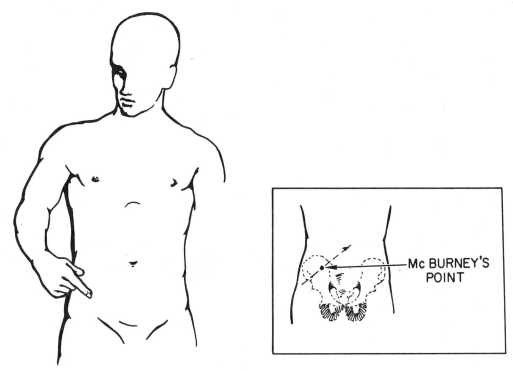

FIGURE 29–1 The patient is pointing to McBurney's point — an important finding in the diagnosis of acute appendicitis.

PROBABLE HOSPITAL COURSE

1. If the surgeon is certain of the diagnosis, the patient will be scheduled for surgery soon after admission.

2. If there is some doubt about the diagnosis, the surgeon may elect to defer surgery for several hours. During this period of time, the patient will not be allowed water or anything by mouth and will be examined at frequent intervals until the diagnosis of appendicitis is confirmed or ruled out.

Many conditions may mimic appendicitis, particularly in the female patient. Some of these conditions, and their usual course, are:

a. *Mesenteric Adenitis.* Low-grade abdominal pains, fever, and occasional vomiting may persist for 3 to 5 days, gradually subsiding thereafter. The condition is benign and self-limited, and requires no specific therapy. Tenderness is often vague and poorly localized.

b. *Ureteral Stone.* Characterized by severe colicky abdominal pains, which wax and wane, and are sometimes accompanied by reflex paralytic ileus, vomiting, and fever. If the stone passes into the urinary bladder, pain rapidly subsides and the patient recovers. Persistence of pain and the development of high fever may signal the onset of hydronephrosis or pyonephrosis due to obstruction of the ureter.

c. *Ruptured Ovarian Cyst.* Small amounts of blood in the pelvis may cause lower abdominal pain and tenderness. This usually subsides in 3 to 5 days without specific therapy.

d. *Ectopic Pregnancy.* This may present as lower abdominal pain. Should rupture occur, the patient may go rapidly into shock due to intra-abdominal bleeding. The nurse should check the vital signs carefully. Any significant change should be brought to the doctor's attention immediately. Increase in abdominal pain, the development of abdominal distention, or the change in location of the pain may also signify progression of the disease.

The nurse should never hesitate to notify the doctor of any change in the patient's condition which disturbs her.

e. *Abdominal Pain of Unknown Etiology.* Represents a potentially lethal situation and even the most subtle change of condition may be the signal of more serious problems to follow.

PREPARATION FOR SURGERY

Generally speaking, the early inflamed appendix presents little in the way of preparation from the point of view of fluids, electrolytes, and nutrition, all of which are usually normal. The following is all that is necessary:

1. Complete history and physical examination.

2. *Psychological Preparation.* The patient undergoing *emergency surgery* often harbors very serious fears. He is acutely ill to begin with and may even be concerned that the condition is worse than appendicitis. He may have heard of fatal cases of a *ruptured* appendix. He is often rushed out of his home in the middle of the night to undergo appendectomy by a surgeon he may not previously have known. Similar fears on his family's part compound his own anxieties. The referring physician and surgeon are often so busy in the "routine" evaluation and scheduling of the patient for surgery that the patient's fears escape their attention.

Thus, emergency surgery constitutes a unique situation as far as patient fears are concerned. Realization of these problems by the nurse affords her an excellent opportunity to share in the psychological preparation of the patient for appendectomy. A few words to boost the patient's confidence in his doctors is perfectly ethical and appropriate, provided this is done with honest intention and without casting any aspersions on other doctors. The relative safety of the operation should be stressed, allowing for the fact that it still is a major operation.

3. *Skin Prep.* The entire abdomen from nipple line as far as and including the pubis is cleanly shaven on the ward. (See Introduction.)

4. *Enema.* A soapsuds or Fleet enema may be ordered at the discretion of the surgeon. This is frequently omitted in acute appendicitis.

5. *Levin Tube.* Unnecessary unless the patient is vomiting.

6. *Blood.* Unnecessary.

7. *Premedications.* These are variable, but may be somewhat as follows:

a. Nembutal, 100 mg. I.M. 90 minutes preoperatively.

b. Atropine, 0.6 mg. I.M. 45 minutes preoperatively.

c. Demerol, 75 mg. I.M. 45 minutes preoperatively.

8. *Operating Room Skin Prep.* The entire abdomen and pubic area are thoroughly washed with pHisoHex and rinsed, then painted with tinted Zephiran. (There are other equally acceptable skin preps.)

9. *Position.* Horizontal supine position. (See Introduction.)

10. *Special Medications.* None.

PATHOLOGY

1. *Acute Appendicitis.* The early stage is manifested by a swollen, turgid, and reddish-purple appendix.

2. *Gangrenous Appendicitis.* This is a more advanced stage of the process. The appendix is black, oozes purulent material, and is on the verge of perforation.

3. *Perforated Appendix.* In the final stage, the appendix perforates, spilling its contents into the peritoneal cavity. If the contents are localized, an appendiceal abscess forms. If no localization has occurred, generalized peritonitis will be present. This may be fatal.

GENERAL RATIONALE AND SCHEME

The inflamed appendix must be removed for fear of its perforating.

Scheme

1. The abdomen is opened and explored; the diagnosis is confirmed and other significant pathological processes are excluded.
2. The blood supply to the appendix is ligated.
3. The appendix is amputated and the stump is cauterized and sterilized.

PROCEDURE

1. *Skin Incision.* The two most commonly used incisions are the right paramedian and McBurney's incision (Fig. 29–1).

2. *Draping Incision.* Because of the possibility of pus being present within the peritoneal cavity, the skin should be draped with towels or abdominal packs prior to the opening of the peritoneum.

3. *Opening Peritoneum.* If purulent fluid escapes, it should be cultured and the excess suctioned.

4. *Delivering Appendix.* The surgeon searches for and delivers the cecum and its attached appendix into the wound.

5. *Dividing Blood Supply.* The mesoappendix contains the appendiceal artery or arteries. These are clamped, divided, and ligated.

6. *Draping Cecum.* An abdominal pack is placed around the base of the appendix to cover the cecum.

7. *Amputating Appendix.* The appendix is clamped near its base and doubly ligated. It is then amputated. The stump may be inverted into the cecum and oversewn with a purse-string suture, or its exposed surface may be cauterized and sterilized with carbolic acid and alcohol. The cecum is then returned to the right iliac fossa.

8. *Closure.* The peritoneum is usually closed with 0 chromic catgut as a running suture. If a paramedian incision has been used, the rectus muscle is then returned to its bed and the anterior fascia is closed with interrupted sutures of catgut or silk. If McBurney's incision has been used, the internal and external oblique muscles are closed, usually with catgut. A drain is used if an appendiceal abscess is found.

SURGICAL HAZARDS

1. *Hemorrhage from Appendiceal Artery.* Very rarely, a large branch of the appendiceal artery may be divided before ligating. Bleeding can be profuse but is usually easily controlled by the surgeon.

2. *Rupture of an Intact Appendix.* The inflamed appendix is very friable. Through careless handling at times, in spite of meticulous technique, the appendix can be torn or ruptured, resulting in spillage of contaminated material into the peritoneal cavity.

3. *Injury to Ureter.* A retrocecal appendix may lie close to the right ureter. Poor lighting, improper exposure, or attempts to control hemorrhage may result in injury or ligation of the right ureter.

EARLY POSTOPERATIVE MANAGEMENT

The patient is returned to the recovery room until sufficiently reactive from the anesthetic. The routine management is discussed in Chapter 4 of Part I, and this should be carefully reviewed at this time. The usual course of the postappendectomy patient is smooth, and few problems are to be anticipated.

1. *Pulmonary Problems.* If spinal anesthesia has been used, pulmonary difficulties are rare, since the lower abdominal incision used will not interfere with respirations.

2. *Pain and Restlessness.* The patient is generally quite comfortable and needs very little in the way of narcotics. Often 50 mg. of Demerol every 4 to 6 hours will suffice.

3. *Nausea and Vomiting.* When these occur, a mild antiemetic drug may be prescribed. The nausea and vomiting are due to the anesthetics and premedications and are quite transient.

4. *Urinary Retention.* A lower abdominal incision may be quite painful when contraction of the abdominal wall is attempted in the act of micturition. This frequently results in acute urinary retention and catheterization may be necessary.

5. *Care of the Wound.* For routine appendectomy, the wound drains very little blood and no recovery room care is necessary. If a ruptured appendix was treated with drainage, the dressing may need reinforcing in the recovery room.

6. *Shock.* Rarely, the appendiceal artery ligature may slip and intra-abdominal bleeding may begin. Shock is usually slow in onset and very insidious as the appendiceal artery is relatively small. Any persistent change in the vital signs should be carefully noted and reported to the surgeon.

7. In the case of a ruptured appendix with generalized peritonitis, the following measures may be necessary in the immediate postoperative period:
   a. Semi-Fowler's position at all times to encourage drainage of pus into the pelvis.
   b. Nothing by mouth.
   c. Careful intake and output chart.
   d. Intravenous fluids containing antibiotics.
   e. Wound dressing changes p.r.n.

8. Wound sepsis is a common occurrence after appendectomy, particularly in advanced cases. This complication is usually heralded, on the third or fourth day after surgery, by increasing wound pain and a fluctuating temperature. The wound should be inspected frequently for swelling, local tenderness, and the beginning of fluctuance. Any drainage should be cultured.

STUDY QUESTIONS

1. What are the typical clinical features of appendicitis?

2. What conditions may mimic appendicitis? What is mesenteric adenitis?

3. Do you think the male or female patient is more apt to have a pathologic condition other than appendicitis mimicking this disease? Why?

4. Are there any known factors predisposing to appendicitis?

5. Why are laxatives dangerous for any severe abdominal pain?

6. Can appendicitis be treated medically? May antibiotics be used?

7. Make a list of activities the nurse should carry out in the preoperative preparation of the patient.

8. What factors may predispose the patient undergoing appendectomy to fear? How would you help to minimize these fears?

9. What is McBurney's incision? What other incisions may be used?

10. Where is McBurney's point? What is the cecum? What is the mesoappendix?

11. Why is the amputated appendiceal stump cauterized and sterilized? What chemicals are commonly used for this procedure?

12. Sketch a rough cross section through the lower abdominal wall, labeling all layers.

13. A 22-year-old female is under observation with acute lower abdominal pain. You have noted a gradually rising pulse rate and the patient appears pale. What likely diagnosis comes to your mind? Should the surgeon be notified of this changing pulse rate?

14. Advanced generalized peritonitis secondary to ruptured appendicitis presents certain signs and symptoms. Can you list some of them? What are some of the modes of therapy used for generalized peritonitis?

15. Review the immediate postoperative nursing care of:
   a. A patient with an uncomplicated appendectomy
   b. A patient who has undergone appendectomy with drainage of an appendiceal abscess

Operation: Colostomy

TYPICAL HISTORY

A 70-year-old male has noted intermittent abdominal cramps, constipation alternating with diarrhea, and weight loss for several months. Three days prior to admission he noted the onset of complete intestinal obstruction and abdominal distention which worsened steadily.

PHYSICAL EXAMINATION

An elderly, emaciated male is admitted experiencing acute abdominal distress.

Significant Findings

1. There is severe abdominal distention with dyspnea and cyanosis due to elevation of the diaphragm.
2. The patient is dehydrated and emaciated, with hypotension and tachycardia due to excess loss of body fluids.
3. The rectal examination is negative; no stool is found in the rectum.
4. Pallor is noted.

DIAGNOSTIC STUDIES

1. Flat and upright abdominal x-ray studies. There is distention of the large and small bowel with obvious gas-fluid levels in the small bowel.
2. WBC is 19,000 per cu. mm.
3. Hematocrit reading is 31 per cent.
4. Electrolyte values include a low sodium level of 131 mEq. per liter and a low potassium level of 2.4 mEq. per liter.
5. BUN level is 60 mg. per cent.

PROBABLE HOSPITAL COURSE

1. The great danger of large bowel obstruction is the possibility of perforation of the cecum. Surgery is, therefore, *relatively urgent* in acute large bowel obstruction as it provides the only certain way of relieving the obstruction.

242

2. A period of 12 to 24 hours is used both for ruling out conditions that can be treated conservatively as well as for repairing the fluid and electrolyte damage created by the obstruction. There are three conditions which do not require surgery but which may mimic a surgical large bowel obstruction:

> *Sigmoid Colon Volvulus.* Treated by inserting a rectal tube through a sigmoidoscope into the sigmoid colon. Rapid decompression and improvement will follow.
> *Fecal Impaction.* Treated with use of oil retention enemas and mechanical disimpaction.
> *Paralytic Ileus.* Treated with use of long intestinal tube and rectal tube.

3. Assuming an organic cause for the obstruction (e.g., carcinoma of the descending colon), rapid repair of fluid and electrolyte deficits is carried out with use of intravenous fluids, following which the patient is scheduled for a decompressing colostomy. During this period of preparation, a Levin or long intestinal tube is inserted and connected to a suction apparatus. Careful replacement of all intestinal fluid loss must be carried out by the intravenous route.

PREPARATION FOR SURGERY

1. A *Levin tube or long intestinal tube* is inserted according to surgeon's preference.
2. A large-bore intravenous needle or intracatheter should be inserted for I.V. fluid therapy.
3. *Blood.* The patient's blood is typed and cross-matched for one unit of whole blood.
4. *Skin Prep.* From nipples as far as and including the pubis. (See Introduction.)
5. *Enema.* Not necessary.
6. *Premedications.* Routine.
7. *Special Medications.* None.
8. *Psychological preparation* is as for any emergency. In addition, the surgeon will probably discuss the nature of a temporary colostomy with the patient. It is not often certain preoperatively whether a permanent colostomy will be required. Consequently, the details of the patient's future condition often cannot be outlined for him prior to the colostomy.
9. *Operating Room Skin Prep.* From the nipples as far as and including the pubis. (See Introduction.)
10. *Position.* Horizontal supine. (See Introduction.)

PATHOLOGY

1. Quite frequently, the large bowel is so distended that the nature of the obstructing process cannot be determined at the time of the emergency colostomy. Following decompression (in 2 to 3 weeks), a barium enema study is done and the pathological condition determined.
2. Common causes of large bowel obstruction are (a) an annular, constricting carcinoma of the colon, and (b) severe diverticulitis with or without perforation and abscess formation.

GENERAL RATIONALE AND SCHEME

Acute large bowel obstruction is relieved by creating a temporary opening in the bowel *proximal* to the point of obstruction. It is hazardous to attempt removal of the obstructing lesion until the bowel has been decompressed and then adequately prepared with enemas and antibiotics.

Scheme

The simplest and most effective method for decompressing an obstructed large bowel is a *transverse loop colostomy.*
1. Abdomen is opened.
2. A loop of transverse colon is delivered into the wound.
3. A glass rod is used to keep the loop outside the abdominal cavity (Fig 30–1).
4. The incision is partially closed around the colostomy.

PROCEDURE

1. *Skin Incision.* The surgeon may choose an upper abdominal *transverse or vertical paramedian incision.* (See Introduction.)

2. *Draping Skin.* This is important, as inadvertent spillage of stool may occur during delivery of colon or during trochar decompression.

3. *Opening Abdomen.* As soon as the peritoneum is opened, there may be leakage of some serous exudate. The greatly distended colon may project into the incision.

4. *Exploration.* This may be difficult or impossible because of distention of the colon.

5. *Identifying the Colon.* The *taeniae coli* are used as identifying landmarks.

6. *Delivering the Colon.* A loop of transverse colon is carefully delivered into the incision. It is held in place by a glass rod which is placed through an incision made in the mesocolon (Fig. 30–1). A rubber tubing is connected to the glass rod, thus securing the loop of colon.

7. *Partial Wound Closure.* The peritoneum and fascia are loosely sutured around the limbs of the colon.

8. *Decompression.* If the colon is so dilated that imminent rupture is feared, a trochar may be thrust into the colon and suction applied to decompress the bowel (Fig. 30–1). Following decompression, a large catheter is left in the colon and held in place with pursestring sutures.

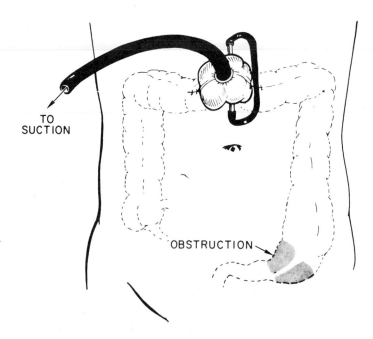

TO SUCTION

OBSTRUCTION

FIGURE 30–1 Tube decompression of the transverse colon for obstruction of the distal bowel. Note the glass rod and tubing which prevents return of the bowel into the abdomen.

SURGICAL HAZARDS

The thin distended colon is always subject to rupture during manipulation. Spillage of liquid stool could then lead to peritonitis, wound sepsis, or both.

EARLY POSTOPERATIVE MANAGEMENT

1. *Levin Tube.* Routine management.

2. *Colostomy Catheter.* If a catheter has been inserted into the colon, it is connected to low suction. This catheter is easily blocked with fecal particles. It should be gently irrigated frequently to prevent its being obstructed.

3. *Fluid Balance.* The fluid and electrolyte losses which have occurred because of the obstruction will continue to require aggressive attention in the early postoperative period. Any signs of hypotension, tachycardia, or *oliguria* may suggest impending *hypovolemic shock* and will require urgent and careful attention. Careful management and recording of intake and output every 8 hours is required.

4. *Management of the Colostomy.* The surgeon probably will remove the colostomy catheter the day after surgery. If the colostomy was not opened during surgery, the surgeon will open it with a cautery the following day. In many cases the colostomy will function within 24 to 48 hours after surgery. The profuse discharge of liquid stool may excoriate the skin if permitted to remain on the abdominal wall. Frequent dressing changes and protection of the skin with zinc oxide minimize skin irritation. The glass rod and tubing, which serve to prevent retraction of the colostomy into the abdomen, must be kept secure until removal 4 to 5 days after surgery.

5. As soon as the abdomen has softened, indicating intestinal decompression, the patient is given a solid diet, and preparations are begun for further evaluation of the cause of the obstruction.

STUDY QUESTIONS

1. What is volvulus of the colon? How is it treated?

2. What type of patient is liable to develop large bowel obstruction from a fecal impaction? What is the nurse's role in the management of this patient?

3. List five causes of acute paralytic ileus. How is this condition usually managed?

4. Review and describe the various types of intestinal drainage tubes available. In what clinical conditions might each one be used? What are the nursing implications in caring for a patient who has such a tube in place? Are there any potential hazards in the use of these tubes?

5. Describe the surgical steps involved in performing a transverse loop colostomy to your class.

6. Two days after a loop colostomy has been done, the surgeon wishes to open this colostomy with an electric cautery:
   a. What equipment might he need?
   b. What role does the nurse play in aiding the surgeon?
   c. Discuss the nursing management of a loop colostomy.

7. Why is it hazardous to remove the cause of large bowel obstruction at the time of the colostomy?

8. Following a transverse loop colostomy for large bowel obstruction, the patient requests information from you. Some of his questions are:
   a. Will a special diet be required?
   b. Will a "bag" be used? For how long?
   c. Will the colostomy be a permanent condition?
How would you handle each of these questions? Discuss these answers with your class.

9. What is the purpose of the glass rod and rubber tubing, used for a transverse colostomy? What complication may arise if the rod and tubing accidentally become disconnected?

10. How is the colostomy stoma managed once it has been incised or opened with a cautery?

11. What psychological support might the nurse give to the colostomy patient in the early postoperative period?

12. Design a nursing care plan for the preoperative and postoperative needs of a patient with a colostomy.

31 THE PATIENT WITH DIVERTICULITIS OF THE COLON

Operation: Sigmoid Colon Resection

TYPICAL HISTORY

A 72-year-old obese male has noted the occurrence of intermittent attacks of diarrhea alternating with constipation and associated with lower abdominal cramps of several months' duration. These episodes are becoming increasingly more severe. There has been no associated weight loss, loss of appetitie, or weakness. He has noted occasional streaks of bright red blood in his bowel movements over the past several months.

PHYSICAL EXAMINATION

A well-developed, somewhat obese male complains of lower abdominal distress, particularly in the left lower abdomen. The general physical examination is unremarkable except for some tenderness in the left lower quadrant.

Significant Findings

1. The patient is obese.
2. There is tenderness in the left lower quadrant with some guarding of the left rectus muscle.

DIAGNOSTIC STUDIES

1. WBC is 9,000 with a normal differential.
2. Hematocrit reading is 41 per cent.
3. Barium enema shows diverticulosis and diverticulitis of the sigmoid colon.
4. Stool for guaiac is 1 to 2 positive.
5. Sigmoidoscopic examination reveals some narrowing and spasm of the rectosigmoid colon with erythema of the mucosa.

PROBABLE HOSPITAL COURSE

1. The patient is suffering from chronic low-grade diverticulitis, which is progressively worsening. He is not now suffering from an acute exacerbation of his illness, but the chronicity and increasing severity of the symptoms suggest that an acute process may soon develop. Consequently, the surgeon will probably elect to do a resection of the involved sigmoid colon.

2. Evaluation of the lower intestinal problem is based upon sigmoidoscopic examination and barium enema.

3. Several days may be utilized in preparing the patient for surgery. This preparation may include:
   a. *Transfusions* of whole blood or packed cells if anemic.
   b. *Vitamin* administration, particularly vitamins C and K.
   c. *Bowel Prep.* A wide variety of routines are employed. In general, a thorough mechanical and chemical preparation is carried out. One such standard routine is the following:
      1) Mechanical prep:
         a) Low-residue diet starting 4 to 5 days preoperatively. This is changed to full liquid diet 48 hours before surgery and to a clear liquid diet on the day prior to surgery.
         b) Daily soapsuds enema.
         c) Laxative each evening.
      2) Chemical prep:
         a) Sulfathalidine for 5 days preoperatively.
         b) Neomycin for 24 to 36 hours preoperatively. (A popular alternative chemical prep is Kantrex, administered in oral doses of one gram every hour for 4 hours, then one gram every 4 hours, beginning 24 to 36 hours before surgery.)

PREPARATION FOR SURGERY

1. A *Levin tube* or long intestinal tube is inserted preoperatively.
2. A *Foley catheter* is inserted preoperatively.
3. *The patient is typed and cross-matched* for three units of whole blood.
4. *Psychological Preparation.* Since it is not altogether possible to rule out the presence of a carcinoma, some preparation must be made for this eventuality. The emphasis is on the known existence of diverticulitis and the probability that a colostomy will *not be involved* in this patient's operation. If there is some likelihood that cancer will be found and a colostomy necessary, this must be mentioned to the patient by the surgeon.
5. A cleansing enema is also given preoperatively.
6. The abdomen is prepped from the nipples as far as and including the pubis. (See Introduction.)
7. Premedications are routine.
8. No specific medications are necessary.
9. *Position.* Horizontal supine. (See Introduction.)

PATHOLOGY

The bowel in acute or chronic diverticulitis usually is thick and rubbery, and the diverticulitis often is limited to the sigmoid area of the colon. The diverticulitis may appear as a narrowed, thickened segment of bowel or may resemble an actual mass in the colon which may be very difficult to distinguish from a carcinoma. The surgeon must distinguish this mass from a carcinoma, and he uses the following criteria for doing so:
a. The x-ray appearance.
b. The sigmoidoscopic appearance.
c. The absence of any involved mesenteric nodes at the time of exploration.
d. The absence of puckering of the serosa of the bowel.

GENERAL RATIONALE AND SCHEME

Advancing and increasing chronic diverticulitis may lead to acute perforation of a diverticulum which would place the patient in a very precarious situation and which might require a three-stage operation. Consequently, the bowel should be resected before the condition becomes acute.

Scheme

1. The abdomen is opened and explored and carcinoma is ruled out.
2. The area of disease in the sigmoid colon is localized, clamps are placed proximal and distal to this area, and the diseased area is removed.
3. A primary end-to-end anastomosis of the two healthy ends of the colon is made, and the abdomen is closed.

PROCEDURE

1. A left paramedian muscle-retracting incision is made in the usual fashion. (See Introduction.)

2. The skin edges are appropriately draped to prevent contamination from the open bowel.

3. The abdomen is explored; carcinoma is excluded.

4. A *self-retaining retractor* is usually put in place to allow for good exposure of the pelvic area of the colon.

5. The *lateral and medial peritoneal reflections* of the sigmoid colon are divided, care being taken not to injure the ureters. The mesentery to the sigmoid colon is incised and all large blood vessels leading to the diseased area of the colon — the sigmoidal arteries — are clamped, divided, and ligated with heavy ligature.

6. *Division of Sigmoid Colon:*

a. Clamps are placed on the proximal and distal sides of the sigmoid colon so that the diseased area of bowel is confined between the clamps.

b. The diseased area is then excised and handed to the nurse.

7. *The Colon Anastomosis:*

a. The two clamps are approximated, thereby bringing the two openings of the bowel together.

b. The anastomosis is carried out like any other intestinal anastomosis: usually it consists of a two-layer closure, one of nonabsorbable material such as silk and the other of absorbable material such as catgut.

8. The defect in the mesentery of the colon is now closed with a running catgut suture, usually 3–0 or 4–0. This is done to prevent a loop of small intestine from invaginating into the defect, causing internal hernia with obstruction of the bowel.

9. Closure of the abdominal incision is done routinely.

SURGICAL HAZARDS

1. *Excessive Blood Loss.* This may be caused by injury to the sigmoid arteries or veins or injury to the large sacral veins in the hollow of the pelvis.

2. *Damage to Ureters.* Good lighting and exposure are necessary to prevent injury or ligation of the nearby ureters, particularly the left ureter, which is usually close to the sigmoid colon.

3. *Damage to Urinary Bladder.* The inflamed sigmoid colon is often adherent to the dome of the bladder and must be carefully separated from the bladder so as to avoid entrance into the bladder. Blood in the urinary catheter signifies that injury to the bladder has occurred and this may lead to the formation of a urinary fistula.

4. *Intraperitoneal Contamination.* If the bowel prep has not been adequate, massive contamination of the peritoneal cavity can occur due to leakage of loose bowel movement during the anastomosis. The use of drapes, proper suctioning, and proper clamping of the bowel is necessary to avoid this complication.

POSTOPERATIVE MANAGEMENT

The early postoperative management is usually quite smooth and uncomplicated.

1. *Vital Signs.* These should be monitored very closely for detection of shock due to either excessive blood loss or under-replacement of blood lost in the operating room.

2. *Management of Foley Catheter.* Particular attention should be paid for the presence of blood in the urine. If this is found, the surgeon should be notified, as it may indicate that the bladder was injured during the operation. Blood-tinged urine for 12 to 24 hours after colectomy is not unusual (the retractors cause contusions of the bladder).

3. *Dressings.* Occasionally, the surgeon will drain the abdominal cavity with a Penrose drain; in this case, one would expect to find some blood present on the dressing. Should the dressing soak through, the surgeon should be notified and the dressing reinforced. If a drain was not used, one should not expect to find a significant amount of bleeding into the dressing. If such occurs, the surgeon should be notified promptly.

4. The Levin tube may be removed 1 to 2 days after surgery, at which time the patient is started on clear liquids. He should be ambulated as soon as possible after surgery, and active leg exercises to prevent pulmonary embolism should be encouraged.

5. If no complications occur, the patient's diet will be rapidly advanced over a 4 to 5 day period, and he should be ready for discharge 7 to 10 days after surgery.

6. Complications to be anticipated after colectomy include:

a. A significant incidence of *pulmonary embolism*, particularly in elderly, obese patients undergoing pelvic dissection.

b. *Wound infection,* a common accompaniment of any bowel resection, regardless of the preoperative bowel prep and the meticulousness of the surgical technique.

c. *Leaking anastomosis,* with resulting pelvic peritonitis. This grave complication, which fortunately is uncommon, can come on rather insidiously. It is often heralded 5 to 7 days after surgery by a slowly rising pulse, temperature elevation, increasing abdominal discomfort, and abdominal distention. Any late fever, tachycardia, abdominal distention, or pain should signal the possibility of an anastomotic leak and call for a careful assessment of the patient.

CONTROVERSIAL ASPECTS OF DIVERTICULITIS SURGERY

1. Not all physicians agree on the value of sigmoid colectomy for sigmoid diverticulitis. Some prefer to reserve surgery for the complications of the disease — namely, perforation, obstruction, or massive bleeding. It is argued that these complications are rare and that most patients respond quite well to medical management of acute diverticulitis. Those who favor elective resection, as described in this chapter, feel that *repeated episodes* of acute diverticulitis are harbingers of an impending perforation and that a one-stage elective colectomy prevents a three-stage procedure for rupture or obstruction in the future.

2. Diverticulitis accompanied by rupture almost always calls for a three-stage approach generally scheduled as follows:

Stage 1: Pelvic drainage and transverse colostomy.

Stage 2 (about 6 months later): Colectomy with end-to-end anastomosis.

Stage 3 (about 6 weeks later): Closure of colostomy.

Some surgeons feel that a one-stage colectomy can be safely carried out, provided that (1) the rupture is well walled-off in the mesentery of the colon, and does not extend over too wide an area, and (2) the proximal and distal bowel walls are healthy. They favor this approach in an effort to save the patient from the disabling 6 to 10 month three-stage procedure. Most surgeons are impressed with the pitfalls of diverticulitis surgery and continue to adhere unreservedly to the three-stage approach.

STUDY QUESTIONS

1. In what way does the management of acute perforated diverticulitis differ from the management of chronic diverticulitis without perforation?

2. Describe the three-stage procedure for managing a patient with acute perforated diverticulitis. What psychological problems might you anticipate? How would you approach this patient?

3. What criteria does the surgeon use for distinguishing diverticulitis from cancer of the sigmoid colon preoperatively? Can this distinction always be made with certainty prior to surgery?

4. Describe a routine bowel prep prior to bowel surgery. What is the nurse's role in ensuring an adequately prepared bowel?

5. What are some of the dangers of prolonged use of intestinal antibiotics for sterilizing the bowel? How would you recognize these dangers?

6. Can you name some of the particular instruments used for sigmoid colon surgery?

7. Describe the Balfour retractor.

8. Describe the suture material used for an anastomosis of two ends of bowel.

9. Describe the anatomic relationship of the two ureters and bladder to the sigmoid colon with particular respect to the *operative hazards* of sigmoid colon surgery.

10. A 72-year-old male has undergone an extensive resection of the sigmoid colon for severe diverticulitis. During the course of the operation, an inflamed mass of bowel was found adherent to the bladder which required extensive dissection for removal from the bladder. Immediately postoperatively, a small amount of blood is noted in the Foley catheter and in the drainage bag. What is the nurse's role in the management of this problem?

11. Do you think that all cases of acute diverticulitis require surgical intervention? If not, what is the medical therapy for acute diverticulitis?

12. The surgeon often orders a low-residue diet in preparing his patient for bowel surgery. What is a low-residue diet and in what way is it beneficial in preparing a patient for this type of surgery?

13. Define and describe acute staphylococcus enterocolitis, paying particular attention to its clinical manifestations and its etiology.

14. Seven days after a sigmoid colectomy, the patient begins to vomit and develop abdominal pain and fever. The vomitus has a coffee-grounds appearance. What might these developments signify? How would you assess the problem?

Operation: Abdominoperineal Resection

TYPICAL HISTORY

A 64-year-old male has noted the occurrence of diarrhea and bloody bowel movements for 4 months, as well as lower abdominal cramps, a weight loss of 15 pounds, anorexia, and fatigue. His past history is otherwise unremarkable.

PHYSICAL EXAMINATION

The patient is a well-developed, poorly nourished male with signs of recent weight loss. The general physical examination is unremarkable, except that the rectal examination reveals a large, fungating, firm tumor in the rectum.

Significant Findings

1. Pallor is noted.
2. Emaciation is evident.
3. A rectal tumor is palpated on rectal examination.
4. The liver is not enlarged.

DIAGNOSTIC STUDIES

1. Hematocrit level is 34 per cent.
2. Barium enema reveals a filling defect in the lower section.
3. Stool guaiac is strongly positive.
4. Sigmoidoscopy is positive, revealing a large ulcerated tumor of the rectum.
5. Liver scan is normal.

PROBABLE HOSPITAL COURSE

1. The diagnosis is confirmed by sigmoidoscopy and biopsy of the rectal tumor. The patient is prepared for sigmoidoscopy according to the surgeon's prescription. Usually all that is necessary is the administration of a low enema 1 hour prior to the examination.

2. A barium enema may also be ordered. For low-lying rectal tumors, this examination is often unnecessary but may be ordered to delineate the extent of the tumor as well as to allow a search for coexisting colonic tumors or polyps. If the tumor lies low enough in the rectum, the barium enema may be normal.

3. If the surgeon is concerned about involvement of the ureters, an intravenous pyelogram may be done.

4. Several days may be utilized in preparing the patient for surgery. The following steps may be taken:

    a. Transfusions of whole blood or packed cells.

    b. Infusions of albumin.

    c. A bowel prep.

    d. Administration of vitamins, particularly C and K.

PREPARATION FOR SURGERY

1. Levin tube or long intestinal tube inserted preoperatively.

2. Foley catheter inserted preoperatively.

3. Type and cross-match six units of blood.

4. *Psychological Preparation.* The patient or his family must be informed about the colostomy which will be necessary. If the surgeon chooses to inform the patient preoperatively, a great deal of anguish can be prevented by describing the function of a modern sigmoid colostomy. Stress should be placed on the following facts:

    a. No bags or other appliances will be needed.

    b. The colostomy will *not* be incontinent.

    c. Very little care is necessary.

    d. There is no odor attending a sigmoid colostomy.

    e. Clothing is not stained by a colostomy.

5. Cleansing enema preoperatively.

6. Prep from nipples as far as and including the pubis. Prep perineum, perianal area, and buttocks. (See Introduction.)

7. Routine premedications.

8. *Special Medications.* None.

9. *Position.* Horizontal supine. (See Introduction.)

PATHOLOGY

The curability of a rectal tumor will depend on how well localized it is to the rectum. Areas of possible spread that must be evaluated are:

    a. The liver.

    b. The omentum.

    c. The para-aortic nodes.

    d. The pelvic nodes.

    e. The outside layer of the rectum (serosa).

    f. The bladder or vagina.

If the tumor has not spread through to the serosa, and if all node-bearing tissue is negative, the cure rate may be as high as 60 to 70 per cent.

GENERAL RATIONALE AND SCHEME

The rectum, the lower sigmoid colon, and all surrounding nodes and lymphatics, in addition to the anus and perianal tissue, must be excised in order to effect complete removal of a rectal carcinoma. The scheme is as follows:

    1. *Abdominal Phase:*
    a. Opening of abdomen.
    b. Exploration.
    c. Division of sigmoid colon.
    d. Creation of sigmoid colostomy.
    e. Closure of abdomen.
    2. *Perineal Phase:*
    a. Closure of anus.
    b. Excision of anus, rectum, and lower sigmoid colon through anal opening.
    c. Closure of perianal tissue.

PROCEDURE

Abdominal Phase

    1. *Skin and Fascial Incision.* The most commonly used incision is a left lower abdominal paramedian incision from level of umbilicus to pubis. (See Introduction.)
    2. *Draping Skin.* In view of the fact that the bowel will be opened, drapes are used to protect the skin and subcutaneous tissues.
    3. *Exploration.* The peritoneal cavity is opened:
    a. The tumor is palpated to determine its size and whether it is fixed or freely moveable. A fixed tumor may indicate spread to the bony structures of the pelvis and sacrum, and is inoperable.
    b. Pelvic peritoneum, bladder, para-aortic nodes, omentum, and liver are palpated to determine spread of the tumor outside the proposed area of resection.
    4. *Obtaining Good Exposure.* This procedure is carried out deep within the confines of the bony pelvis. Good lighting and exposure are absolutely necessary for safe and effective surgery. Some of the steps used for obtaining good exposure are:
    a. *A Self-retaining Retractor.* This should be of a proper size to accommodate itself to the particular abdominal wall.
    b. *Deep Trendelenburg Position.* This permits the loops of small bowel to gravitate toward the respiratory diaphragm, thus exposing the pelvic cavity.
    c. *Packs.* Moist abdominal packs are used to maintain the loops of small bowel out of the pelvis.
    d. *Evisceration.* Occasionally, the loops of small bowel are removed from the abdominal cavity. To keep them moist, they may be placed in a watertight plastic or rubber bag (e.g., Lahey bag).
    5. *Dissection of Sigmoid Colon and Rectum*
    a. The surgeon detaches the mesentery of the sigmoid colon and rectum, dividing the posterior peritoneum and the blood supply.
    b. Care is taken to avoid injury to the ureters which descend in proximity to the colon and rectum.
    c. The bladder is detached from the surface of the rectum.

6. *Division of Sigmoid Colon*
a. Clamps are placed on the mid-sigmoid colon and the colon divided.
b. The proximal end will be brought out of the abdomen as a sigmoid colostomy.
c. The distal end will be removed along with the rectum.
7. *Sigmoid Colostomy* (Fig. 32–1).
a. The proximal colon is brought out of the abdomen either through the abdominal incision or through a separate opening in the left lower quadrant.
b. A clamp is left on the colostomy to prevent retraction of the bowel into the abdominal cavity. Alternatively, the colon is sutured to the opening in the abdominal wall.
8. *Closure of Abdominal Incision.* This is done in routine fashion.

Perineal Phase

1. *Positioning.* The patient is kept in the Trendelenburg position and his legs are placed in stirrups. Some surgeons prefer to use the Sims' position. (See Introduction.)

2. *Prepping.* The perineum, the upper thighs, and the buttocks are prepped in the usual fashion and the patient is adequately draped. (See Introduction.)

3. *Closure of Anus.* A large pursestring suture is used to close the anus, thus preventing fecal spillage during the dissection.

4. *Excision of Anus, Rectum, and Lower Colon*
a. An elliptical incision is made around the anus.
b. This is deepened through the muscles of the perineal floor until the pelvic cavity is opened.
c. The lower colon, the rectum, and the anus are then removed.

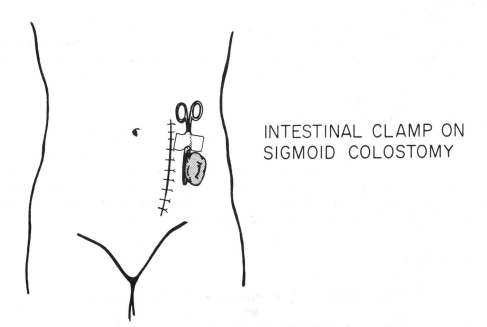

INTESTINAL CLAMP ON
SIGMOID COLOSTOMY

FIGURE 32-1 Following abdominal phase of abdominoperineal resection. Clamp is left on colostomy for 24 to 48 hours. Some surgeons "mature" the colostomy at the time of surgery by suturing it to the opening in the abdominal wall. A clamp is not used in such a case.

5. *Closure of Perineum.* Large Penrose drains are placed in the pelvic cavity and through and through sutures are used to close the perineal defect around the drain. Some surgeons prefer to use sump catheters to promote easy egress of serum and blood collecting in the pelvic basin.

SURGICAL HAZARDS

1. *Excessive Blood Loss.* This may occur as a result of injury to the sigmoid arteries or veins or injury to the large sacral veins in the hollow of the pelvis.

2. *Damage to Ureters.* Good lighting and exposure are necessary to prevent injury or ligation of the nearby ureters.

3. *Damage to Urinary Bladder.* Blood in the urinary catheter signifies injury to the bladder. This may lead to formation of a urinary fistula.

EARLY POSTOPERATIVE MANAGEMENT

1. *Vital Signs.* An abdominoperineal operation is one of the most shocking of procedures in general surgery. Blood loss may approach 1500 to 2000 cc.; often the amount lost is underestimated and therefore transfusion is insufficient. A rapid pulse and hypotension are indicative of the degree of shock involved. These vital signs must be watched carefully. Any significant trend in the direction of further deterioration must be called to the surgeon's attention. Several questions must be kept in mind at all times:
   a. Are the pulse and blood pressure stable?
   b. Is there any cyanosis about the lips or in the nail beds?
   c. Are the abdominal and perineal dressings dry?
   d. Is the urine output adequate?
2. *Dressings*
   a. The perineal dressing is apt to require early changing, as the drains will produce saturation of the dressing from old blood in the pelvis. The amount of drainage, color of blood, and frequency of dressing changes may alert the nurse to the development of an inordinate amount of fresh bleeding. If sump catheters have been used, they are attached to low continuous suction.
   b. If the abdominal dressing requires changing, care must be taken to avoid disturbance of the colostomy clamp.
3. *Pain.* There is often a great deal of pain associated with this procedure, particularly after the first 24 hours. Demerol, I.M., 100 mg. doses, may be required.
4. *Management of Levin Tube or Miller-Abbott Tube.* Routine management is observed.
5. *Immediate Care of the Colostomy.* Ischemia of the colostomy due to deficient blood supply is an early and serious complication of abdominoperineal resection. The nurse should check the viability of the colostomy frequently during the first day after surgery.

STUDY QUESTIONS

1. What are the Seven DANGER Signals of cancer?

2. What sign might this patient present and why?

3. What is the stool guaiac test for occult blood?
   a. What is the nature of the chemical reaction involved?
   b. How is the test interpreted?
   c. List six diseases which can cause a positive test for occult blood in the stool.

4. What is the nurse's role in preparing a patient for sigmoidoscopy? Can you describe the various positions the patient may be placed in, as well as the equipment needed for the examination?

5. Following a sigmoidoscopy and rectal biopsy, what possible complications may develop?

6. A patient, preoperative for an abdominoperineal resection, asks you whether he will require a colostomy. What is your reaction to his question? How would you respond?

7. Summarize the steps of an abdominoperineal resection for your class. List:
   a. All the special instruments that may be required.
   b. Some of the surgical hazards involved.

8. What danger is involved in changing the abdominal dressing on the day following an abdominoperineal resection?

9. Discuss the early management of a sigmoid colostomy as far as the nurse's role in patient education is concerned. What is the most significant hazard in colostomy irrigation? How is this prevented?

10. What is the purpose of gastric decompression in the patient who has had an abdominoperineal resection?

11. Would a Levin tube or a tube gastrostomy be indicated here? Discuss the advantages and disadvantages of each.

VASCULAR SURGERY

33 INTRODUCTION

The modern surgical nurse is exposed to an increasing number of patients undergoing surgery for vascular diseases. Only two decades ago the patient with advanced vascular insufficiency was faced with loss of life or limb as a result of impaired blood flow to vital organs. Direct surgical attack on the vascular tree was essentially unheard of except in the research laboratory. Here pioneer investigators sought ways and means to perform surgery on major vessels, completely or partially occluded by emboli, thrombi, and atherosclerotic plaques. Technical success in opening and closing blood vessels was marred by sepsis, hemorrhage, and intravascular thrombosis. With the advent of powerful antibiotics and anticoagulants, some of the complications of vascular surgery were obviated, and clinical application of vascular surgical research became feasible.

It soon became evident that while atherosclerosis was a generalized phenomenon, affecting the entire vascular tree, *segmental* narrowing or occlusion threatened specific organs and was amenable to local vascular procedures. The development of arteriography enhanced our knowledge of segmental vascular disease as localized narrowings could be visualized by x-ray. It then remained for investigators to develop artificial prostheses to replace worn out vessels, and vascular surgery moved from its infancy to a state of rather common application in general hospitals.

The important highlights, then, in the development of vascular surgery may be outlined as follows:

a. Early development of the techniques of opening and closing arteries.
b. Development of powerful antibiotics, and, especially, anticoagulants.
c. The evolution of the concept of segmental atherosclerotic disease affecting arteries.
d. Development of suitable vascular prostheses.
e. Refinements in vascular surgical techniques, coupled with the invention of the Fogarty catheters.

DISEASES AMENABLE TO VASCULAR SURGERY

Arterial

Segmental disease of the circulatory system amenable to vascular surgery may be summarized as follows:

Coronary Artery Disease. Atherosclerotic narrowing of the coronary vessels has been treated with *gas endarterectomy* with varying results. The procedure is extremely hazardous and unpredictable and remains, at present, a research tool. More widely used are coronary vein by-pass procedures, which seem to offer a better solution to the problem.

258

Aortic Arch Disease

Extracranial Cerebral Vessels. Atherosclerotic narrowing of the carotid and vertebral arteries may lead to cerebral syndromes and, ultimately, strokes. Endarterectomy and by-pass arterial grafting have successfully revascularized the brain particularly in cases of transient ischemic attacks in which a completed stroke has not occurred.

Subclavian-axillary Vessels. Ischemia of the upper extremity due to stenosis, thrombosis, or embolism of the subclavian-axillary arterial tree has been solved with by-pass grafting, embolectomy, and thrombectomy.

Brachioradial Vessels. Injury or embolism to the brachioradial arteries is frequently amenable to vascular surgery and may prevent the loss of a hand.

Descending Aorta. Coarctation of the aorta as well as dissecting aortic aneurysms are successfully treated, although mortality from dissection remains high.

Superior Mesenteric Artery. Narrowing or occlusion of the superior mesenteric artery may result in ischemia to the bowel with threatened intestinal gangrene. Thrombectomy and endarterectomy of this vessel may be successful if accomplished before gangrene supervenes.

Renal Artery

Renal Artery Embolism. Usually a consequence of rheumatic heart disease, it may result in kidney infarction. Early diagnosis and embolectomy may save the affected kidney.

Renal Artery Stenosis. Atherosclerotic narrowing of the renal artery may result in renal ischemia and the development of hypertension. Endarterectomy or by-pass grafting may relieve the hypertension.

Abdominal Aorta. Occlusive disease, aneurysms, and emboli may be successfully treated.

Iliofemoral Arteries. Occlusive disease, aneurysms, and emboli may be successfully treated.

Femoropopliteal Arteries. Occlusive disease, aneurysms, and emboli are successfully treated.

Vasospastic diseases involving upper or lower extremity vessels may be successfully treated with cervical and lumbar sympathectomies respectively.

Venous

Phlebitis. Under certain circumstances, venous ligation is indicated to prevent recurrent pulmonary emboli.

DIAGNOSIS OF VASCULAR SYNDROMES

HISTORY

A carefully taken history of the patient alerts the clinician to the type of vascular impairment and the particular organ system involved in the disorder. *Vasospastic* conditions are characteristically transient and recurrent. The symptoms wax and wane, often aggravated by emotional crises and a cold environment. On the contrary, *vaso-obstructive* disorders generally worsen with time and show far less periodicity.

The history defines the time sequence of events, dividing vascular syndromes into acute and chronic. Major embolic and thrombotic phenomena are among the most acute and catastrophic events in medicine. An extremity may suddenly develop exquisite pain, coldness, and numbness. Within minutes, marked pallor and mottling supervene, and the arm or leg takes on a cadaveric appearance. If surgery is not performed within several hours of events, irreversible tissue damage and gangrene are inevitable. More chronic disorders, such as intermittent claudication, are measured in years and only rarely lead to gangrene. The history is valuable here, particularly in determining the degree of disability produced by claudication as well as the rate of deterioration over the years.

Many conditions that aggravate vascular disease are suggested by the history. These include:

1. Diabetes mellitus.
2. History of hypercholesterolemia.
3. Family history of vascular disease.
4. History of hypertension.
5. Previous trauma.
6. Consumption of cigarettes.

Since vascular disease is widespread in the circulatory tree, its local manifestations should alert the clinician to more covert arterial disease in other parts of the body. Symptoms of neurological, cardiac, renal, and hepatic disease must be sought by careful, thorough study of the patient's history.

PHYSICAL EXAMINATION

Vascular diseases can cause widespread impairment of organ function, and a thorough physical examination must be done for each patient. Physical findings should be recorded on a vascular flow sheet, which becomes part of the patient's permanent record (Fig. 33–1). In addition, a careful *vascular examination* is carried out as follows:

1. *All* accessible pulses are carefully examined. These pulses include:
   a. Carotid.
   b. Axillary, brachial, and radial.
   c. Abdominal aorta.
   d. Iliac.
   e. Femoral and popliteal.
   f. Dorsalis pedis and posterior tibial.

When examining a pulse it is important to determine:

   a. *Degree of pulsation or pulse volume:* Does the vessel have a feeble or a bounding pulse sensation?
   b. *Softness or hardness of the wall of the vessel:* Roll the vessel gently against surrounding tissues. Is the vessel soft and compressible, or hard, irregular, and incompressible?
   c. *Occlusion pressure of vessel:* How much pressure does it take to temporarily occlude the vessel? This may be a reflection of the patient's blood pressure or a function of the suppleness of the vessel wall.
   d. Presence or absence of a *thrill* or *bruit:* Any sensation of vibration or murmur within a vessel almost always signifies proximal stenosis.

2. Affected extremity is examined for:
   a. Relative *temperature* compared to nonaffected extremity.
   b. *Color.* The color of an ischemic extremity will often vary with changes in its position.
      1) *Pallor on elevation* of a leg usually indicates some degree of peripheral vascular insufficiency.
      2) *Rubor on dependency* of a leg is also a sign of peripheral vascular disease.
   c. *Nail and hair changes.* Thickening and cracking of nails and loss of hair are consistent with peripheral vascular disease.
   d. *Venous filling time.* The affected extremity is raised to empty its veins of all blood. The extremity is now lowered to a dependent position and observed until the veins begin to fill with blood. The time it takes for blood to begin filling the vein is known as *venous fill time.* Normal fill time is up to 20 seconds.

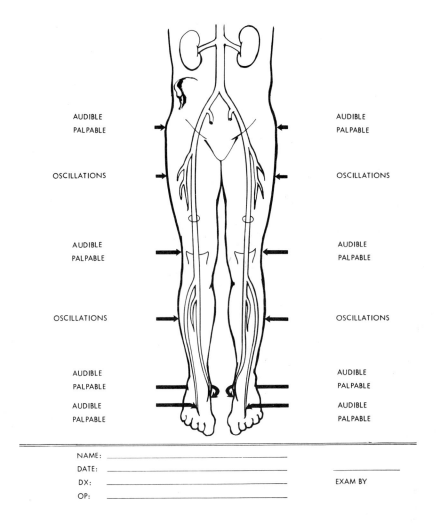

AUDIBLE
PALPABLE

OSCILLATIONS

AUDIBLE
PALPABLE

OSCILLATIONS

AUDIBLE
PALPABLE

AUDIBLE
PALPABLE

AUDIBLE
PALPABLE

OSCILLATIONS

AUDIBLE
PALPABLE

OSCILLATIONS

AUDIBLE
PALPABLE

AUDIBLE
PALPABLE

NAME: _____
DATE: _____
DX: _____   EXAM BY
OP: _____

FIGURE 33–1 Typical vascular chart used to record the results of examinations of the lower extremities.
Pulses may be graded on a 0 to +4 scale. All oscillometric findings are recorded, and all arteriographic findings
"colored in."

e. Edema, moisture, dryness, fissuring, and scaling of the skin of the affected extremity are
   also evaluated.
   3. Examination of the eyegrounds with an ophthalmoscope may reveal narrowing and
sclerosis of retinal vessels.

ARTERIOGRAPHY

The introduction of radiopaque dye into the vascular tree permits x-ray visualization of many
vascular diseases. Arteriography has been used for many years. Recently, more sophisticated
techniques have made this diagnostic tool a highly refined method of evaluating vascular disease.

Methods

Percutaneous Needle Arteriography. A large-bore (e.g., #17), short-tapered arteriography needle is inserted through the skin into the artery to be visualized. A bolus of radiopaque dye is injected manually or with a pressure injector into the vessel and single or serial films are taken. This method can be used to visualize carotid, femoral, brachial, and aortoiliac vessels. Some of the more common sites of injection are as follows:

Carotid Angiography. Injection is made directly into the carotid artery in the neck.

Brachial Angiography. Injection is made directly into the brachial artery in the antecubital fossa.

Femoral-popliteal Angiography. Injection is made directly into the femoral artery in the groin.

Aortoiliac Angiography. Injection is made into the abdominal aorta through the left flank.

Percutaneous Retrograde Angiography. A bolus of dye may be injected under some pressure into a vessel and a certain degree of retrograde flow will occur, allowing visualization of more proximal vessels. For example, the left axillary artery is entered and 30 cc. of dye injected retrograde, visualizing the more proximal subclavian and carotid system. Retrograde visualization of the iliac vessels via the femoral route is also feasible.

Percutaneous Catheter Angiography. The most sophisticated types of angiography today involve the use of various angiographic catheters that are introduced into a major vessel and passed up to more proximal levels where the individual vessels can be catheterized and studied.

Retrograde Femoral Angiography. In this technique the femoral artery is punctured with an appropriate arterial needle. The inner stylet is removed and a guide wire passed into the vessel through the needle. The needle is now removed, permitting the guide wire to remain within the vessel. An appropriate arteriographic catheter is now threaded over this guide wire and it is directed, along with the guide wire, up the iliac vessel, and into the aorta. Here, under fluoroscopic control, and by careful manipulations, the catheter can be introduced into the renal or mesenteric vessels for visualization of these areas only.

Retrograde Axillary Angiography. Using a similar technique, a catheter may be introduced through the axillary vessel, into the subclavian, and then into the arch of the aorta. Here the extracranial cerebral vessels, the upper extremity vessels, and the aortic arch may be catheterized and visualized. The catheter may then be passed down the aorta for visualizing any part of the thoracic or abdominal aorta.

Risks

Angiography is not without its risks and should be done only by experienced vascular surgeons or arteriographers. It is reserved for situations in which safer procedures are not available for diagnosing vascular problems and only when knowledge derived from the procedure will be of major value in charting the further course of medical or surgical therapy.

Intravascular Thrombosis. A needle or catheter introduced into a major vessel can be the nidus around which clot formation and subsequent major vessel thrombosis can occur. If not recognized and treated aggressively, loss of limb may follow.

Dislodgment of Calcified Plaques. Diseased vessels may be traumatized by the tip of a needle or catheter. Calcific emboli may be shed into the more distal vessel where occlusion may result.

Major Hemorrhage and Hematoma Formation. Unexpected bleeding tendencies or a traumatic entrance into a vessel may result in postcatheter bleeding from a vessel. This is more prone to occur in catheter angiography, in which a larger hole is created in the vessel. The hematoma may be the site of subsequent sepsis.

Nerve Damage. Trauma to nearby nerves may occur at the time of puncture. This may result in palsy of an extremity or permanent paresthesia. Wrist drop from axillary arteriography is a real hazard, particularly if a large and unrecognized hematoma occurs and causes pressure against the axillary nerves.

Cerebrovascular Accident. This can occur following carotid or retrograde axillary angiography and is due to clot formation and calcific emboli.

Preparation

Very little preparation is needed for angiography. Most procedures can be done under local anesthesia with minimal sedation. Morphine and scopolamine may be ordered one to two hours prior to the procedure. The only skin prep consists of shaving around the area where the needle or catheter will be introduced.

Knowledge Obtained

Modern vascular surgery is not possible without proper angiographic control. X-ray visualization of the vascular tree can determine the degree of obstruction to blood flow, the length of obstruction, the adequacy of collateral flow, and the extensiveness of atherosclerotic disease in nearby vessels. Physical examination can frequently determine the approximate level of obstruction to blood flow. However, only by adequate angiography can one determine the feasibility of vascular surgery. Frequently angiography reveals an inoperable problem because of the extensiveness of the disease process, particularly when large and small vessels are diseased.

TREATMENT OF VASCULAR SYNDROMES

CONSERVATIVE

Many vascular problems are managed without drastic procedures and without the need for surgical intervention. This is particularly true of nondisabling claudication of the extremities. The patient is frequently reassured and asked to put up with a moderate degree of discomfort in the hope that time will permit the development of adequate collateral blood flow, thus decreasing symptoms. Various exercises have been devised to aid in the speedy development of collateral circulation. These so-called Buerger's exercises are of questionable value. Some forms of vasospastic conditions are at least partially relieved with mild vasodilator drugs. Transient ischemic brain syndromes may respond to oral anticoagulation.

SYMPATHECTOMY

Cervical sympathectomy may aid the patient suffering from Raynaud's disease of the upper extremities. Lumbar sympathectomy may be of some value in the treatment of ischemic ulcers of the legs and feet. There seems to be very little value in the use of lumbar sympathectomy for lower extremity claudication.

VASCULAR SURGERY

Many procedures have been devised for revascularizing an ischemic limb or organ. These procedures include:
1. Embolectomy, thrombectomy, or both.
2. Thromboendarterectomy:
a. with closure of the artery.
b. with patch graft.
c. with onlay graft.
3. End-to-end grafting.
4. By-pass grafting.

POSTOPERATIVE MANAGEMENT

Vascular surgery is usually a lengthy and, at times, very shocking procedure. This is particularly true of thoracic and abdominal aortic surgery. The patient is often elderly and often has diffuse vascular disease involving vital end organs such as the brain, heart, and kidney. Mortality and morbidity are therefore considerably higher in patients undergoing vascular procedures than in most other forms of elective surgery. These patients must be carefully monitored in a well-staffed and well-equipped room until most of the significant complications have been overcome and the patient is on his way to recovery.

Thrombosis is perhaps the most serious specific complication of vascular surgery because its occurrence negates the very goal achieved by the operation. Moreover, if thrombosis of a graft is not treated by immediate reoperation, retrograde and antegrade thrombosis of the collateral circulation may occur and actually render the limb worse than its preoperative state. It is not our purpose here to discuss the various technical and physiological factors that predispose to postoperative intravascular thrombosis. What is most important for the nurse to ascertain is the status of the limb the moment the surgery has been completed. This baseline information may be invaluable as a comparison with what follows subsequently in the course of the patient's recovery. If distal pulses have been restored immediately, it is a relatively easy task to check these pulses every hour and to report loss of a pulse immediately. However, it frequently happens that pulses do not return for 24 hours to an affected limb. Other more subtle ways of following the circulatory status must be relied upon. Color, sensation, venous fill time, capillary flush, and nail-bed cyanosis are all important clues to the circulatory status of the patient. These changes may be subtle, and it is only by careful and frequent observations under adequate lighting that serious delays in recognizing thrombosis may be avoided.

Hemorrhage, either early or delayed, is another serious complication of vascular surgery. This is particularly apt to occur if anticoagulation is used postoperatively. Early hemorrhage is usually due to faulty hemostatic technique and may occur a few hours after surgery. It may be massive and may require immediate return to the operating room. If possible, a blood-pressure cuff may be applied proximal to the hemorrhage and may be life-saving. Delayed hemorrhage may occur days to weeks after the operation and is usually associated with infection. Any patient showing sustained temperature elevation in the late postoperative period should be observed carefully for signs of delayed hemorrhage.

Other frequent complications of vascular surgery include acute renal failure, myocardial and cerebral thrombosis, wound infection due to hematoma formation, venous thrombosis, and pulmonary embolism. For these and many other reasons the postoperative vascular patient is best observed in the intensive care unit until safely beyond the time when these events are likely to occur.

THE PATIENT WITH RAYNAUD'S DISEASE

34

Operation: Cervicodorsal Sympathectomy

TYPICAL HISTORY

A 31-year-old female, in otherwise excellent health, enters the hospital with painful ulcers on her fingertips, which are generally cold, pale, and cyanotic. There are small areas of gangrene associated with intractable infections on the volar aspect of her fingers. She has been under careful observation by her physician for Raynaud's disease for the past 10 years. The condition began with cold, clammy hands, often aggravated by exposure to cold or by anxiety. Soon the patient noted pallor of her fingertips on exposure to cold. Her fingertips eventually became numb and very painful. Vasodilators were used over the years with only moderate and unpredictable success. Because of increasing infection, ulceration, and small patches of gangrene, she now enters the hospital for elective surgery.

PHYSICAL EXAMINATION

The patient is a well-developed, well-nourished, and very tense female complaining of painful, tender fingertips and cold, clammy hands.

Significant Findings

1. The hands are cold, pale, and somewhat cyanotic, particularly at the fingertips.
2. The volar surfaces of the fingertips display small ulcerations, patchy scars, and small areas of gangrene (Fig. 34–1). They are extremely tender to palpation.
3. The axillary, brachial, and radial pulses are equal and excellent.
4. The fingertips are tapered and the nails are fissured.

DIAGNOSTIC STUDIES

1. Since the major pulses are intact, there is no need to evaluate the arterial tree with angiography. *Lack* of pulses would suggest a vaso-obstructive process and would necessitate angiographic analysis of the aortic arch and the axillary-brachial arterial tree.
2. Underlying collagen diseases are always suspected in so-called Raynaud's phenomenon. The surgeon will order a complete evaluation in order to rule out such diseases as lupus erythematosus, progressive systemic sclerosis, rheumatoid arthritis, dermatomyositis, and other systemic collagen diseases which can provoke peripheral vasoconstriction. The entire chemical and

265

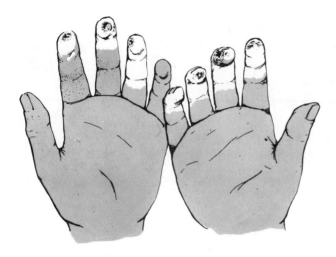

FIGURE 34-1 Raynaud's disease. Digital vasospasm often leads to painful ulcerations of the fingertips.

immunological analysis of these conditions is beyond the scope of this book, and the student is referred to articles dealing with the underlying causes of vasoconstrictive disease in any appropriate medical book.

PROBABLE HOSPITAL COURSE

Once the work-up has been completed, the surgeon must decide whether cervicodorsal sympathectomy will be of value in relieving this chronic vasoconstrictive process. The treatment of any underlying disease always takes precedence over the vasoconstrictive process itself. Physicians trained in immunological diseases are often consulted in an effort to determine whether an immunological problem underlies the Raynaud's phenomenon.

Cervicodorsal sympathectomy is likely to relieve vasospasm in carefully selected cases. Vaso-*obstructive* diseases, whether due to intrinsic arterial disease or secondary to extrinsic vascular compression (e.g., thoracic outlet syndromes), are not likely to be benefited by sympathectomy.

GENERAL RATIONALE AND SCHEME

Peripheral blood vessels are under continuous control of the sympathetic nervous system. Under normal conditions, the sympathetic nervous system causes only the amount of vasoconstriction necessary to keep the extremities warm, dry, and comfortable without oversupplying the parts with too much blood. As environmental conditions change, the normal waxing and waning of sympathetic stimuli alternately vasoconstrict or vasodilate the peripheral vessels according to the subtle needs of the body for heat transfer and maintenance.

Raynaud's disease is not well understood. Whatever its cause(s), it appears to result in an *inappropriate over-reaction* of various segments of the sympathetic nervous system, leading to prolonged periods of peripheral vasoconstriction with all its attendant sequelae. The effects, as in this case of prolonged vasoconstriction, can include digital arterial thrombosis with small areas of gangrene, subcutaneous fibrosis, and intractable, painful infections.

Cervicodorsal sympathectomy effectively denervates the upper extremity of all extrinsic vasoconstrictor influences arising in the sympathetic nervous system and permits the return of normal vasodilation. The result is a warm, well-vascularized, comfortable extremity. Infection rapidly subsides, ulcers heal, and small areas of gangrene and fibrosis disappear. The results are permanent in the majority of patients, although return of vasoconstrictor influences, again not well understood, may lead to a recurrence of the disease.

Scheme

1. The cervicodorsal nerve chain is approached through the route favored by the surgeon.
2. The thoracic ganglia (from T2 to T6) are resected, along with half of the stellate ganglion (C8-T1).
3. The wound is closed.

PROCEDURE

Originally this procedure was performed by neurosurgeons, who approached the cervicodorsal chain through a posterior neck incision. This incision does not lend itself well to a dissection of the thoracic ganglia and is no longer recommended. An anterior cervical approach carries with it the same disadvantage and leaves an unsightly scar. The most popular approach today, described in the following, is the transaxillary, transpleural approach.

1. The patient is placed in a horizontal, supine position with the appropriate arm extended and supported on an arm board.
2. The axilla and anterolateral chest cage are shaven and prepped in the usual fashion.
3. The incision, made transversely in the axilla, overlies the third rib and extends from the protruding lateral border of the pectoralis major muscle to the protruding border of the latissimus dorsi muscle.
4. Small bleeders are ligated with plain, fine catgut.
5. Wound towels are applied according to the surgeon's preference.
6. The serratus anterior muscle overlying the rib is split, and the periosteum overlying the third rib is incised with a scalpel and dissected from the rib with a periosteal elevator.
7. About 4 inches of exposed third rib are resected. A rib spreader is used to improve exposure.
8. The pleura is incised and the lung is permitted to collapse. The cervicodorsal chain is thus made visible along the angle of the ribs posteriorly. With good lighting and with sufficient separation of the ribs, the view of the cervicodorsal chain is usually excellent.
9. The ganglionated chain is grasped with a nerve hook, the large, dumbbell-shaped *stellate ganglion* is identified, and ganglia T2 through T6 are traced. A hemoclip is used to clip *rami communicantes* entering and leaving the chain. The stellate ganglion is hemisected, preserving the upper half of the ganglion. The lower half is removed along with ganglia T2 through T6.
10. The ribs are approximated over a chest tube and held with heavy sutures. The chest is expanded and the chest tube is placed on underwater seal drainage. The muscular tissue is approximated with heavy suture, the skin with fine silk suture.
11. The chest tube is secured to the skin with a suture and a dressing is applied.

SURGICAL HAZARDS

1. *Occasional brisk bleeding from an intercostal artery:* If injury to an intercostal vessel is not noted, it may cause troublesome postoperative bleeding.
2. *Damage to the underlying lung when the thoracotomy incision is made:* This could lead to a persistent pneumothorax postoperatively.

3. *Damage to the thoracic aorta or subclavian artery:* Though such damage is improbable, it could occur, with massive intra-operative bleeding as a result.

POSTOPERATIVE MANAGEMENT

The patient is brought to the recovery room until reactive from her anesthesia. She is then transferred back to the surgical ward for follow-up care.

1. The chest tube is on underwater seal, and all connections should be checked carefully.

2. Fluctuations in the water bottle may continue for a few hours and then cease. Since an air leak from the lung is not expected, the fluctuations will disappear as soon as residual intrathoracic air has dissipated.

3. Some surgeons will connect the water bottle to mild negative pressure, whereas others are satisfied with dependent underwater seal. The surgeon should make his own choice clear if it is not already indicated in his orders.

4. Bleeding into the water bottle should be minimal, perhaps less than 100 to 200 cc's over the first 8 hours postoperatively and then gradually diminishing. Any further bleeding is distinctly abnormal and merits the surgeon's attention.

5. The hand is checked to make certain that circulation is intact. The radial pulse should be palpable and the hand warm, pink, and dry.

6. The nurse should check the patient's pupils to see if *Horner's syndrome* has developed. Its presence should not cause any alarm.

7. Breath sounds are evaluated as soon as the patient arrives on the floor and frequently for the first few hours thereafter. There may be some decreased breath sounds on the operative side due to splinting, but the sounds should be audible. If not, or if they become inaudible, the surgeon should be notified.

8. There are no special intravenous procedures for this type of patient. She may be started on light liquids the moment she is awake and will progress to a full liquid or solid diet the following day. Nausea and vomiting from the anesthetic agents are the only limitations to full alimentation after sympathectomy.

9. The chest tube will probably be clamped the day after surgery and a chest x-ray ordered. If the lung remains expanded for 24 hours after clamping of the chest tube, the tube will be removed, and the patient will generally be discharged the following day.

STUDY QUESTIONS

1. Distinguish *Raynaud's disease* from *Raynaud's phenomenon.*

2. Discuss Raynaud's disease and its relationship, if any, to the following:
   a. ergot poisoning
   b. nicotine
   c. diabetes
   d. hypertension
   e. age, sex, race
   f. thoracic outlet syndromes
   g. collagen diseases

3. What causes the cyanosis in Raynaud's disease?

4. Describe the anatomy of the cervicodorsal sympathetic chain and present sketches to your class.

5. What is the stellate ganglion and what does it innervate?

6. Describe the functions of the sympathetic nervous system and the heat-regulating mechanisms of the body. How are these functions affected by sympathectomy?

7. What is Horner's syndrome and what causes it?

8. Discuss the management of a chest tube. What causes fluctuations in a chest tube? If fluctuations are still occurring 24 hours after sympathectomy, what might this mean?

THE PATIENT WITH ISCHEMIC ULCERS AND REST PAIN

35

Operation: Lumbar Sympathectomy

TYPICAL HISTORY

A 67-year-old male has noted increasing cramps in the calves of his legs on walking. These cramps are relieved when he rests or sits. More recently, he has noted coldness of both feet and a small area of ulceration on the great toe on the right foot. This ulcer has resulted in severe, steady rest pain that keeps him awake at night. He smokes two packs of cigarettes daily. His general health has been normal otherwise.

PHYSICAL EXAMINATION

A thin, well-developed male is admitted in acute distress.

Significant Findings

The peripheral pulses, particularly in the right leg and foot, are markedly diminished. The right foot is extremely pale, but develops erythema when placed in the dependent position. There is a small ulceration on the great toe of the right foot. This ulcer has a sharp, punched-out appearance, and a gray, shaggy base covered with a yellow membrane.

DIAGNOSTIC STUDIES

The patient with peripheral vascular disease is studied both clinically and by special x-rays to determine the nature of his arterial disease, as well as the appropriate treatment. The most important single study in evaluation is the clinical examination, which includes a careful history and physical examination. This procedure alone might well determine the specific treatment given to the patient. Angiography is almost always indicated in the evaluation of patients with peripheral vascular disease. Multiple x-rays of the aortic, iliac, femoral, and popliteal arteries are obtained by passing a catheter into the aorta and injecting radiopaque dye. Depending on the type and location of any vascular obstructions, along with the age and general condition of the patient, the surgeon will decide on sympathectomy or direct vascular surgery as the most appropriate treatment for his patient.

PROBABLE HOSPITAL COURSE

Provided his general condition will tolerate major surgery, the patient is taken to the operating room as soon as the studies are completed.

PREPARATION FOR SURGERY

1. Levin tube is unnecessary.
2. The patient is typed and cross-matched for two units of whole blood.
3. The abdomen is prepped from the nipple line as far as and including the pubis, and laterally to the flank on the appropriate side. (See Introduction to Section I.)
4. A cleansing enema is given preoperatively.
5. Laboratory work is routine.
6. *Premedications.* Routine.
7. *Special Medications.* None.
8. Operating room skin prep extends from the nipple line as far as and including the pubis and laterally to the flank. (See Introduction to Section I.)
9. *Position.* Either horizontal supine or in the right kidney position. (See Introduction to Section I.)

PATHOLOGY

The lumbar chain is usually approached through a flank incision and generally shows no particular pathologic process; the pathologic process is limited to the peripheral vascular system and is not directly approached in lumbar sympathectomy.

GENERAL RATIONALE AND SCHEME

Vasospastic phenomena are often superimposed on organic arterial disease of the lower extremities; it is the vasospasm which is amenable to treatment by lumbar sympathectomy. The lumbar sympathetic chain lends arterial tone to the lower extremity. When it is divided, maximum vasodilatation occurs, affording maximum blood supply to the affected extremity. When feasible, direct vascular surgery is done. Lumbar sympathectomy is losing favor as a primary treatment for vascular obstructive disease except in cases in which no other procedure is possible. The syndromes most amenable to good results from sympathectomy include (1) vasospastic diseases, (2) ischemic ulcers with rest pain, and (3) certain forms of causalgia.

Scheme

1. A flank incision is made in the midpart of the abdomen extending out to the flank.
2. The peritoneum and intraperitoneal structures are reflected medially.
3. The lumbar sympathetic chain is located in the groove between the vertebral column and the psoas muscle.
4. The lumbar chain, including ganglia 2, 3, and 4, is excised.
5. Bleeding is controlled.
6. The skin incision is closed.

PROCEDURE

1. *Skin Incision.* This is a right horizontal abdominal flank incision. (See Introduction.)
2. The abdominal musculature, including the external oblique, the internal oblique, and the transversus abdominis, is split in the direction of the fibers.
3. The properitoneal fat, the peritoneum, and the intraperitoneal structures are now reflected medially, elevating the entire peritoneal sac away from the quadratus lumborum and the psoas muscle.
4. The lumbar sympathetic chain is palpated in the groove between the vertebral column and the psoas muscle.
5. The surgeon is cautious to avoid injury or misidentification of nearby nerves or ureter.
6. Lumbar ganglia 2, 3, and 4 must be excised to afford complete sympathectomy.
7. Small hemostatic clips are placed on the nerve fibers which run from the sympathetic chain to the spinal column, as these often contain small blood vessels which may bleed profusely and are difficult to control.
8. The lumbar chain is divided and removed.
9. Careful hemostasis must be obtained; at times this requires the use of Gelfoam or Surgicel.
10. The transversus abdominis, the internal oblique, and the external oblique muscles are closed with either a running 2–0 chromic catgut suture or interrupted silk sutures.
11. The skin is closed in the usual manner and a heavy dressing applied.

SURGICAL HAZARDS

1. *Damage to Ureter.* The retroperitoneally located ureter runs along the anterior surface of the psoas muscle and can be confused with the sympathetic chain. This must be carefully identified and preserved during the procedure. Postoperative drainage of urine through the incision would suggest injury to the ureter. Postoperative flank pain should suggest hydronephrosis secondary to a ligature on the ureter. Either event should be promptly reported to the surgeon, who may then order an intravenous pyelogram.
2. *Uncontrollable Hemorrhage.* This may occur as the result of avulsion of one of the lumbar veins which pass superior to and over the lumbar sympathetic chain. These must be carefully avoided or clipped.

3. *Damage to the Genitofemoral Nerve.* This nerve passes over the psoas muscle. Damage caused by a retractor may result in postoperative neuralgia.

4. *Inadvertent Opening of the Peritoneal Sac.* This can occur during reflection of the sac medially and may result in damage to the intestine or in postoperative ileus. If such inadvertent opening of the sac occurs, it should be sutured immediately.

POSTOPERATIVE MANAGEMENT

The patient is returned to the recovery room until sufficiently reactive from the anesthetic. The usual course of the post sympathectomy patient is smooth, and few problems are to be anticipated.

1. The dressing should be checked for postoperative hemorrhage, although this is unusual following this operation.

2. Ileus may occur, usually 24 to 48 hours following surgery. The abdomen should be palpated and percussed for hypertympany for 2 to 3 days after surgery. The development of ileus may require a Levin tube, and the earlier this is known, the smoother the recovery.

3. *Acute Urinary Retention.* The incision is often very painful, and postoperative urinary retention may occur. This is relieved, if necessary, with use of a Foley catheter.

4. Appropriate foot care for patients with vascular insufficiency should be instituted at once.

5. The patient is ambulated the day after surgery, and a smooth postoperative course is expected.

STUDY QUESTIONS

1. What is the relationship, if any, between heavy smoking and peripheral vascular disease? Discuss this relationship specifically with respect to *Buerger's disease.*

2. What are the risks of angiography?

3. What is an oscillometer? What are its uses in estimating the degree of peripheral vascular disease?

4. Should a patient with known peripheral vascular disease develop acute leg pain, what is the probable diagnosis?

5. Discuss the anatomy and physiology of the lumbar sympathetic chain with your class.

6. Describe the foot care which should be carried out by the nurse on any patient with severe peripheral vascular disease. List all the measures for obtaining proper foot care and the rationale for each one.

7. Describe some of the tests which may be carried out by the surgeon preoperatively on a patient with peripheral vascular disease. How do these tests help the surgeon determine the appropriate therapy?

8. Diagram the operative site which contains the sympathetic chain and place in this diagram all the structures which might be confused with the sympathetic chain.

9. What is postsympathectomy neuralgia? What causes this syndrome?

10. Acute postoperative hypotension in a postsympathectomy patient may be due to many causes. List as many as you can, describing the appropriate therapy for each one.

11. What is the difference between arterial embolism and arterial thrombosis?

12. What causes postsympathectomy paralytic ileus? How is this condition recognized and how is it treated? What are the physical signs that usually accompany severe postoperative ileus?

13. What psychological problems may the patient with peripheral vascular disease be suffering from, particularly with respect to his legs and feet? How are these factors anticipated and dealt with?

14. Why are elastic stockings contraindicated in the immediate postoperative period?

15. List four complications that might arise in the immediate postoperative period and the measures that would be employed to treat them.

THE PATIENT WITH PERIPHERAL VASCULAR DISEASE

36

Operation: Femoral-popliteal By-pass Graft

TYPICAL HISTORY

A 51-year-old male, who had smoked heavily for several years, noted the onset of pain and coldness in his right foot about 3 weeks prior to admission. Review of his recent past history reveals that he has suffered from *intermittent claudication* for about 2 years which is more marked in the right leg than in the left. He is not a diabetic and denies any family history of diabetes. He states that he is unable to sleep because of the painful foot and is forced to hang his foot over the side of the bed at night to get relief.

PHYSICAL EXAMINATION

A well-developed, thin male is admitted, in obvious distress, holding his right foot over the side of the bed.

Significant Findings

1. The right foot is pale, cold, and somewhat cyanotic.
2. The right femoral pulse is adequate; no other pulses are felt below the femoral pulse.
3. There is no hair on the lower third of the right leg and foot.
4. The toenails are markedly hypertrophied and cracked.
5. When dependent, the foot becomes deep bluish-red.

DIAGNOSTIC STUDIES

1. An angiogram is performed in order to view the aorta and the iliac, femoral, and popliteal vessels. The outflow vessels into the calf and foot must also be evaluated very carefully. The presence of a narrowed femoral artery with distinct blockage in *the lower third* is revealed. The remainder of the femoral and popliteal arterial system in the right leg is good.
2. Glucose tolerance test is negative.
3. Electrocardiogram shows changes consistent with arteriosclerotic heart disease but without active process.

PROBABLE HOSPITAL COURSE

The patient with peripheral vascular disease may be handled in one of four ways depending on the local and general findings:

Conservative Management. The patient is advised to stop smoking completely and at once. He is told to bathe his feet daily, to powder them dry, and to apply lanolin daily to prevent skin breakdown. This is the usual form of therapy offered to the patient with mild vascular disease in which the only symptom is intermittent claudication and in which there are no skin changes suggesting imminent loss of tissue.

Sympathectomy. This is offered to patients whose prime complaints are coldness or numbness of the extremity. In addition, some vascular surgeons feel that sympathectomy should be done before or during direct vascular surgery to prevent any postoperative vasospasm which might result in thrombosis of a graft.

Direct Vascular Surgery (see "Rationale"). When ischemia threatens the survival of a limb, and when it can be proven by arteriography that a localized block exists in a major vessel of the extremity, some form of direct vascular surgery is offered.

Amputation. This is a last resort for patients in whom the possibility of improvement by any of the other means is too remote to allow the patient's life to be risked.

In the present patient, angiography has revealed obstruction of a main vessel to the extremity. Consequently, he is prepared for direct vascular surgery. If the surgeon feels that lumbar sympathectomy should precede the operation on the femoral artery, he may choose to perform it on the current admission and readmit the patient about a month later.

PREPARATION FOR SURGERY

1. Levin tube not necessary.
2. Type and cross-match for two units of whole blood.
3. *Enema.*   Fleet or soapsuds enema is given on the evening prior to surgery.
4. A large-bore intravenous needle or intracatheter should be inserted for emergency intravenous therapy or transfusions.
5. *Skin Prep.*   This includes the right groin and the entire right lower extremity.
6. *Premedications.*   Routine.
7. *Special Medications.*   None.
8. *Psychological Preparation.*   Vascular surgery involves the risk of loss of limb or even of life. The patient must be carefully selected for this type of surgery, and it should be thoroughly explained to him that his only alternative is to have the limb amputated. In other words, vascular surgery is performed only on those patients whose disease threatens limb survival or in whom *disabling claudication* is present.
9. *Operating Room Skin Prep.*   From groin as far as and including the entire leg.
10. *Position.*   Horizontal supine.

PATHOLOGY

The patient who is selected for direct vascular surgery usually demonstrates discrete atherosclerotic blockage of his femoral artery. There is some involvement of the proximal and distal arteries as this is a generalized disease. If significant involvement of the entire vessel is found, and if small "run-off" vessels in the lower calf are diseased, vascular surgery will be impossible.

GENERAL RATIONALE AND SCHEME

In vascular surgery, an attempt is made to remove or by-pass discrete blockage in the femoral artery. There are two main approaches:
a. *Endarterectomy.*   This consists of opening the artery over the blockage and reaming out the blocked area. Endarterectomy is limited to very short, discrete segmental obstructions.
b. *By-pass.*   This consists of establishing a detour or by-pass graft around the area of blockage. The by-pass graft may employ a saphenous vein direct from the patient's body or an artificial graft of Dacron or Teflon. The use of a vein graft is generally considered preferable.

Scheme

1. The medial thigh is opened through a lengthy vertical incision.
2. A saphenous vein graft is anastomosed proximal and distal to the obstruction in the femoral artery.
3. The incision is closed.

PROCEDURE

1. *Skin Incision.*   This extends from below the inguinal ligament in the downward direction to the knee along the medial aspect of the thigh.

2. The femoral artery is located medial to the sartorius muscle, and the sheath of the artery is carefully opened, thus exposing the full length of the femoral artery.

3. The blockage in the femoral artery is noted, as well as the state of health of the proximal and distal arteries.

4. If it is decided to establish a graft, a saphenous vein is retrieved from the same leg, its tributaries are ligated, and the vein is reversed.

5. Rubber catheters are placed around the proximal and distal femoral arteries for control should a vascular clamp slip off the vessel during the procedure.

6. The patient is given intravenous heparin to prevent thrombosis during clamping of the vessel. (As an alternate method, the surgeon may choose to inject heparin directly into the femoral artery via small polyethylene catheters.)

7. Small nontraumatizing vascular bulldog clamps are placed across the femoral artery proximal and distal to the points of anastomosis for the graft.

8. Small elliptical openings are made in the femoral artery and the graft is sutured in place.

9. The clamps are released and blood begins flowing immediately around the area of obstruction (Fig. 36–1).

10. Distal pulses are checked to be certain that a thrombus has not formed distal to the graft.

11. The incision is closed and a light dressing is applied.

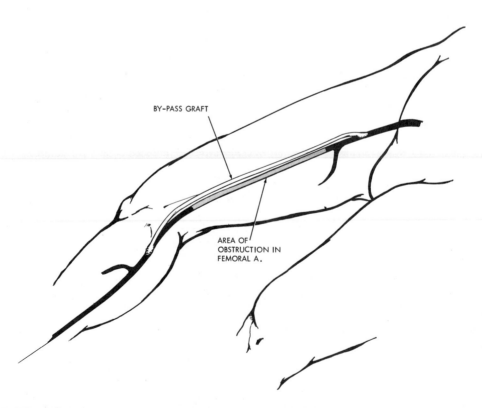

BY-PASS GRAFT

AREA OF
OBSTRUCTION IN
FEMORAL A.

FIGURE 36–1 Saphenous femoral-popliteal by-pass graft in place, going around the femoral artery obstruction.

SURGICAL HAZARDS

1. Injury to the femoral nerve or femoral vein.
2. Massive hemorrhage from loss of control over the opened femoral artery.

POSTOPERATIVE MANAGEMENT

The patient is returned to the recovery room until sufficiently reactive from the anesthetic. The usual postanesthesia management is carried out. In addition:

1. The head of the bed is elevated on 6 inch shock blocks to encourage increased blood flow in the leg and foot.

2. The circulation in the feet is checked every 2 hours. Any noticeable change is called to the surgeon's attention at once. A good examination of foot circulation should be carried out as soon as the patient arrives on the floor. If one or more pedal pulses are palpable, postoperative observations are quite simple, in that the continued presence of a pedal pulse assures the staff that the graft is patent.

Difficulties arise when the pedal pulses have not been restored by the graft. The nursing staff must then judge the continued patency of the graft by more subtle parameters -- color, temperature, and the presence or absence of touch and pin-prick sensations, for instance. The pulses may be audible with a Doppler device. Above all, it is important to compare the general postoperative appearance of the foot with that evident immediately after surgery; in this way graft function can be carefully evaluated.

3. The patient is allowed fluids by mouth as soon as he is reactive from the anesthetic.

STUDY QUESTIONS

1. Define endarterectomy, by-pass graft, autogenous graft.

2. What is the relationship of smoking to peripheral vascular disease? What is the relationship of diabetes to peripheral vascular disease?

3 Describe the vascular anatomy of the lower extremity.

4. What is intermittent claudication?

5. Why does a patient with severe peripheral vascular disease obtain some relief from his pain by hanging his foot over the side of his bed?

6. Describe the locations of all pulses in the lower extremity which can be palpated clinically.

7. Why was a glucose tolerance test performed in this patient?

8. Describe the essential steps in the performance of a by-pass graft.

9. Describe the makeup and function of a bulldog vascular clamp.

37

THE PATIENT
WITH THE
LERICHE SYNDROME

Operation: Aorto-iliac By-pass Graft

TYPICAL HISTORY

A 56-year-old non-diabetic male, with a history of excess cigarette consumption, enters the hospital for evaluation of increasing fatigue and pains in his legs of several months' duration and impotency of recent onset. He is very vague about the leg problem, describing increasing fatigue of both lower extremities and "a heavy feeling in the thighs and lower legs." These symptoms began rather insidiously several months ago when he noticed some discomfort and heaviness when walking on the golf course. He paid little attention to it at first, thinking he was just "out of shape." However, the symptoms worsened, and he noticed that he was unable to walk any great distance without developing cramps and pain in his buttocks, thighs, and calves. He still made little of his symptoms until the rather sudden development of impotency about one month prior to admission. He had previously suffered no difficulty in maintaining an erection and was at a loss to explain this new problem. He first consulted a urologist, who referred him to a vascular surgeon.

PHYSICAL EXAMINATION

The patient is a well-developed male, in no acute distress, and appearing in excellent health.

Significant Findings

1. Extreme pallor of both lower extremities.
2. Absence of pulses in both lower extremities. The femoral pulses are absent as well.

DIAGNOSTIC STUDIES

1. Blood cholesterol and lipoproteins are normal.
2. Blood sugar is normal.
3. An aortogram reveals a complete occlusion of the distal aorta and proximal iliac arteries, with excellent collateral flow into the femoral arteries.

PROBABLE HOSPITAL COURSE

This patient is suffering from the Leriche syndrome, a condition first described by Leriche in 1940. The syndrome consists of claudication and leg pains involving the buttocks, thighs, and calves, often coming on suddenly and associated with inability to maintain an erection. The condition is due to thrombotic occlusion of the distal aorta and proximal iliac vessels. The impotency is due to inadequate arterial flow to the penis, caused by hypogastric arterial obstruction. The vascular insufficiency in the lower extremities can be relieved by an aorto-femoral by-pass procedure, but the impotency is usually not overcome.

Providing the patient's general condition will tolerate surgery, he will be scheduled for the operation soon after admission. It is important to perform an intravenous pyelogram to check the location of the ureters and to test renal function. A bowel prep is usually done because injury to the inferior mesenteric artery during dissection for by-pass surgery can produce ischemia in the large bowel, necessitating a colectomy.

PREPARATION FOR SURGERY

1. A Levin tube is inserted preoperatively to decompress the stomach. This may be replaced with a tube gastrostomy at the end of the procedure.
2. A Foley catheter is inserted preoperatively.
3. Type and cross-match for 8 units of whole blood.
4. The abdomen is prepped from the nipples to and including the mid-thighs.
5. *Special Medications.* None.
6. Routine premedications.
7. *Position.* Horizontal supine.

PATHOLOGY

The essential lesion of the Leriche syndrome is atherosclerotic narrowing of the distal aorta and proximal iliac arteries with, at times, thrombotic occlusion secondary to a low flow state. As with any vascular problem, all types of secondary occlusive states may be found at the time of surgery, and a complete evaluation of the peripheral vasculature must then be made. The obstructed vessels will result in the enlargement of collaterals running to the lower extremities. These collaterals develop from the intercostal arteries, the lumbar arteries, and the mesenteric vessels. The lower abdominal aorta and iliac vessels may be totally occluded or severely stenotic.

GENERAL RATIONALE AND SCHEME

The low flow state to the lower extremities secondary to stenosis or occlusion of the distal aorta predisposes the legs to further deterioration and eventual gangrene. In addition, the low flow state may result in deep phlebitis at a later date. For these reasons, some type of by-pass procedure with an artificial graft is indicated.

Scheme

1. The abdomen is opened through a long midline incision and a general exploration is made.
2. The extent of vascular obstruction is determined and, if feasible, an aorto-femoral by-pass graft is carried out (Fig. 37–1).

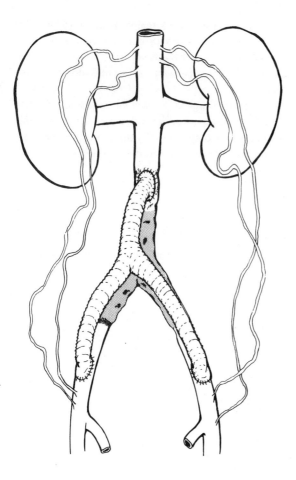

FIGURE 37-1 An aorto-iliac Dacron by-pass graft in place.

3. Often, a tube gastrostomy is performed because of the anticipated prolonged postoperative ileus.

4. The wound is closed in the usual fashion without drains.

PROCEDURE

1. A long midline incision is made from the ziphoid process to the pubis. Bleeders are controlled with catgut or silk ties, and wound towels are applied to the wound edges.

2. The peritoneum is incised and, through general exploration, associated diseases (e.g., cancer, gall stones) are ruled out.

3. The posterior peritoneum overlying the distal aorta and iliac vessels is incised. The surgeon must be careful to avoid injuries to the ureters.

4. The aorta and iliac vessels are carefully palpated to determine the extent of the disease process and to establish the nature of the vascular procedure to be carried out.

5. The aorta is freed just below the renal arteries, and an umbilical tape is placed around that segment of the aorta in which there is a good pulse.

6. Umbilical tapes are also placed around the iliac arteries at a level where there is a good pulse.

7. The patient is given intravenous heparin by the anesthesiologist.

8. A vascular clamp is applied to the aorta and two clamps are placed on the iliac vessels to interrupt the flow of blood temporarily.

9. An artificial graft of pre-clotted Teflon or Dacron is measured and cut for size.

10. An incision is made in the anterior wall of the aorta in an area of good pulsation, and a button or ellipse of tissue is removed. The proximal end of the graft is then sutured to the opening in the aorta with one or more running sutures of 3–0 or 4–0 mersilene. When this anastomosis is complete, the clamp on the aorta is temporarily opened and blood allowed to rush into the graft with the distal ends clamped. Blood will pour through the interstices of the graft in spite of the latter's pre-clotted condition. The anastomosis is reinforced with interrupted sutures if this is thought necessary by the surgeon.

11. An opening is made in the anterior wall of one of the iliac arteries, a small ellipse of arterial wall is removed, and one limb of the vascular prosthesis is sutured end-to-side with a running 4–0 or 5–0 suture. Just prior to completing the anastomosis, the surgeon carries out retrograde flush from the clamped iliac artery, followed by proximal flush from the aorta. The anastomosis is then completed. With a clamp on the opposite free limb of the graft, the aortic and iliac clamps are removed and circulation is restored to one side.

12. A similar anastomosis is carried out with the opposite limb, again with retrograde and proximal flush.

13. The posterior peritoneum is closed over the graft with a running 2–0 chromic catgut suture.

14. Prior to wound closure, the surgeon may perform cholecystectomy (if stones are present) or appendectomy.

15. The wound is closed in the usual manner without drains.

SURGICAL HAZARDS

1. Injury to a ureter.
2. Dislodgement of calcific emboli into either or both kidneys.
3. Dislodgement of calcific emboli into either femoral-popliteal artery.
4. Massive hemorrhage from the aorta, iliac arteries, or veins.
5. Ischemia to the colon, necessitating colectomy.

CONTROVERSIAL ASPECTS

Most surgeons feel aorto-iliac occlusive disease should be treated with aorto-femoral by-pass or aorto-iliac by-pass as described here. Some surgeons feel that a short block can more easily and safely be treated with aorto-iliac endarterectomy, in which the aorta and iliac arteries are opened, an endarterectomy performed, and the openings in the vessels closed without a grafting procedure. The technical aspects of this controversy, while interesting, are not appropriate for this type of textbook.

POSTOPERATIVE MANAGEMENT

Following a short period of recuperation in the recovery room, the patient is taken to the intensive care unit, where he will remain for 2 or 3 days for careful monitoring. Like all extensive abdominal procedures involving moderate to large amounts of blood loss, prolonged anesthesia, and lengthy exposure of the intestines to the air, aorto-iliac by-pass surgery is very shocking to the system and results in a very labile cardiopulmonary and renal status for 2 or 3 days. In addition, the presence of atherosclerotic occlusive disease in the aorto-iliac region suggests occult vascular disease in the heart, brain, kidneys, and intestines. These vital organs, which are potentially compromised by vascular insufficiency, cannot long sustain the low blood flow states of surgical or postoperative shock without suffering the risk of irreversible damage. The intensive care unit nurse is left with the grave responsibility of careful monitoring of all vital systems; in addition, she must anticipate and recognize the early warning signs and symptoms of clinical deterioration. Thus, along with the usual postoperative management of any major surgical patient, the nurse should develop an approach to the major vascular surgical patient which embodies a logical, step-by-step sequence of observations designed to monitor the entire patient with emphasis on his vascular system.

There is no single correct way to formulate this approach, but the following points should be noted:

1. *The Vital Signs.* A systolic blood pressure of 100 mm of mercury is acceptable *if* the preoperative pressure was not in the hypertensive range and provided the operating surgeon does not prefer some other minimum. Below 90 systolic threatens thrombosis of the vascular prosthesis as well as thrombosis in any other stenotic vessel supplying other vital organs in the body.

Blood pressure trends may be just as important. Serial drops in blood pressure on the order of 10 mm Hg or more on two or three separate readings should suggest an imminent problem and, under these conditions, one ought not to wait until the pressure reaches 100 systolic before notifying the attending physician.

Pulse rate is a bit more difficult to pin down in this context. One expects a moderate tachycardia on the order of 110 to 120 simply from the massive alarm reaction to the degree of surgery. A pulse above 130 should be cause for some concern, particularly if it is on the rise and associated with a slippage in blood pressure.

Pulse rhythm is best observed on a cardiac monitor. Sinus arrhythmias should cause no concern, but any other rhythm not previously present demands an immediate explanation. The hypotension associated with cardiac tachyarrhythmias, possibly tolerable in other circumstances, can ruin a vascular prosthesis and must be treated before the hypotension supervenes.

Temperature elevations of up to 101 or 102 degrees are to be expected in the immediate postoperative period and in most cases are of no significance. Temperatures of 103 degrees or higher usually signify major pulmonary atelectasis and should be investigated promptly. In addition to predisposing to pneumonia, major atelectasis could lead to anoxia and aggravate pre-existing cardiac problems, with all the attendant sequelae.

As is the case with pulse rate, *respiratory rate* is usually elevated and, if under 30 respirations per minute, is tolerable. Many patients are on controlled ventilation for 24 hours and consequently the underlying rate is masked.

2. *Cerebral Function.* The state of the carotid pulses, as documented in the preoperative physical examination, should be known by the intensive care nurse. She should palpate the carotid vessels and listen to them with a stethoscope at least once every 8 hours and report any abnormalities or changes to the next nurse taking charge of the patient. The level of consciousness of the patient, facial function, strength of extremities, and the size and reaction of pupils should be monitored as well, as possible indices of postoperative cerebrovascular accidents.

3. *Cardiac Function.* The vital signs, cardiac monitor, CVP, and the general appearance of the patient are reviewed periodically. Coronary failure, manifested by shock, and myocardial failure, manifested by pulmonary congestion and edema, are encountered very frequently in the early postoperative period when a labile system is placed under possible fluid overload during or shortly after surgery.

4. *Renal Function.* Pre-existing renal artery stenosis is always a possibility. Hypotension may further aggravate the low flow states to the kidney and result in renal failure. Hourly urine

outputs should be monitored and any significant downward trend called to the surgeon's attention. Probably a minimum of 40 cc's of urine per hour should be the lowest acceptable quantity that is passed, unless the surgeon sets some other standards. The urine should be observed for cloudiness, concentration, and blood or other sediment.

  5. *Intestinal Signs.* Intestinal ischemia is often difficult to diagnose. One important sign is early bloody stool, occurring within 12 hours after aortic surgery. This calls for immediate attention by the surgeon, as it may suggest impending infarction of the colon and necessitate an emergency colectomy.

  6. *Signs in the Extremities.* The circulation in the lower extremities is of course checked frequently. If pulses have been restored by the surgery, they must remain palpable throughout the postoperative period. Failure to feel a distinct pulse when one was present before calls for immediate investigation by the surgeon.

  Other details of care, including care of the Foley urinary catheter, management of the tube gastrostomy, ventilator care, and so forth, follow the standard nursing patterns. The truly *vital* parts of the patient's management are the parameters listed above. The authors cannot emphasize enough the importance of *frequent, scheduled, "by-the-numbers" assessments* of these danger areas if catastrophes are to be anticipated and their sequelae prevented or minimized.

STUDY QUESTIONS

  1. Discuss some of the examinations carried out preoperatively in the total assessment of the patient with the Leriche syndrome.

  2. Of what significance is a loud carotid murmur heard preoperatively in terms of postoperative management of an aorto-iliac by-pass graft?

  3. A rising CVP, a falling cardiac output, and oliguria suggest what possible event in the postoperative period?

  4. Describe a nursing care plan for the postoperative management of an aorto-iliac by-pass graft. What factors should be stressed in this plan?

  5. The following urine outputs and CVP's were recorded over a 4-hour period for a patient who has undergone aorto-iliac by-pass graft surgery:

	urine/hour	CVP
hour 1	46 cc	14 cm water
hour 2	20 cc	8 cm water
hour 3	12 cc	3 cm water
hour 4	10 cc	2 cm water

  a. Discuss the possible causes of this situation. Do you think this situation is serious?

  b. What diagnostic tests can be done to further evaluate the above data?

  c. In your opinion, what should be done with this patient if it is determined that a fluid overload is occurring?

    d. If nothing is done with this patient, what sequence of events might soon occur?

    e. What will be the course of action if it is determined that hypovolemia exists?

38

THE PATIENT WITH AN ABDOMINAL AORTIC ANEURYSM

Operation: Resection of Abdominal Aortic Aneurysm

TYPICAL HISTORY

A 63-year-old male has noted the development of increasing intermittent claudication, involving the thighs, calves, and buttocks. These symptoms have been present for several months. He has also noted the onset of diminished sensation in the lower extremities, pallor, and coldness of the feet. He denies any past history of hypertension or diabetes. Except for some low-grade backache in recent weeks, he is asymptomatic and in good general health.

PHYSICAL EXAMINATION

A well-developed, thin male is admitted in no acute distress and in apparent good health.

Significant Findings

1. There is a pulsatile mass in the left lower quadrant of the abdomen near the midline. This mass is globular and firm, and pulsates with each beat of the heart. The femoral pulses are present, but bilaterally decreased. The popliteal pulses are present, but bilaterally decreased.

2. The lower extremities are cold and somewhat pale, with loss of hair from approximately the knee down.

DIAGNOSTIC STUDIES

1. AP, lateral, and oblique x-rays of the abdomen reveal the presence of a calcific aneurysm of the abdominal aorta, confirming the clinical impression.

2. Intravenous pyelogram reveals some displacement of both ureters, particularly the left ureter, by what appears to be a round mass consistent with an aneurysm of the aorta. The kidneys function well otherwise. The ureters are not obstructed.

PROBABLE HOSPITAL COURSE

1. Before resection of the aneurysm is undertaken, the patient's cardiovascular, pulmonary, and renal status must be carefully evaluated, inasmuch as this type of surgery carries a high morbidity and mortality rate. Patients often have arteriosclerosis, involving the heart, the brain, and the kidneys, and complications are prone to occur in these organ systems. Consequently a complete evaluation of these systems will be undertaken. Some of the tests done will include the following:

    a. A *general medical examination* to determine the patient's general status, including his blood pressure and pulse, and clinical evaluation of the heart, the lungs, and kidney function.

    b. A *BUN* or creatinine test is done to determine the excretory function of the kidneys, and a urinalysis is done to determine whether there is any evidence of chronic renal disease. The intravenous pyelogram (IVP) is done to determine the presence of any obstructive uropathy due to the aneurysm, as well as any degree of diminution in excretion due to involvement of the renal arteries.

    c. An electrocardiogram and a chest x-ray are done.

    d. Blood volume and total protein studies as well as electrolyte studies may be done to determine the status of the patient's general metabolic reserves, which will be stressed by the operation.

2. When the general and specific organ systems have been evaluated and surgery is feasible, the patient will be operated upon without further delay.

PREPARATION FOR SURGERY

1. *Psychological Preparation.* Resection of an abdominal aortic aneurysm is associated with a high degree of mortality and morbidity, but it is a life-saving operation and must be carried out if the general condition permits. The patient should be carefully apprised of the nature of his problem by the surgeon. While not attempting to produce any undue amount of morbid thinking on the patient's part, the surgeon is obliged to present to the patient the risks to life and limb involved in this operative procedure. Only after the patient has been so apprised can he make an *informed decision* to undergo the surgery.

2. *Skin Prep.* Includes the entire abdomen from the nipple line as far as and including the pubis. The surgeon may also wish the groin and lower extremities prepared as far as the knees in case further surgery below the common iliac vessels becomes mandatory. (See Introduction.)

3. *Enema.* A soapsuds or Fleet enema may be ordered the evening before or the day of surgery. Some surgeons advocate a formal bowel prep identical to that done for bowel surgery in that occasionally the left colon must be resected at the conclusion of the operation (see Chapter 31).

4. A *long intestinal or Levin tube* is inserted on the evening prior to surgery.

5. A *Foley catheter* is inserted on the day of surgery.

6. The patient is typed and cross-matched for seven or eight pints of blood.

7. *Premedications.* Routine.

8. Special medications:

    a. I.V. heparin may be given at start of surgery.

    b. A mannitol infusion is started at the beginning of surgery.

9. An intracatheter or large-bore cutdown should be placed in both upper extremities in order to insure complete control of the patient's vascular system in the event of massive hemorrhage.

10. The operating room skin prep again extends from the nipple line as far as the pubis, including the groin and, at the discretion of the surgeon, the thighs and knees are also prepped. (See Introduction.)

11. *Position.* Horizontal supine. (See Introduction to Section I.)

PATHOLOGY

Most aneurysms of the abdominal aorta are found below the renal arteries. The aneurysms extend to a greater or lesser degree into the common iliac vessels. The aneurysm is usually associated with a good deal of periaortic inflammation, causing adherence of the inferior vena cava and iliac veins to the arteries. At times, the ureters are also adherent to the periaortic inflammation, and must be carefully dissected from the aortic aneurysm in the course of the operation. Signs of recent periaortic hemorrhage may be present in the form of hematomas, indicating the precarious nature of these aneurysms and their tendency to bleed and rupture. The size of the aneurysm may vary from 2 to 3 cm in diameter to as much as 10 to 15 cm in diameter. There is usually marked associated atherosclerosis, partially obstructing the iliac and external iliac vessels.

GENERAL RATIONALE AND SCHEME

Experience has proven that once an aneurysm becomes symptomatic, the threat to the patient's survival is sufficiently high to warrant excision of the aneurysm. The mortality and morbidity associated with elective resection of an aortic aneurysm is considerably lower than that associated with emergency resection for a ruptured aneurysm. Consequently, as soon as the diagnosis of aortic aneurysm is made, and particularly when it is symptomatic, it should be removed. An occasional small asymptomatic aneurysm may sometimes be followed by the surgeon if the general condition of the patient would produce a formidable operative risk.

Scheme

1. The abdomen is opened through a long left vertical incision or a midline incision from the xiphoid process to the pubis, curving around the umbilicus.

2. The posterior parietal peritoneum is reflected laterally, exposing the aortic aneurysm.

3. Surrounding structures are carefully dissected free from the aneurysm.

4. Clamps are placed proximal to the aneurysm on the aorta and distal in the iliac vessels.

5. The aneurysm is removed.

6. An artificial graft, usually of Dacron or Teflon, is inserted in place of the aneurysm, and sutured.

7. The posterior peritoneum is closed.

8. The abdomen is closed.

9. A tube gastrostomy may be established.

PROCEDURE

1. *Skin Incision.* This is usually a left paramedian, muscle-retracting incision, extending from the left costochondral angle to the symphysis pubis. Frequently a long midline incision is chosen. It is more rapidly opened and closed.

2. *Opening Abdomen.* This is accomplished in the usual fashion, and a general abdominal exploration is carried out to be certain there is no pathologic process contraindicating aortic resection.

3. *Mobilizing Right Colon.* The right side of the colon is dissected from its lateral attachment to the abdominal wall and reflected medially, thereby exposing the inferior vena cava and right ureter.

4. *Eviscerating Small Intestine.* The mobilized small intestine is placed in a Lahey bag and delivered from the abdominal cavity in order to provide further room for the remainder of the procedure.

5. The posterior parietal peritoneum overlying the aneurysm is now incised and the outline of the aneurysm cleared by careful dissection around it.

6. The aneurysm is carefully dissected from its attachment to the inferior vena cava, if this is possible.

7. The aorta proximally and the common iliac arteries distally are encircled with Penrose drains or cotton tapes. This step allows the surgeon control of the entire vascular system involved should inadvertent hemorrhage occur.

8. The inferior mesenteric artery is clamped, divided, and ligated with a ligature of 0 chromic catgut or a double ligature of 2–0 silk.

9. The lumbar vertebral arteries which exit from the posterior wall of the aorta are clamped, divided, and ligated.

10. Noncrushing clamps, such as Pott's, are applied to the common iliac arteries and the aorta proximal to the aneurysm. A Y-graft of Dacron or Teflon is obtained, correct measurements are made, and any excess length is removed from the graft (Fig. 38–1).

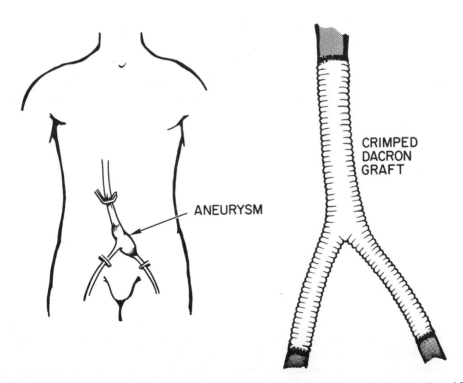

ANEURYSM

CRIMPED DACRON GRAFT

FIGURE 38–1 Note the clamps isolating the aneurysm of the distal aorta. On the right, the crimped Dacron graft has been inserted.

11. The aneurysm is excised and the proximal end of the graft sutured to the proximal aorta. The distal ends of the graft are sutured to the iliac vessels at a level of normal tissue. The small bowel is returned to the abdominal cavity and the abdominal wound closed in the usual fashion; stay sutures may be used to provide further support of the abdominal wall.

12. Prior to closure of the abdomen, a tube gastrostomy is done.

SURGICAL HAZARDS

The resection is a major vascular operation associated with many serious hazards.

1. *Massive Hemorrhage.* The abdominal aorta is diseased and weakened by the athero-sclerotic process. Any rough handling of tissue can result in a tear in the abdominal aortic wall, with massive bleeding. There is also a great hazard of injury to the iliac vessels or the inferior vena cava; these are quite thin-walled and often adherent to the aortic aneurysm.

2. *Injury to One or Both Ureters.* The ureters are often close to and adherent to the abdominal aneurysm and must be carefully freed. Otherwise injury may result.

3. *Injury to Nearby Structures.* The duodenum, the renal arteries, the renal veins, the kidneys, and the spleen are all subject to injury during the course of the operation.

4. *Renal Shutdown.* Blood loss occurring during the operation may be associated with a hypotensive episode. In a patient with chronic renal disease such an episode may be accompanied by tubular necrosis of the kidneys and renal shutdown. Many surgeons feel that the use of an osmotic diuretic such as mannitol, given intravenously during the operation plus maintenance of normal blood pressure by careful infusion of fluids and blood to meet the patient's needs, will diminish or offset the development of postoperative renal shutdown.

IMMEDIATE POSTOPERATIVE MANAGEMENT

The patient is returned to the recovery room until sufficiently reactive from the anesthetic. The routine management is discussed in previous chapters and should be carefully reviewed at this time. Certain specific problems are prone to develop following aortic resection and must be carefully watched for. These include:

a. Continued intra-abdominal bleeding or under-replacement of lost blood may result in severe and significant postoperative hypotension and tachycardia. As mentioned previously, renal failure may ensue. Consequently, the vital signs must be carefully observed for 12 to 24 hours following surgery until the patient's condition stabilizes. Any significant fall in the blood pressure or elevation in the pulse must be reported to the surgeon at once.

b. Intravenous infusions must be maintained throughout the postoperative period so that the patient obtains an adequate quantity of fluids. A careful intake and output chart is kept and the necessary fluids ordered by the surgeon given at the proper rate.

c. The Foley catheter is connected to dependent drainage and the hourly output of urine is measured. The surgeon will usually designate the minimum amount of urine per hour necessary, and if this is not obtained the surgeon should be notified at once. Any blood in the Foley drainage bag should also be reported to the surgeon at once.

d. The Levin or long intestinal tube is connected to low suction and managed in the usual fashion. If a tube gastrostomy was done, the management is similar to that of a Levin tube.

e. The hemoglobin and hematocrit determination is usually ordered on the evening following surgery. As soon as results are available, the surgeon should be notified. Three to four units of blood should be kept available at all times postoperatively until released by the surgeon, and the nurse should make certain that this blood is available in the blood bank throughout the postoperative period until so released.

f. Circulation in the lower extremities is checked every hour. The pulses should be palpated and the warmth of the skin determined.

g. The wound is usually dry and the abdominal cavity not drained and, consequently, there should be little difficulty in the management of the wound during the first 24 hours.

h. Pulmonary complications are prone to develop because of the painful incision, the age of the average patient undergoing this type of surgery, and the length of time under anesthesia. The anesthesia department will often *assist* or *control* the patient's respirations during the first few postoperative hours.

i. Broad-spectrum antibiotics will usually be ordered by the surgeon to be given in the immediate postoperative period. These should be given in adequate doses around the clock.

STUDY QUESTIONS

1. What are the typical clinical features of an abdominal aortic aneurysm?
a. An aneurysm which is intact, but expanding?
b. An aneurysm which has ruptured?

2. Why is aortography usually unnecessary in the diagnosis of abdominal aneurysm?

3. How is the diagnosis of abdominal aneurysm suspected and confirmed by the surgeon?

4. Are there any known factors predisposing to the development of an abdominal aortic aneurysm?

5. Make a list of preoperative activities the nurse should carry out in preparing the patient for such surgery.

6. What is a Lahey bag? What is its function?

7. What are the possible consequences of a period of prolonged hypotension in the immediate postoperative period?

8. Why is an accurate intake and output chart necessary in the immediate postoperative period?

9. In the immediate postoperative period following resection of an abdominal aortic aneurysm, the patient complains of a cold left foot. On examination the left foot is, indeed, cold, pale, and cyanotic. The right foot appears to be unremarkable. What is the probable cause of coldness in his left foot? What is the treatment? Do you think it would be wise for the nurse to treat this cold foot symptomatically with a hot water bottle?

10. Review the basic nursing care and safety factors of which the nurse must be aware when caring for a patient who is receiving oxygen therapy by:
   a. Nasal catheter
   b. Oxygen tent
   c. Bird or Emerson respirator

11. What is a tube gastrostomy? Why is it usually done following resection of an aortic aneurysm?

12. Discuss central venous pressure monitoring. How is it done? What is its rationale? What are its pitfalls?

39   THE PATIENT WITH POPLITEAL ARTERY EMBOLISM

Operation: **Popliteal Artery Embolectomy**

TYPICAL HISTORY

A 45-year-old female with longstanding rheumatic heart disease developed the sudden onset of a painful, cold, numb right leg and foot. The patient denied any previous symptoms in either leg. Her heart disease has been well compensated with only minimal dyspnea on exertion and no chest pain. Several years ago she had been told that she had a heart murmur and an irregular cardiac rhythm.

PHYSICAL EXAMINATION

A well-developed, thin female is admitted, in obvious acute distress and complaining of pain in her right leg and foot.

Significant Findings

1. The right foot is pale and cold and shows patches of cyanosis alternating with pallor. There is a rather sharp line of demarcation between a normally warm leg and the colder section. This line of demarcation is located at the midcalf.
2. The right femoral pulse is excellent in quality although a grossly irregular rhythm is present. No other pulses are palpable below the femoral pulse.
3. There is normal distribution of hair on the toes and no nail changes are present.

DIAGNOSTIC STUDIES

1. Oscillometric studies of the extremities will confirm the presence of good oscillations in the thigh with absence of oscillations in the calf. This strongly suggests an acute embolism or thrombosis to the distal femoral or popliteal artery.

2. A right femoral arteriogram is performed under local anesthesia. This demonstrates a complete obstruction at the distal femoral artery. If multiple, timed x-rays are taken, distal fill into a normal popliteal artery will occur via a few collateral vessels. Since the disease is acute in onset, very few collaterals will have had time to develop.

3. Chest x-ray will reveal an enlarged heart consistent with the patient's known rheumatic heart disease. An electrocardiogram may show atrial fibrillation.

PROBABLE HOSPITAL COURSE

Acute embolism or thrombosis in a major vessel produces acute ischemia and threatens the survival of the affected limb. The lower extremity is particularly apt to suffer irremediable damage or gangrene since adequate collateralization does not exist below the knee. Direct vascular surgery should be performed as soon as the patient's general condition can tolerate it.

After confirmation of the diagnosis, and while waiting to operate on the patient, it is wise to start intravenous heparin (e.g., 10,000 units stat.) to prevent distal and proximal thrombosis. Propagation of the clot into smaller inaccessible vessels is thereby prevented. Lumbar blocks are time-consuming and not of any great value. Their use in this situation is not to be recommended. Similarly, *vasodilators are not to be used.* What little value they may have in warming the skin is deceptive and may lead to a false sense of security. Like the lumbar blocks, vasodilators are time-consuming as well. Dissolution of fresh clots with intra-arterial fibrinolysins is still experimental and is largely unpredictable.

PREPARATION FOR SURGERY

1. Levin tube not necessary.
2. Type and cross-match for four units of blood.
3. Enema not necessary.
4. A large-bore intravenous needle or intracatheter should be inserted for emergency intravenous therapy or transfusions.
5. *Skin Prep.* This includes the pubis, right groin, and entire right leg to the ankle.
6. *Premedications.* Routine.
7. *Special Medications.* Heparin is given preoperatively and during the operation. A heparin antagonist, such as protamine, should also be available since it may be necessary to neutralize the effects of the heparin at the conclusion of the procedure.
8. *Operating Room Skin Prep.* Right groin and entire leg.
9. *Position.* Horizontal supine; the surgeon may wish to flex the knee 10 degrees and externally rotate the leg. This relaxes the gastrocnemius muscle and affords better exposure and visualization of the popliteal vessel behind the knee.

PATHOLOGY

Rheumatic heart disease is frequently associated with atrial fibrillation. The lack of efficient contractility in the left atrium predisposes to clot formation within this heart chamber. Patients with atrial fibrillation may, at any time and with no warning, dislodge a clot into the left ventricle and then into the general circulation. The clot, or embolism, may lodge anywhere in the arterial tree, producing an acute vascular accident (Fig. 39–1). Some of the more common embolic syndromes associated with atrial fibrillation include:

a. *Cerebrovascular accidents* due to carotid and/or vertebral emboli.
b. *Superior mesenteric embolism* with acute ischemia to the small intestine.
c. Renal artery embolism with infarction of kidney.
d. Aorto-iliac embolism with acute ischemia to both legs.
e. Axillobrachial emboli.
f. Femoropopliteal emboli.

Associated with an acute obstruction of a major vessel is a diffuse spasm of the entire nearby vascular tree. This spasm, plus the acutely diminished flow of blood, results in early proximal and distal thrombosis involving, at times, the entire vascular tree of the affected extremity. The limb is sometimes kept alive in a borderline state by the rapid dilatation of collateral vessels which bring some blood supply around the point of obstruction. In acute processes involving major vessels, collateral blood supply is usually inadequate for survival of the extremity.

GENERAL RATIONALE AND SCHEME

Embolectomy can be an extremely gratifying and successful form of vascular surgery providing that it is performed soon enough and providing that the vessel explored is a healthy vessel. Removing the clot and flushing out the proximal and distal vessel can reinstitute pulsatile flow to the vessel and permit normal circulation to resume.

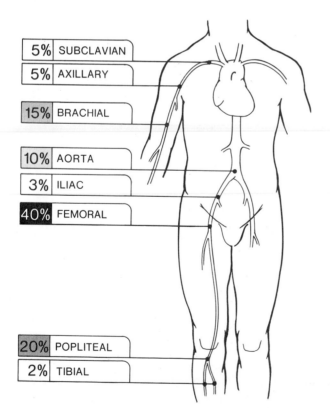

5%	SUBCLAVIAN
5%	AXILLARY
15%	BRACHIAL
10%	AORTA
3%	ILIAC
40%	FEMORAL
20%	POPLITEAL
2%	TIBIAL

FIGURE 39–1 Common sites for peripheral emboli. What visceral sites for emboli are not depicted here?

Scheme

1. The distal thigh and proximal calf are opened through the vertical incision.
2. The area of obstruction is palpated in the vessel.
3. An arteriotomy is performed and the clot removed.
4. The proximal and distal vessels are flushed.
5. The vessel is closed and normal circulation resumed.
6. The incision is closed.

PROCEDURE

1. *Skin Incision:* This will vary somewhat depending upon the surgeon's estimate of the location of the clot. Often a small incision is initiated below the knee, in the medial calf. The incision may have to be extended later above the knee if the clot is higher than that appreciated by arteriography. Alternatively, many surgeons prefer to open the common femoral artery and extract more distal or proximal emboli with a Fogarty embolectomy catheter.

2. The incision is made along the posterior border of the tibia, below the medial condyle. The deep fascia along the posterior edge of the tibia is incised.

3. The medial head of the gastrocnemius muscle is retracted inferiorly, away from the tibia. Retracting the popliteal vein, which is now in view, will expose the popliteal artery. If further exposure is necessary, the medial head of the gastrocnemius muscle may be incised at its insertion on the medial condyle of the femur. This will not produce any untoward problems postoperatively.

4. The popliteal artery is carefully palpated. The sudden abrupt cessation of pulsation will define the precise point of obstruction. Care is taken during exposure of this vessel not to injure any nearby collateral vessels.

5. Rubber catheters or gauze tapes are placed proximal and distal to the embolism so as to obtain safe control of the vessel in case unexpected hemorrhage should occur.

6. If the patient has not already received heparin, it should now be given intravenously by the anesthetist. The circulating nurse should note the time when the heparin was administered.

7. Small "bulldog" vascular clamps are now gently applied to the popliteal artery proximal and distal to the embolism.

8. A small vertical or transverse arteriotomy incision is now made directly over the embolism. This should be made with a small scalpel blade, such as No. 15. If necessary, the incision is extended, using right-angle vascular scissors.

9. The embolism is extracted with a smooth forceps.

10. An appropriate size Fogarty embolectomy catheter is inserted into the distal vessel and passed down into the lower leg. The balloon is expanded with water and the catheter is gently extracted. Distal clots are thereby removed. Further efforts are made with the balloon and irrigating catheters until the surgeon has satisfied himself that adequate *retrograde bleeding* is occurring.

11. The proximal bulldog clamp is momentarily released and a strong pulsatile flow of blood is noted. This flushes out any residual clot in the proximal popliteal vessel.

12. Vascular clamps are re-applied and the arteriotomy incision is rapidly closed with a running, over-and-over, fine, nonabsorbable suture. Nylon or mersilene suture on a fine, small, atraumatic, tapered needle is favored. If it appears that suturing a small popliteal artery may result in narrowing of the vessel, a *vein onlay patch graft* may be used.

13. Just before completing the suturing, the clamps are removed and, once again, adequate retrograde and forward flow is noted.

14. After the clamps have been released, some bleeding occurs for a few moments through the suture line. This usually stops spontaneously and rarely needs further suturing. If bleeding is generalized, the surgeon may elect to give the patient protamine to neutralize the effects of heparin.

15. Distal pulses are checked. If there is any doubt about return of circulation, an arteriogram can be done in the operating room prior to closure.

16. The incision is closed in layers and a light, sterile dressing is applied. Drains may be used.

SURGICAL HAZARDS

1. Injury to the femoral nerve or vein.
2. Massive hemorrhage from loss of control over the opened *popliteal* artery. This is very unusual.

POSTOPERATIVE MANAGEMENT

This procedure may be done under general or spinal anesthesia. If the patient's general condition is precarious, it may also be done under local anesthesia with supplementary intravenous sedation or tranquilization. Providing a great deal of blood has not been lost, it is not a particularly traumatizing or shocking procedure and usually does not take a great deal of time to perform.

The patient is returned to the recovery room until sufficiently reactive from the anesthetic. The usual postanesthesia management is carried out. In addition:

1. The head of the bed is elevated on 6-inch shock blocks to encourage increased blood flow in the leg and foot.

2. The circulation is checked in *both* feet. The nurse should satisfy herself that she can feel all pulses on admission to the recovery room. If there is any doubt about this, the surgeon should be consulted at once. Both the surgeon and the nurse should agree on what the circulatory status is in the immediate postoperative period. If pulses are *not* palpable, the nurse should carefully note color, temperature, capillary flush, and sensation in both feet. Pallor or cyanosis of the nail beds is also a helpful sign. An ultrasonic Doppler device may be used to hear a pulse that is not palpable.

3. Thereafter, circulation is checked every 2 hours. Any change must be called to the surgeon's attention immediately. Loss of a previously palpated pulse will mean immediate return of the patient to the operating room.

4. The dressing is checked for inordinate bleeding. Since the patient is in fibrillation, capable of experiencing further emboli, the surgeon will maintain full anticoagulation in the postoperative period. This can lead to excess postoperative bleeding.

5. A tourniquet should be at or near the bedside for use in the rare instance of massive bleeding from a ruptured arteriotomy site. This is placed about the thigh proximal to the incision and carefully inflated until bleeding just stops.

6. The patient is allowed fluid by mouth as soon as she is reactive from her anesthetic.

7. The patient is allowed a diet of solid foods the day after surgery and is usually ambulated immediately. When the patient's anticoagulants have been adjusted, she can be discharged from the hospital (in most cases 5 to 7 days after surgery).

STUDY QUESTIONS

1. Define: embolus, thrombus. Locate the sites where peripheral arterial emboli are most often found. What organs are involved? What clinical syndromes are to be expected as a result of emboli at these sites?

2. What are some of the causes predisposing to systemic arterial embolization?

3. Seven days after a coronary occlusion, a patient suddenly notes severe and generalized abdominal pain. The white count rises sharply. The abdomen becomes tender and distended. The patient rapidly becomes hypotensive and cyanotic. What is the most likely diagnosis? How is this situation treated?

4. Severe left flank pain followed by gross hematuria in a patient with rheumatic heart disease and atrial fibrillation may signal the onset of what acute vascular syndrome? How can the diagnosis of this condition be confirmed or excluded? How is this syndrome treated?

5. Discuss the relative values of *heparin* and *Coumadin* in the management of acute arterial embolism. Do you think Coumadin has any use here at all?

6. Discuss the Fogarty embolectomy catheter. Obtain one from the operating room and demonstrate its use to your class. Compose a comprehensive nursing care plan for a patient who is to undergo popliteal embolectomy.

THE PATIENT WITH GANGRENE OF THE FOOT

40

Operation: Midthigh Amputation

TYPICAL HISTORY

A 70-year-old male has had pain and coldness in his right foot for several months. He is also a diabetic, taking large quantities of insulin daily. A sympathectomy was done 4 months prior to the present admission with some increase in the warmth of his foot but no significant diminution in the amount of pain or disability. He now enters with cyanosis of the entire right foot and gangrene of the first two toes.

PHYSICAL EXAMINATION

A thin, elderly male, complaining of severe, steady right foot pain. On several examinations during his hospital course it is found that he holds his right foot in a dependent position over the side of the bed.

Significant Findings

1. Wet gangrene is noted in the right great toe and right second toe.
2. The right femoral pulse is diminished but palpable. The popliteal pulse is absent, as are any further distal pulses.
3. The right foot from about the midcalf region down is cold.
4. The remainder of the examination is unremarkable.

DIAGNOSTIC STUDIES

The patient does not appear to be a candidate for any further attempts to improve circulation in his foot. The presence of gangrene in an elderly diabetic male would appear to eliminate the possibility of vascular surgery. However, the surgeon may utilize every means short of amputation initially and may elect occasionally to do an arteriogram. Should this reveal localized blockage in the superficial femoral artery, direct vascular surgery may be possible.

The patient's general condition should be evaluated by chest x-ray, electrocardiogram, and determination of fasting blood sugar and BUN prior to amputation.

PROBABLE HOSPITAL COURSE

The mortality rate from what might appear to be a simple technical operation is rather imposing because of the patient's age, general condition, and diabetic status. Such a patient will often succumb because of poor wound healing and sepsis. Consequently, every attempt must be made to plan the level of amputation properly so that further surgical intervention will not be necessary. It is, of course, very tempting for the surgeon to attempt amputation through the midaspect of the foot or below the knee so that the patient may be rehabilitated more easily with use of a prosthetic device. However, experience has shown that in a patient who has no popliteal pulse and who is diabetic and elderly, there is little likelihood of healing below the knee. Consequently, the surgeon will usually perform a midthigh amputation. Some of the tests which must be performed during the hospital stay to prepare this patient for surgery are as follows:

1. The diabetic often has urinary tract infection. This should be evaluated and treated prior to surgery.
2. His diabetic state should be brought into maximum control by careful titration of the amount of insulin needed and the correct diet.
3. Much psychological preparation must be given this patient before surgery is done.
4. The leg should be wrapped in sheets from the knee down, and the thigh and groin prepped daily with pHisoHex to minimize the number of skin bacteria.
5. The patient's heart, lungs, and kidneys should be evaluated and any necessary steps taken to put them in maximum condition prior to surgery.

PREPARATION FOR SURGERY

1. *Levin Tube.* Not necessary.
2. The patient is typed and cross-matched for one unit of whole blood.
3. *Skin Preparation.* As described, the leg should be wrapped from the knee down and the thigh washed daily with pHisoHex. On the evening prior to surgery, the entire right groin and thigh down to the knee are prepped in the usual fashion. (See Introduction.)
4. *Enema.* A Fleet or soapsuds enema is given on the evening prior to surgery.
5. *Premedications.* Routine.
6. *Special Medications.* None.
7. *Psychological Preparation.* This is extremely important in the patient undergoing amputative surgery. Loss of a limb or a segment of a limb represents partial destruction of the body image and there is foreknowledge of permanent disability to follow. From a medicolegal point of view, it is also extremely important for the patient to understand the absolute necessity of amputation. It is frequently necessary to allow the patient to have many sleepless, pain-filled nights before he is emotionally and intellectually convinced of the need for amputation. It is often said that the patient must come to the surgeon for amputation, rather than the converse.
8. *Operating Room Skin Prep.* This extends from the groin as far as and including the knee. (See Introduction.)
9. *Position.* Horizontal supine. (See Introduction.)

PATHOLOGY

In the elderly diabetic, the peripheral vasculature is usually markedly diseased throughout its course and there is small possibility of direct surgical intervention to repair the artery. In the present patient, sympathectomy has failed to dilate the vessels sufficiently, a situation which is, again, indicative of his poor general vasculature.

GENERAL RATIONALE AND SCHEME

In most cases, failure to amputate a gangrenous extremity will finally cause overwhelming sepsis, septicemia, and death. In addition, the painful extremity will be the cause of many sleepless nights for the patient. Consequently, when all other means of increasing circulation of the foot have been utilized to no avail, amputation must be done.

Scheme

1. A circular incision is made above the knee.
2. The incision is carried down through the muscles.
3. The femur is amputated with a saw.
4. The vessels and nerves are ligated.
5. The amputated stump is closed.
6. A noncompression dressing is applied.

PROCEDURE

1. *Skin Incision.* The surgeon incises the skin over the distal femur, attempting to leave large anterior and posterior flaps for easy closure over the amputated femur.

2. The incision is now deepened through the anterior and posterior fasciae of the thigh. The flexor, extensor, and adductor muscles are severed, bleeding being controlled with chromic catgut ties and ligatures.

3. The femoral vein and artery are found in the medial aspect of the thigh; they should be doubly ligated with suture ligatures of heavy chromic catgut so as to prevent massive hemorrhage. (However, often these vessels are occluded and only a small amount of bleeding will occur.) The sciatic nerve should be divided as high up in the thigh as possible to prevent the development of a painful postoperative neuroma.

4. When the femur is approached, a periosteal elevator is used to remove all periosteum from the distal femur.

5. The femur is amputated as high up in the wound as possible to avoid a painful bony protuberance against the skin flaps.

6. The sharp edges of the stump of the femur should be smoothed with a rat-tooth file.

7. At the completion of the amputation, the wound is thoroughly irrigated with sterile saline and bleeding controlled with chromic catgut ties.

8. The posteroanterior fasciae are approximated with interrupted chromic catgut ties. Large Penrose drains are brought out through the medial and lateral aspects of the incision. Some surgeons do not use drains.

9. The skin is closed with fine interrupted wire sutures which can be left for 3 to 4 weeks.

10. A noncompression, heavy dressing is applied to the stump.

SURGICAL HAZARDS

There are no particular common surgical hazards following the operation. Occasionally a large amount of bleeding may occur from the femoral artery or vein, but this should be anticipated and prevented by careful dissection.

POSTOPERATIVE MANAGEMENT

The patient is returned to the recovery room until sufficiently reactive from the anesthetic. He is kept in the horizontal supine position. The usual postanesthesia management is carried out. In addition:

1. The patient often suffers from obstructive uropathy due to his age and will often need a Foley catheter for several days. This should be connected to dependent drainage and managed in the usual fashion.

2. Sepsis is very common in amputative surgery. Consequently, if the dressing soaks through in any fashion, however minimal, the surgeon should be notified.

3. Narcotics are given in small doses to control the pain.

4. The dressing should be checked for constrictiveness and loosened accordingly.

5. Pulmonary embolism is a genuine hazard following amputative surgery in the elderly. An anti-embolism stocking should be fitted to the unaffected extremity. Early physiotherapy is encouraged, and the patient should be ambulated with a walker the day after surgery.

STUDY QUESTIONS

1. List the various levels of amputation in the lower extremity, describing the indications for each level of amputation.

2. Discuss some of the prostheses available for lower extremity amputees.

3. Discuss some of the psychological problems which your patient may have in the preoperative as well as the postoperative period following a midthigh amputation and how you would manage them.

4. Describe the essential steps in the midthigh amputation procedure.

5. What is the danger involved in use of a constricting dressing on the stump following this procedure?

6. List some of the causes of death following midthigh amputation in an elderly, arteriosclerotic patient. How would you anticipate and prevent these?

THE PATIENT WITH CAROTID ARTERY INSUFFICIENCY

41

Operation: Carotid Artery Endarterectomy

TYPICAL HISTORY

A 71-year-old male has noted transient episodes of lightheadedness and recurrent attacks of weakness in his left arm and leg. On one occasion, he was found in a semicomatose condition, was unable to speak, and had definite paralysis on the left side of his body. This gradually improved and, apart from his mild episodes of lightheadedness and recurrent weakness in the left side of his body, he has been well otherwise.

PHYSICAL EXAMINATION

A well-developed, thin male is admitted in no acute distress.

Significant Findings

1. There is a diminution in the pulse caliber of the right common carotid artery in the neck.
2. There is some palsy in the left arm and leg.
3. There is a bruit over the right common carotid artery.
4. The remainder of the physical examination is unremarkable.
5. In a substantial number of patients with transient cerebral ischemic attacks due to extracranial vascular disease, there are no significant findings in the neck.

DIAGNOSTIC STUDIES

1. Plain x-rays of the head and neck may be taken in an attempt to demonstrate calcification in an atherosclerotic plaque in the carotid arteries. These x-rays are often unremarkable.
2. A *carotid arteriogram* is done. In this test, which is similar to a femoral arteriogram, a catheter is inserted into the aortic arch via the femoral artery and radiopaque dye is injected. Any aneurysm or stenosis of the artery will be visualized by x-ray study.

PROBABLE HOSPITAL COURSE

Assuming that the patient's general condition would make major vascular surgery feasible, the patient will be taken to the operating room soon after the diagnosis of carotid insufficiency is made, and direct surgery of the common carotid artery will be carried out.

PREPARATION FOR SURGERY

1. Levin tube is not necessary.
2. The patient is typed and cross-matched for three to four units of whole blood.
3. *Skin Prep.* This will extend on the side of the neck involved from the face down to the clavicles. (See Introduction to Section III.) The lower leg should also be prepped in the event that the surgeon might wish to retrieve a saphenous vein for onlay grafting.
4. *Fleet Enema.* Not necessary.
5. *Premedications.* Routine.
6. *Special Medications.* None.
7. *Operating Room Skin Prep.* Encompasses the entire neck on the side of the operation. (See Introduction.) The lower leg is also prepped.
8. *Position.* The patient is placed in the semi-Fowler's position with the head hyperextended and turned to the side opposite the operative site. (See Introduction to Section III.)

PATHOLOGY

In most cases, the atherosclerotic occlusive disease process will be localized to the bifurcation of the common carotid artery where it divides into the internal and external carotid arteries. Plaquing usually narrows the internal carotid artery near its origin from the common carotid artery. Multiple lesions are frequent, occurring in more than 75 per cent of patients with carotid artery insufficiency. The lesions may produce complete or incomplete occlusion. The plaques are often ulcerated and are covered with atheromatous debris rich in agglutinated platelets and fibrin deposits. These loose aggregates are probably responsible for recurrent embolic episodes in the brain.

GENERAL RATIONALE AND SCHEME

Until a few years ago, cerebral vascular insufficiency was thought to be inoperable and, indeed, most patients were treated expectantly and often died of a cerebral vascular accident. Within recent years it has been discovered that at least 50 per cent of cerebral vascular accidents are due to major vessel disease in the neck. In most cases, this involves disease of the carotid arteries which are easily accessible to surgical intervention and treatment.

The obstructive process usually occupies a small segment of the common carotid artery where it bifurcates into the external and internal carotid arteries. This area may be opened and the atherosclerotic plaque removed (thromboendarterectomy); or, if the vessel wall proximal and distal to the obstruction appears to be diseased also, a by-pass graft may be put in place so as to completely by-pass the area of obstruction. The decision as to the exact nature of the operation will be determined by the surgical findings.

Scheme

1. An incision is made in the lateral aspect of the neck over the bifurcation of the carotid artery.

2. Tapes are placed proximal and distal to the area of obstruction to secure the vessels adequately should bleeding occur.

3. The vessel wall is opened and the lesion removed.

4. The vessel wall is closed.

5. The skin incision is closed.

PROCEDURE

1. *Skin Incision.* A vertical skin incision is made, following the course of the sternomastoid muscle.

2. The sternocleidomastoid muscle is visualized and retracted laterally, exposing the common carotid sheath.

3. Several centimeters of common carotid artery are mobilized proximal and distal to the bifurcation.

4. Umbilical tapes are placed around the artery proximal and distal to the lesion for control should bleeding occur.

5. At this point, tolerance to complete carotid occlusion must be determined. If the patient tolerates temporary occlusion of the carotid artery, then the operation can be carried out without an internal shunt. If, by clinical examination or electroencephalographic tracings, the patient does not appear to tolerate temporary clamping of the carotid artery, then an internal shunt consisting of an artificial tubular graft placed proximal and distal to the obstruction must be used before endarterectomy is attempted. Many surgeons routinely use such shunts, acting on the belief that no test of ability to tolerate temporary carotid occlusion is trustworthy.

6. A small incision is made, overlying the obstructed area in the carotid artery.

7. Using endarterectomy spatulas, the plaque of atherosclerotic occlusive material is removed.

8. The arteriotomy opening is now closed with a running 5-0 silk suture. A small patch of saphenous vein may be retrieved from the ankle and used as a vein onlay patch graft.

9. The incision is closed in the usual fashion and a small dressing applied. A small Penrose drain may be used for 24 hours.

SURGICAL HAZARDS

1. Uncontrollable hemorrhage may result from rough handling of diseased vessels in the neck.

2. There may be damage to the mandibular branch of the facial nerve or the hypoglossal nerve, both of which are found in this vicinity.

3. Acute cerebral vascular accident may occur during anesthesia, secondary to occlusion of the artery in a patient whose remaining carotid artery or vertebral arterial system is also insufficient.

POSTOPERATIVE MANAGEMENT

The patient is returned to the recovery room until sufficiently reactive from the anesthetic. General postanesthesia management is carried out. In addition:

1. Careful neurological observations must be made in the immediate postoperative period. These include:

   a. Checking patient's level of consciousness. This is most feasible if the operation has been done under local anesthesia. However, even under general anesthesia, the gag and lid reflexes as well as the patient's response to painful stimuli may be monitored. Any change in the patient's level of consciousness should be reported to the surgeon immediately.

   b. Measuring the size and reaction of pupils.

   c. Measuring for motion or lack of motion of the extremities.

   d. The Babinski response.

2. If the dressing soaks through, the surgeon should be notified immediately.

3. The patient is kept in a low semi-Fowler's position to minimize venous oozing in the neck.

4. The patient is allowed clear liquids when reactive from the anesthetic.

5. The patient may be ambulated the day after surgery and allowed to resume a solid diet. He can be discharged from the hospital in 5 to 7 days.

STUDY QUESTIONS

1. Describe a typical cerebral vascular accident, discussing the signs and symptoms.

2. Is there any treatment for acute cerebral vascular insufficiency apart from surgical correction of the carotid arteries?

3. Describe the rationale for the use of anticoagulants in people who have had a cerebral vascular accident.

4. Define thromboendarterectomy, internal vascular shunting, external vascular shunting.

5. Describe the make-up and function of a Pott's vascular clamp.

6. Describe the essential steps in the performance of carotid thrombo-endarterectomy.

7. Outline the postoperative nursing care plan for 24 hours for a patient who has had carotid endarterectomy.

8. What complications might be anticipated in this patient postoperatively?

THE PATIENT WITH PULMONARY EMBOLISM

42

Operation: Inferior Vena Caval Plication

TYPICAL HISTORY

A 74-year-old male underwent an inguinal hernia repair with no apparent operative complications. On the eighth postoperative day, he complained of a swollen, painful calf. Anticoagulants were started but gave only minimal relief of symptoms. Four days after the start of therapy, the patient developed severe left chest pain and coughed up blood. His condition appeared to be deteriorating.

PHYSICAL EXAMINATION

The patient is a well-developed but cyanotic and dyspneic male.

Significant Findings

1. Cyanosis and dyspnea are noted.
2. There is hypotension (90/60) and tachycardia (120).
3. Pleural friction rub and rales over left posterior chest are found.
4. The right thigh and calf are enlarged, mottled, and tender.
5. Homans' sign is strongly positive on the right.

DIAGNOSTIC STUDIES

1. EKG indicates right heart strain (cor pulmonale).
2. Chest x-ray reveals possible opaque area in left lung base, with some fluid collection.
3. WBC is 15,000 per cu. mm.
4. Clotting time is 34 minutes.
5. Pulmonary scan demonstrates an extensive area of diminished perfusion in the left lower lung field.

PROBABLE HOSPITAL COURSE

1. Thrombophlebitis is generally treated medically with anticoagulants.
2. The occurrence of a pulmonary embolism after adequate anticoagulation therapy is thought by some to be a strong indication for surgical intervention.
3. If surgery is indicated, the patient is rapidly prepared and taken to the operating room in the hope of preventing a second, possibly fatal, pulmonary embolism.

PREPARATION FOR SURGERY

1. *Skin Prep.* The entire right flank from the costal margin to the iliac crest is prepped laterally. The prep is extended anteriorly across the entire abdomen, including the pubis. (See Introduction to Section I.)
2. *Levin Tube.* Not necessary.
3. Type and cross-match for three units of blood.
4. *Enema.* Not necessary.
5. *Premedications.* Routine.
6. *Special Medications.* The anticoagulant may have to be neutralized to prevent operative bleeding.
   a. For heparin neutralization use protamine or Polybrene.
   b. For Coumarol or Dicumarol neutralization use vitamin K. This may take 24 to 48 hours.
7. *Position.* Right kidney position. (See Introduction to Section I.)

PATHOLOGY

1. The blood clots are usually limited to the iliac, femoral, and popliteal veins and are therefore not usually seen at the level of the inferior vena cava.
2. Occasionally, the vena cava is distended and turgid and, if opened, will be found to contain formed blood clots.

GENERAL RATIONALE AND SCHEME

Blood from the lower extremities drains ultimately into the inferior vena cava and thence into the right heart and lungs. An embolism consists of a fragment of blood clot which is dislodged from its source in the leg, passes up the vena cava into the heart, and finally lodges in the lung; here it obstructs the flow of normal blood and a pulmonary infarction occurs. Failure to control embolization with anticoagulation is an indication for venous interruption. Plication of the inferior vena cava prevents further emboli from moving toward the heart.

Scheme

1. The flank is opened and the inferior vena cava is exposed.
2. A teflon clip is placed on the vena cava (Fig. 42–1).
3. The flank is closed.

PROCEDURE

1. *Skin Incision.* A right transverse or oblique incision is made from the level of the anterior iliac crest to just below the umbilicus. (See Introduction to Section I.)
2. *Deepening Incision.* The aponeurosis of the three abdominal muscles (external oblique, internal oblique, and transversus) is split.
3. The *peritoneum* is reflected medially, exposing the inferior vena cava near the vertebral column.
4. The *vena cava* is dissected from the surrounding tissues. Two large umbilical tapes are passed around the vena cava.
5. The vena cava is partially occluded with a teflon clip.
6. The three muscles are reapproximated with suture.
7. The skin incision is closed.

SURGICAL HAZARDS

1. *Massive Hemorrhage.* Injury to the vena cava or the lumbar veins can result in massive venous hemorrhage which is extremely difficult to control.
2. *Injury to Ureter.* The right ureter lies close to the inferior vena cava and is easily damaged, particularly when the operative field is obscured by poor lighting or bleeding.
3. *Dislodging Further Emboli.* At any time during the operation, a fatal embolism may be dislodged from its source. Except for careful and speedy surgery, nothing can be done to prevent this potential complication. The situation is always extremely hazardous until the vena cava has been securely ligated.

POSTOPERATIVE MANAGEMENT

1. If the original pulmonary embolism was large, the patient will remain extremely ill from the effects of the embolism. The cardiopulmonary status is treated with:
   a. Oxygen.
   b. Intermittent positive pressure breathing (IPPB).
   c. Frequent suctioning.
   d. Bronchodilators.
   e. Support of cardiovascular tree with vasopressors.
2. Should he survive the embolism, rapid improvement in his general condition is to be expected.

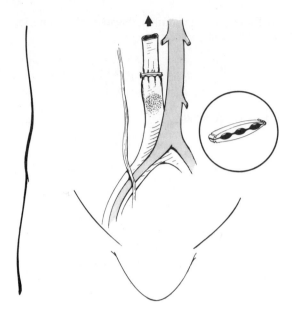

FIGURE 42-1 A partially occluding teflon clip on vena cava, preventing a caval embolism (faintly visible below clip) from reaching lungs.

3. The patient is maintained in the Trendelenburg position with 6 inch blocks under the foot of the bed.

4. The legs are kept firmly wrapped in Ace bandages from toes to groin. The pedal pulses are checked frequently in the first 24 hours.

5. If anticoagulation has been resumed, the nurse should check the dressing frequently for bleeding.

STUDY QUESTIONS

1. What factors may be predisposing to postoperative thrombophlebitis? What is the nurse's role in the prevention of phlebitis?

2. While on anticoagulation therapy, a patient develops gross hematuria and reports this to the nurse. What is the probable cause of this hematuria? How should the nurse handle the situation?

3. What is a pleural friction rub?

4. The clotting time is used to measure the effects of heparin anticoagulation. What test is used to measure the effects of Coumadin anticoagulation? Discuss the nature of this test.

5. Explain to your class the rationale for inferior vena cava plication in the control of pulmonary embolism.

6. Do you think this operation is highly successful?

7. What other operation can be done to prevent the development of pulmonary embolism? What are its advantages and disadvantages over caval ligation?

8. Describe the operative steps in inferior vena cava plication.

9. Discuss some of the immediate postoperative complications of inferior vena cava plication.

10. What nursing measures are employed in the immediate postoperative period to decrease the incidence of bilateral leg swelling?

11. Outline a nursing care plan covering the first 24 hours following an uncomplicated vena caval plication.

12. Discuss the management of deep thrombophlebitis from a medical point of view, paying particular attention to the indications and contraindications and to the use of heparin.

13. What is the significance of a positive Homans' sign? A negative Homans' sign?

THE PATIENT WITH VARICOSE VEINS

43

Operation: Ligation and Stripping of Varicose Veins

TYPICAL HISTORY

The 42-year-old mother of four children noted the development of painful swollen veins in her legs during her third pregnancy. Following this pregnancy, the symptoms subsided, only to worsen again during her fourth pregnancy. On one occasion, a small, red, tender area was seen overlying one of the veins. The patient states that the symptoms did not subside following her last pregnancy. The veins produce a dull ache and a tired sensation, particularly by the end of the day. She denies any swelling of her ankles or legs.

PHYSICAL EXAMINATION

The patient is a well-developed, well-nourished female in no acute distress.

Significant Findings

1. There are enlarged tortuous veins on the front and inner sides of both thighs and legs.
2. Brownish pigmentation is seen on the inner sides of both ankles.
3. There is no swelling of the legs or ankles.
4. The remainder of the examination is unremarkable.

DIAGNOSTIC STUDIES

There are no specific x-ray or laboratory procedures available to evaluate varicose veins; the diagnosis is made clinically. It is important for the surgeon to rule out insufficiency of the deep femoral veins of the legs. This is done by the use of various *tourniquet tests* which will not be described here.

PROBABLE HOSPITAL COURSE

Once deep vein insufficiency has been ruled out and proper indications for surgery have been met, the patient will be operated upon.

PREPARATION FOR SURGERY

1. Levin tube not necessary.
2. Type and cross-match not necessary.
3. *Skin Prep.* This includes the lower abdomen, the pubis, the perineum, and the entire thighs and legs.
4. *Premedications.* Routine.
5. *Special Medications.* None.
6. *Operating Room Skin Prep.* Extends from lower abdomen as far as and including ankles.
7. *Position.* Horizontal supine.
8. The varicose veins are marked out with indelible ink preoperatively.

PATHOLOGY

Varicose veins represent a tortuosity of the greater or lesser saphenous sytems of the leg. Loss of venous tone results in backflow of venous blood. This, in turn, causes the dilatation of veins which is seen clinically. The exact cause of the condition is obscure; it may be caused by an inherited weakness of connective tissue throughout the body. Predisposing factors include:
1. Obesity.
2. Pregnancy.
3. Pelvic masses.
4. Erect position.

GENERAL RATIONALE AND SCHEME

Varicose veins, if untreated, may gradually worsen. The symptoms of dull aching leg pain will tend to increase. In addition, episodes of acute phlebitis due to stasis of blood and clotting in the dilated veins will gradually increase in frequency and severity and will eventually cause stasis ulcerations, particularly in and about the ankles. Varicose ulcers, due to hemorrhage under the skin, are another complication of varicose veins.

Scheme

1. Skin incisions are made in both groins and ankles.
2. Internal strippers are passed the full length of the veins and the veins are removed.
3. Accessory "feeders" are directly excised by various incisions in the legs and thighs.
4. Compression dressing is applied.

PROCEDURE

1. *Skin Incision.* The main incision is an oblique one below the inguinal ligament overlying the saphenofemoral junction.
2. The saphenofemoral junction is located. Tributaries of the saphenous vein in the thigh and groin are ligated and divided.
3. The saphenous vein is ligated and divided at its junction with the femoral vein.
4. The distal end of the greater saphenous vein in the ankle is obtained, ligated, and divided.
5. An internal stripper is passed the full length of the vein, fixed to the proximal vein, and then removed through the distal incision, carrying the entire saphenous vein with it.
6. Accessory feeding veins in the thighs and legs (marked prior to surgery) are located through separate incisions, ligated, and divided.
7. All incisions are closed in the usual fashion.
8. A compression dressing (such as Ace bandages) is applied the full length of the extremity.

SURGICAL HAZARDS

1. Injury to the femoral vein, with hemorrhage or postoperative deep phlebitis.
2. Damage or ligation of femoral artery with loss of limb is a rare complication and results from faulty knowledge of the anatomy or careless surgery.

POSTOPERATIVE MANAGEMENT

The patient is returned to the recovery room until sufficiently reactive from the anesthetic. The general management of the postoperative patient is carried out. In particular:
1. The patient should be kept in the recumbent position for 24 hours.
2. Urinary retention should be anticipated and the patient catheterized if this develops.
3. The patient is allowed liquids by mouth as soon as alert.
4. If the dressings soak through, the surgeon should be notified at once.
5. The patient is ambulated 24 hours after surgery, resumes a house diet, and is discharged in 3 to 5 days.

STUDY QUESTIONS

1. Name three predisposing causes of varicose vein formation.

2. Discuss the complications of untreated varicose veins.

3. Distinguish acute superficial and deep phlebitis. Which is more serious? What is the treatment of each?

4. Why must the surgeon make certain his patient has adequate deep femoral veins before ligation and stripping of superficial veins?

5. Describe the *Trendelenburg test* for venous insufficiency. What help can the nurse afford the surgeon in the performance of this test?

6. Why do patients with varicose veins develop superficial phlebitis? Stasis ulcers?

7. Describe the basic steps in ligation and stripping of varicose veins.

8. What role does injection therapy play in the treatment of varicose veins?

9. Discuss the early postoperative management and nursing care of a patient who has undergone stripping of varicose veins.

10. Describe the construction of *internal* and *external* vein strippers.

44

THE PATIENT WITH BLEEDING ESOPHAGEAL VARICES

Operation: Portacaval Shunt

TYPICAL HISTORY

A 48-year-old male, with a background of alcoholism, was found to have cirrhosis of the liver 4 years prior to this admission. On at least two earlier occasions, he was hospitalized for moderate upper gastrointestinal bleeding. A previous upper G.I. series confirmed the presence of esophageal varices, and his liver function tests confirmed the diagnosis of cirrhosis of the liver.

Three days prior to admission, he began vomiting bright red blood and he passed large, liquid, black bowel movements. He was admitted in shock through the emergency room.

PHYSICAL EXAMINATION

A well-developed male is admitted, vomiting bright red blood and passing black liquid stools.

Significant Findings

1. Extreme pallor, coldness, and clamminess of extremities are noted.
2. Blood pressure is 70/40; pulse, 120 and weak.
3. There is bloody vomitus on face and chin.
4. There is black, tarry stool on rectal examination.
5. The stigmata of cirrhosis of the liver are present:
a. Erythema of both palms.
b. Severe acne rosacea with "liver spiders."
c. Liver palpable three fingers below the right costal margin.
d. No axillary or pubic hair.
e. Distended veins on the abdominal wall.

DIAGNOSTIC STUDIES

1. Hematocrit level is 16 per cent, hemoglobin, 7 gm.
2. Stool is positive for guaiac, plus 4.
3. Flat and upright films of the abdomen are negative except for some haziness on the film.
4. Liver studies reveal the following abnormalities:
a. Bromsulphalein retention (BSP), 45 per cent.
b. Cephalin flocculation, 4 plus.
c. Thymol turbidity, 4.
d. Alkaline phosphatase, 2 units.
e. Total bilirubin, 3 mg. per cent.
f. Total proteins, 5 gm. with albumin 3 gm. and globulin 2 gm.
g. Prothrombin time, 50 per cent.
5. Upper G.I. series when patient's condition was stabilized revealed esophageal varices; there was no evidence of duodenal ulcer.

PROBABLE HOSPITAL COURSE

1. The patient appears to be bleeding massively from esophageal varices. The first order of business is to control the shock, which will require a significant number of blood transfusions given through large-bore intracatheters or cutdowns. A Levin tube is inserted into the stomach and connected to nasogastric suction in order to permit monitoring of the amount of continued blood loss. If bleeding cannot be controlled by these conservative measures, emergency surgery will be necessary. The patient's chances for recovering from the operation are far improved if the bleeding can be controlled and surgery postponed until the condition stabilizes.

Bleeding may also be controlled by the introduction of a *Sengstaken* or *Blakemore tube* into the stomach and esophagus. This tube consists essentially of three tubes in one (Fig. 44–1). They are described as follows:

a. *One* of the tubes is a gastric suction tube which acts very much in the manner of a Levin tube.

b. The *second* tube is connected to a long sausage-like balloon which is placed in the esophagus and expanded with approximately 40 mm. of mercurial pressure, monitored by a sphygmomanometer at the bedside, so as to provide tamponade of any bleeding vessels in the midesophagus.

c. The *third* tube is connected to a gastric balloon which is expanded with 200 to 300 cc. of water and pulled up against the gastroesophageal junction in an attempt to provide tamponade of the vessels in this region. The tube is diagnostic in that bleeding from below the balloon (namely, in the lower stomach or duodenum) will not be controlled; if the bleeding is from the lower esophageal varices, it will be controlled. In addition, the tube is therapeutic in that it temporarily stops the bleeding and allows the patient's condition to stabilize before any surgery is contemplated.

Another method of controlling esophageal bleeding on a temporary basis consists of gastric cooling. In this procedure, a large balloon shaped like the stomach is inserted into the stomach and a gastric coolant is passed through this balloon. The rationale of this treatment is that local hypothermia tends to cause sludging of blood within the veins and considerably minimizes or stops the bleeding. Again, this is a temporary procedure and should be followed by definitive therapy.

2. Assuming that the bleeding subsides, the surgeon must then evaluate the patient as to his eligibility for surgery. There is a high mortality associated with portacaval shunting and consequently very definite criteria must be met before a patient is submitted to this operative procedure. These criteria will not be described in detail here but, basically, they have to do with

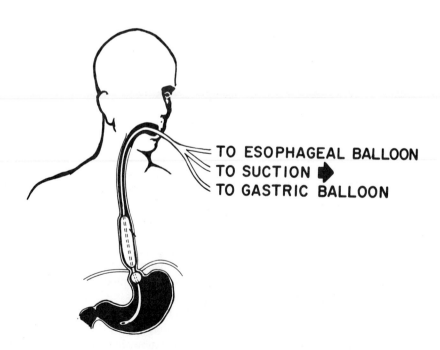

TO ESOPHAGEAL BALLOON
TO SUCTION ▶
TO GASTRIC BALLOON

FIGURE 44–1   Blakemore tube in place. Note position of gastric and esophageal balloons.

the total liver reserve which the patient has and which is manifested by the results of liver function tests. In general, the criteria for surgery are these: serum albumin of greater than 3 gm.; a prothrombin time which, although initially low, is able to be returned to normal levels with parenteral administration of vitamin K; and total bilirubin of less than 3 mg. If these criteria are met, the patient is generally considered to be a good candidate for portacaval shunting. If the surgeon elects to perform a portacaval shunt on his patient, he will take several days to properly prepare him for this operation. These preparations are described in the subsequent section.

PREPARATION FOR SURGERY

1. *Psychological Preparation.* Portacaval shunting does nothing to add vitality to the already injured liver. It merely by-passes the mechanical block set up against the return flow of blood to the liver from the portal vein. If the patient continues to drink alcohol following this operation, he will invariably worsen the state of his liver and will die. Consequently, every effort must be made to make the patient understand that the operation will fail in respect to survival time should he continue to drink postoperatively.

This psychological preparation should take advantage of various departments within and without the hospital including, perhaps, psychiatric help, social service help, as well as aid from the clergy. Preparation of the patient for his rehabilitation will continue in the postoperative period but should not be minimized preoperatively.

2. The patient's blood volume must be returned to as near the normal as possible, and preferably with the use of fresh whole blood and plasma.

3. Various defects due to his cirrhosis should be adjusted. These include:
   a. *Hypoproteinemia,* which is corrected with serum albumin infusions.
   b. *Low prothrombin time,* which is corrected with parenteral administration of vitamin K.
   c. *Electrolyte deficiencies,* particularly hyponatremia, which is corrected with hypertonic saline infusions.
   d. *Nutritional deficiencies* associated with liver cirrhosis and which are partially corrected with a high carbohydrate, low protein diet.

4. The intestinal tract must be prepared in a special way for portacaval shunting. The retained old blood within the small and large intestines is decomposed by intestinal bacteria and converted to ammonium by-products, which are transmitted to the liver. The sick liver is unable to chemically convert these ammonium compounds into less toxic forms and cerebral encephalopathy results — "liver coma." The two basic ways of handling this situation preoperatively are:
   a. Cathartics and enemas to rid the intestinal tract of old blood.
   b. Per oral neomycin, which tends to minimize the overgrowth of *ammonium-producing* bacteria within the intestinal tract.

5. A long intestinal tube, such as a Miller-Abbott tube, is placed within the small intestine in order to deflate the intestine. This allows more room for the extensive surgery which will be performed.

6. A Foley catheter is inserted on the day of surgery.

7. The patient is typed and cross-matched for eight to ten units of whole blood.

8. Premedications are routine.

9. *Special Medications.* There are usually none, provided the proper preparation of the patient has already been made.

10. The skin preparation should extend from the nipples as far as and including the pubis. (See Introduction.)

11. *Enema.* A soapsuds enema or Fleet enema is given the evening prior to or the day of surgery.

12. A large-bore intracatheter or cutdown should be inserted preoperatively in case massive transfusions of blood are needed during the operation. The surgeon may insert a catheter into the superior vena cava to monitor central venous pressure.

13. The operating room skin prep again extends from the nipple line as far as and including the pubis. (See Introduction.)

14. The position is horizontal supine. (See Introduction.)

PATHOLOGY

When the abdomen is opened, signs of increased portal pressure or portal hypertension are usually in evidence. These consist of distended and dilated veins in the abdominal wall, the omentum, the porta hepatis, the stomach, and the large and small intestines. Thus, surgery is very vascular and a good deal of blood is needed during the operative procedure.

The portal vein will be seen to be greatly distended and if pressure is taken within the vein it will be extremely high, in the neighborhood of 300 mm. of saline. The liver is usually small and hobnailed in appearance, although sometimes the liver appears larger than normal.

GENERAL RATIONALE AND SCHEME

The patient with cirrhosis of the liver and esophageal varices, who has bled massively on one or more occasions, represents a high risk in terms of possible future bleeding episodes. Any one of these bleeding episodes can result in massive exsanguination and death. Surgery for this condition has evolved over the years and several procedures have been tried and discarded because of failure. The operation, portacaval shunt, was designed to solve the mechanical problem of portal hypertension resulting from blocked flow of blood from the portal vein to the liver. The resulting back pressure on the portal vein dilates various veins throughout the entire body, particularly in the lower esophagus, and these tend to break down and bleed. If the blood from the portal vein is shunted through to the inferior vena cava, the portal hypertension is relieved partially or completely, the esophageal varices collapse and future bleeding is minimized or prevented.

The operation does nothing to solve the basic liver disease per se and is merely a mechanical answer to portal hypertension and bleeding. Experience has shown that the mortality from liver failure does not diminish following this operation, but the mortality from exsanguination certainly does.

Scheme

1. The abdomen is opened through a long transverse abdominal incision or a thoraco-abdominal incision.

2. The portal vein and vena cava are dissected in their beds and apposed.

3. A window is placed in the portal vein and vena cava and the two vessels are anastomosed.

4. The abdomen is closed in the usual manner.

PROCEDURE

The operation to be described is the end-to-side portacaval shunt.

1. A long oblique subcostal incision extending from the left of the midline in the epigastrium and running to the right flank is the incision of choice. The incision is deepened to the rectus muscle and oblique muscles, and the abdomen is opened. (See Introduction.)

2. The liver is reflected superiorly and into the pleural space, and the right hepatic flexure of the colon is displaced inferiorly by dividing the phrenocolic ligament.

3. The hepatoduodenal ligament is divided, as well as the lateral ligament of the duodenum, thereby mobilizing the duodenum and reflecting it medially.

4. By mobilizing the head of the pancreas and duodenum medially, the portal vein and inferior vena cava are exposed.

5. The distal end of the portal vein where it inserts into the liver is ligated with a transfixion ligature. The proximal end of the portal vein at its exit from the head of the pancreas is clamped with a Potts-Smith clamp and the portal vein is divided leaving a long segment for anastomosis with the inferior vena cava.

6. A Potts-Smith clamp or a partially occluding Satinsky clamp is now placed on the inferior vena cava so that the medial side of the vena cava is totally occluded. This allows blood to continue through the inferior vena cava so as to prevent a fall in blood pressure which would occur if the inferior vena cava were totally occluded.

7. The end of the portal vein is now brought down to the inferior vena cava, a small elliptical window having been cut previously in the inferior vena cava of approximately the same size as the diameter of the portal vein. An anastomosis is now created between the portal vein and the inferior vena cava (Fig. 44–2).

8. A liver biopsy may now be done by the surgeon. The histologic picture will be used to determine liver function.

9. The abdomen is closed in the usual fashion.

SURGICAL HAZARDS

Portacaval shunt is a major vascular operation associated with many serious hazards:

1. *Massive Hemorrhage.* The distended, dilated, tortuous veins throughout the abdominal cavity and the surrounding edema and possible ascites due to liver failure produce much oozing in

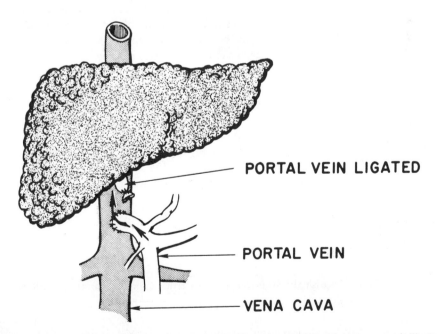

FIGURE 44–2 Portacaval anastomosis is complete. New flow of portal blood into vena cava is illustrated.

the operative site, and a good deal of blood is lost on this account alone. In addition, tearing of the inferior vena cava, renal vein, or portal vein during dissection and anastomosis is also associated with massive hemorrhage.

2. Injury to nearby structures, such as the common duct, the hepatic artery, the pancreas, and the duodenum, is a serious hazard and, because of the amount of oozing and edema which obscure the operative site, injury can occur if meticulous care is not taken in this operative procedure.

3. Rough handling of the veins may result in roughening of the surfaces and early postoperative thrombosis, with consequent failure of function of the new shunt.

POSTOPERATIVE MANAGEMENT

The patient is returned to the recovery room until sufficiently reactive from the anesthetic. Routine management is discussed in previous chapters and should be carefully reviewed at this time. Several important major problems to be watched for in the early postoperative period are as follows:

a. *Under-replacement of lost blood* which may result in hypotension, tachycardia, and shock. To prevent this difficulty from going unnoticed, the Foley catheter should be connected to dependent drainage and all urinary output recorded. In addition, the vital signs should be checked every 15 minutes until stable or until the surgeon gives other instructions. Central venous pressure monitoring is often indicated.

b. *Intravenous infusions* must be maintained throughout the postoperative period so that the patient obtains an adequate quantity of fluids and electrolytes. Careful charting of intake and output is necessary, as the fluid and electrolyte imbalances may be extremely complex and difficult to manage. The surgeon will probably check the electrolyte balance and hematocrit level on the evening of the day of surgery. Intravenous fluid adjustments will be made according to the laboratory results and the patient's general condition.

c. The long intestinal tube is connected to low suction and managed in the usual fashion.

d. Fresh bleeding from esophageal varices is rare after the operation, but the Miller-Abbott tube or long intestinal tube should certainly be checked for this occurrence. If a good deal of bleeding occurs through this tube, the surgeon should be notified at once.

e. Pulmonary complications are prone to develop because of the painful long incision in the upper abdomen. The usual pulmonary precautions should be aggressively undertaken.

f. Because the operation is a long one, the surgeon will probably institute antibiotic therapy in the postoperative period, preferably in the recovery room. This should be given and charted accordingly.

g. The wound is usually dry, as the abdominal cavity is not drained. However, should the abdominal cavity be drained or should oozing occur from the skin surfaces, dressing changes may be necessary in the early postoperative period. The first dressing change should be done by the surgeon and subsequent dressing changes by the supervising nurse.

STUDY QUESTIONS

1. Distinguish the several types of cirrhosis of the liver as to etiology as well as treatment.

2. List the clinical criteria used in the diagnosis of cirrhosis of the liver.

3. List the chemical criteria used in the diagnosis of cirrhosis of the liver.

4. What are the *three* most common causes of massive gastrointestinal bleeding in a young patient, and how are these distinguished?

5. Diagram a portacaval shunt and a splenorenal shunt. What are the indications for the use of these two procedures? State the advantages and disadvantages of each.

6. Discuss the nurse's role in the preoperative preparation of the cirrhotic patient for portacaval shunt.

7. Discuss the main steps in the performance of a portacaval shunt. Explain the design and function of partial occlusion clamps such as the Potts-Smith or Satinsky clamp.

8. Describe to your class the exact nature of portal hypertension and the rationale behind the operation of portacaval shunt.

9. What effect does portacaval shunt have on cirrhosis of the liver?

10. Following portacaval shunting, patients often tend to develop hepatic coma, or heptatic encephalopathy. How is this condition related to a portacaval shunt?

11. Demonstrate the mechanical make-up and function of a Blakemore tube to your class.

12. The patient has been placed on a Blakemore tube for control of esophageal varices. Discuss the nurse's role in the management of a Blakemore tube, paying particular attention to the sphygmomanometer pressures that should be maintained, and describing the dangers in using such a tube if not properly managed.

13. Devise a nursing plan for the postoperative care of a patient who has undergone a portacaval shunt.

GYNECOLOGICAL SURGERY

45

INTRODUCTION

BOUNDARIES, ANATOMY, AND CONTENTS

The gynecological surgeon concerns himself with the anatomical structures of the lower female pelvis and perineum — i.e., the uterus, ovaries, fallopian tubes, pelvic diaphragm, vagina, urinary bladder, and perineum. The perineum has no specific landmarks, but is generally considered to be contained within the upper folds of the thigh extending from the pubic bone anteriorly to the coccyx posteriorly. Operations in the perineal region generally involve the female genital tract, the bladder, and the anus.

SURGICAL APPROACHES

The abdominal aspect of gynecological surgery is usually approached by suprapubic midline incisions, useful for surgery on the uterus, tubes, urinary bladder, and ovaries. Perineal surgery, on the other hand, may involve a variety of cutaneous and/or mucous membrane incisions in the perineum, vagina, or anus, depending on the problem to be solved.

SKIN PREPARATIONS

Preparation for abdominopelvic surgery is not unlike other phases of abdominal surgery, and usually extends from the xiphoid process to and including the pubis. Preparation for perineal surgery usually includes the suprapubic area, the perineum, and the upper third of both thighs. The operating room skin prep should also include washing the vaginal canal with an appropriate antiseptic solution if vaginal surgery is planned, or washing the anal canal if anal surgery is to be undertaken.

POSITION

Abdominopelvic surgery is carried out with the patient in the horizontal, supine position. The usual position for perineal surgery is the lithotomy position.

SPECIAL FEATURES OF GYNECOLOGICAL SURGERY

Abdominopelvic surgery does not carry with it any profoundly new features not already considered under general surgery in Section I. The same problems that attend the opening of the abdomen by the general surgeon face the gynecologist when he performs abdominopelvic surgery.

The gynecologist deals most frequently with the pelvic organs, as well as the sigmoid colon and rectum, the ureters, and the urinary bladder. It is understandable, therefore, that complications of abdominopelvic surgery, in addition to the standard wound problems covered in Section I, will usually revolve around injury to the rectum, bladder, and ureters.

Because of the contamination in the area involved, perineal surgery is always considered to be practiced under conditions of contamination.

Perineal surgery, as well as most forms of abdominopelvic surgery, should always be carried out with a Foley catheter inserted in the urinary bladder preoperatively.

Nonabsorbable suture material is generally avoided in any perineal surgery, as the contamination in the area will often cause marked foreign body reaction and abscesses if such sutures are used.

It is not within the scope of this textbook to deal with all the various psychological aspects of gynecological surgery. Since these aspects certainly should not be minimized, we encourage the reader to refer (as necessary) to texts that deal more specifically with the significant psychological problems that accompany all phases of gynecological surgery.

THE PATIENT WITH ABNORMAL UTERINE BLEEDING

46

Operation: Dilatation and Curettage: Cervical Biopsy

TYPICAL HISTORY

A 47-year-old female in excellent health previously has noted the recent onset of excessive menstrual bleeding (menorrhagia), with formation of blood clots, particularly between periods. Also, her periods are lasting several days longer than normal. She denies any other associated symptoms.

PHYSICAL EXAMINATION

The patient is a well-developed, well-nourished female in no acute distress.

Significant Findings

1. The cervix is slightly scarred, but otherwise unremarkable.
2. The uterus is movable, smooth, round, and nontender.
3. The ovaries and fallopian tubes are normal.

DIAGNOSTIC STUDIES

1. *A Papanicolaou (Pap.) smear* was taken of the uterine cervix and the vaginal vault and was reported back as representing Class III, atypical cells. In this procedure a small amount of secretion is removed from the os of the cervix as well as the vaginal vault; it is smeared and fixed with Pap. smear fixative. Following cytological study, the pathologist is then able to give an opinion whether or not the cells which have been exfoliated from the cervix or uterus exhibit any malignant characteristics. A Class III report is equivocal and is generally followed by dilatation and curettage (D and C) as well as cervical biopsies.

2. *Routine laboratory data* may indicate the presence of mild anemia, but are unremarkable otherwise.

PROBABLE HOSPITAL COURSE

Following the report of an equivocal Pap. smear, the surgeon will often choose to do dilatation and curettage of the uterus as well as to obtain multiple cervical biopsies in order to rule out the presence of any occult malignancy. Preparation for this test is minimal, and the patient should be taken to the operating room soon after admission.

PREPARATION FOR SURGERY

1. Levin tube is not necessary.
2. The pubic and perineal areas are prepped. (See Introduction.)
3. Typing and cross-matching of blood is not necessary.
4. A Fleet enema is given the night before or the day of surgery.
5. *Psychological Preparation.* The patient should be made thoroughly familiar with the nature of the procedure and should understand that it will in no way interfere with her reproductive or sexual capacity.
6. Premedications are routine.
7. No special medications are required.
8. *Position.* Lithotomy. (See Introduction.)

PATHOLOGY

The curettings from the uterus usually show no gross characteristics consistent with carcinoma or benign disease. The diagnosis must be made microscopically.

GENERAL RATIONALE AND SCHEME

In the particular age group of the patient, abnormal uterine bleeding is frequently associated with uterine or cervical carcinoma. It is frequently impossible to determine this without performing dilatation and curettage as well as obtaining cervical biopsies. There are, of course, a number of other causes of abnormal uterine bleeding, including cervical polyps, cervical erosions, endometrial polyps, retention of gestational products, endometritis, subinvolution of the uterus, uterine sarcoma, ectopic pregnancy, and ovarian tumors.

Scheme

1. The bladder is decompressed with a Foley catheter.
2. A thorough pelvic examination is carried out under anesthesia.
3. The cervical canal is dilated.
4. The uterine canal is curetted.
5. Multiple biopsies are taken from several areas of the cervix. Preferably, a cone biopsy will be done.

PROCEDURE

1. The patient is placed in the lithotomy position. (See Introduction.)
2. The perineum, vaginal outlet, and pubic areas are prepped in the usual fashion.
3. A thorough bimanual pelvic examination is carried out at this time, since certain conditions can be diagnosed under anesthesia which cannot be diagnosed when the patient is conscious.
4. The urinary bladder is catheterized and decompressed and the catheter is removed.
5. The cervix is grasped with a cervical snare.
6. A uterine sound is passed into the cervical canal and into the uterine cavity to determine the length of the uterine cavity. This is of importance, particularly since abnormal foreshortening of the uterine cavity could easily result in perforation of the uterus during dilatation.
7. Successively larger dilators are passed into the cervical-uterine canals to dilate the cervix and cervical canal.
8. A sharp or blunt curette, depending on the surgeon's choice, is used to scrape the entire uterine cavity. The curettings are collected on a small sponge and passed on to the nurse, who places them in formaldehyde.
9. Multiple biopsies of the entire face of the cervix are done with a cervical biopsy instrument.
10. If there is any significant bleeding following this procedure, the areas of cervical biopsy are cauterized.

SURGICAL HAZARDS

Too vigorous manipulation with the dilators and curettes can result in perforation of the uterus. This may cause peritonitis or bleeding into the peritoneal cavity.

POSTOPERATIVE MANAGEMENT

The patient is returned to the recovery room for a short period. The only significant aspect of the postoperative management is checking for heavy vaginal bleeding.

STUDY QUESTIONS

1. List some danger signals of cancer. What are the implications for a patient with abnormal menstrual bleeding?

2. Distinguish menorrhagia and metrorrhagia.

3. What are some of the more common causes of abnormal bleeding in the 40 to 50 year age group in women?

4. Discuss the rationale of the Pap. smear test and the chemicals used for the Pap. smear fixation.

5. What are some of the psychological factors which must be taken into consideration by the nurse in preparing the patient for a D and C and a cervical biopsy?

6. Describe the significance of Pap. smears reported as representing Classes I, II, III, and IV.

7. Describe to your class the various dilators and curettes used in performing a D and C.

8. Four hours following D and C, the patient's blood pressure falls significantly and the pulse rises to 130 per minute. She is pale and her skin feels clammy. What is the probable cause of this patient's hypotensive episode? What is the nurse's role in the management of this emergency?

9. An outpatient has been told by her physician that her Pap. smear represents Class IV interpretation. She has been told to enter the hospital for further studies and possible surgery. She is now quite anxious about her impending hospitalization and the nature of the pathology. Being a good friend of yours, she seeks your advice. How would you handle this situation? Explain in detail the reasons for your statements to her.

THE PATIENT WITH AN OVARIAN CYST

47

Operation: Excision of an Ovarian Cyst

TYPICAL HISTORY

The patient is a 42-year-old female who has been in excellent health. She noted recurrent episodes of mild, dull, lower abdominal pain on the right side. There has been no change in her menstrual periods, and no gastrointestinal symptoms have been noted. She denies any weight loss or loss of appetite.

PHYSICAL EXAMINATION

A well-developed, well-nourished female is admitted in no particular distress, but complaining of low-grade intermittent abdominal pain.

Significant Findings

1. A mass is palpable in the right lower quadrant on abdominal examination.
2. A mass in the region of the right ovary and tube is found on pelvic examination. This mass is round, smooth, and freely movable.

DIAGNOSTIC STUDIES

Routine studies are unremarkable.

PROBABLE HOSPITAL COURSE

1. The history and physical examination are consistent with an ovarian cyst or tumor. Consequently, the patient will be booked for laparotomy and evaluation as soon as this can be scheduled. Surgery is indicated not only to eliminate the chronic abdominal pain but also to rule out ovarian carcinoma.
2. If there is any possibility of the presence of a carcinoma of the cecum, a barium enema will be done preceding laparotomy. Once the presence of an intestinal tumor has been ruled out, the surgeon can proceed with laparotomy and resection of the ovarian mass.

323

PREPARATION FOR SURGERY

    1. Levin tube is not necessary.

    2. The abdomen is prepped from the nipple line as far as and including the pubis. (See Introduction.)

    3. The patient is typed and cross-matched for two units of whole blood.

    4. A Fleet or soapsuds enema is given the night before surgery.

    5. Routine premedications are given.

    6. No special medications are needed.

    7. *Operating Room Skin Prep.*   (See Introduction.)

    8. *Position.*   Horizontal supine. (See Introduction.)

PATHOLOGY

The ovary may contain solid or cystic tumors. Should these appear grossly benign, the surgeon can proceed with the removal of the cysts on the side of the disease. Should there be any serious question of malignancy, bilateral oophorectomy and salpingectomy are done as well as hysterectomy because of lymphatic drainage which can cause a tumor to metastasize in either direction.

GENERAL RATIONALE AND SCHEME

It is impossible to determine preoperatively whether a mass lesion of the ovary is benign or malignant. Consequently, in spite of the lack of significant symptoms, a mass of the ovary generally requires exploration. Even a benign cystic lesion of the ovary is subject to surgery, which alleviates the symptoms, which would tend to worsen as this cyst increases in size.

Scheme

    1. The abdomen is opened through a midline, lower abdominal incision.

    2. The cyst, if benign, is excised. Bleeding is controlled with catgut sutures.

    3. The remaining tube, ovary, and uterus are carefully evaluated for disease.

    4. The abdomen is closed in the usual fashion.

PROCEDURE

    1. *Opening Abdomen.*   A vertical, midline, lower abdominal incision is made in the usual manner. (See Introduction.)

    2. *Exploration.*   It is generally difficult to explore the upper abdomen through a lower abdominal incision. Consequently, the abdominal exploration is limited to the pelvic organs. These include the bladder, the uterus, and both tubes and ovaries, as well as the sigmoid colon and rectum. The appendix is also visualized at this time.

    3. The mass lesion in the ovary is evaluated. If its appearance is cystic, smooth-walled, and unilocular — containing only one sac — the surgeon may feel reasonably certain that the lesion is benign. He may elect to merely excise the cyst and preserve part of the ovary. Many factors will determine whether or not this procedure will be done. If, on the other hand, the lesion appears to be malignant, the surgeon will elect to do a total hysterectomy and a bilateral salpingo-oophorectomy.

4. The involved ovary is grasped with a clamp. The cyst is completely excised and bleeding controlled with a catgut ligature.

5. If all goes well, the surgeon may elect to do an appendectomy. If so, this is done in the usual fashion.

6. The surgical site is inspected for hematoma formation to be certain that no further bleeding is occurring.

7. Any blood that has entered the pelvic cavity is aspirated.

8. The abdominal wound is closed in the usual manner, no drains being used.

SURGICAL HAZARDS

1. Injury to the right ureter is always a hazard whenever the right adnexal organs are removed.

2. Occasionally, the mesentery of the tube and ovary may contain large varices which can cause significant bleeding during excision of the cyst. The dissection should be done with great care to prevent any such bleeding.

POSTOPERATIVE MANAGEMENT

The patient usually does quite well postoperatively. She should be given nothing by mouth (NPO) on the day of surgery and thereafter gradually advanced from a liquid diet to a solid diet. The wound usually offers no difficulties, as no drains are used, and it usually heals per primum. Pulmonary complications are minimal following lower abdominal surgery in patients 40 to 50 years of age. If a Foley catheter has been used, it can be removed on the day of surgery or connected to dependent drainage and removed within the next day or two.

STUDY QUESTIONS

1. What are some of the psychological factors which have to be taken into consideration in women undergoing pelvic surgery?

2. What are the dangers in failing to operate on a patient who has a large mass in the ovary?

3. Describe the preoperative preparation of a woman undergoing oophorectomy and salpingectomy, including psychological as well as physiological considerations.

4. Why is a midline incision chosen as opposed to a right paramedian incision when the surgeon is planning to remove a right ovarian tumor?

5. If the tumor of the right ovary is malignant, what other organs will the surgeon usually remove? Why?

6. Describe the operative steps in the removal of an ovary and tube from a surgical nurse's point of view.

7. Prepare a nursing care plan for the postoperative care of this patient. Substantiate your nursing actions by the use of scientific principles.

48

THE PATIENT WITH
A FIBROID TUMOR
OF THE UTERUS

Operation: Hysterectomy

TYPICAL HISTORY

A 47-year-old married female, the mother of three children, has noted an increase in bleeding during her menstrual periods for the past 6 months. For 3 weeks before her admission, she has noticed profuse bleeding. She denies any other symptoms and appears to be in good health otherwise.

PHYSICAL EXAMINATION

A well-developed and well-nourished female, somewhat pale, is admitted in no acute distress.

Significant Findings

1. Pallor is noted.
2. Blood pressure and pulse are normal.
3. Pelvic examination reveals a large, irregular, moveable uterus. The cervix appears to be normal.

DIAGNOSTIC STUDIES

1. WBC is normal.
2. The hematocrit reading is 32 per cent.
3. The hemoglobin is 9 gm. per 100 ml.
4. Routine studies are normal.

PROBABLE HOSPITAL COURSE

The patient probably will receive blood transfusions sufficient to assure a normal level. This will require 2 to 3 days, following which a diagnostic dilatation and curettage (D and C) will be performed. During the course of this procedure, a more thorough pelvic examination can be accomplished under anesthesia and may reveal the nature or the cause of the uterine bleeding. If the surgeon is convinced that the bleeding is secondary to fibromyomata — fibroids — of the uterus, he may undertake at that point to do an abdominal hysterectomy. The diagnosis is not

326

always clear-cut at the time of the initial pelvic examination and diagnostic D and C; consequently, the surgeon will await the return of the curettings from the pathologist before performing a hysterectomy. If the surgeon is not convinced that the fibroids are causing the uterine bleeding, he may wait following the D and C to determine whether or not this will effect a cure of the patient's excessive bleeding. Otherwise, the abdominal hysterectomy will be planned. For many years there has been a trend toward conservatism in the treatment of *benign* uterine bleeding.

PREPARATION FOR SURGERY

1. A Levin tube is not necessary.
2. The abdomen is prepped from the nipples as far as and including the pubis. (See Introduction.)
3. The patient is typed and cross-matched for three units of blood, in the event further bleeding occurs during surgery.
4. A Fleet or soapsuds enema is given the night before or the day of surgery.
5. Routine premedications are given.
6. Special medications. None.
7. In the operating room, a vaginal prep is done because the vagina will be opened at the time of the abdominal exploration.
8. A Foley catheter is inserted and connected to gravity drainage.

PATHOLOGY

The uterus will be found to be enlarged and irregular. The surface will contain multiple and many sized nodules of fibrous and muscular tissue — hence the name, fibromyomata of the uterus. Those which are submucous or located just below the mucous membrane of the uterus often erode the mucous lining, and are responsible for the uterine hemorrhage. Very occasionally, one of these fibromyomata may degenerate into a fibromyosarcoma. However, this is unusual.

GENERAL RATIONALE AND SCHEME

Persistent bleeding from submucous fibroids may, with time, threaten the patient's blood level to the point at which hysterectomy is absolutely necessary. Under most conditions, the surgeon is operating because he cannot rule out a more significant cause of the bleeding such as carcinoma of the uterus. A total abdominal hysterectomy to include the cervix is performed. Otherwise, the cervix, if left within the abdomen, may later develop carcinoma. At the time of the hysterectomy, the surgeon must decide whether or not to remove both ovaries.

Scheme

1. The abdomen is usually opened through a lower abdominal midline incision. (See Introduction.)
2. Exploration is carried out.
3. If both ovaries and tubes are to be removed with the specimen, the ligaments attaching these ovaries and tubes to the lateral abdominal wall are divided. The remaining ligaments

supporting the uterus are divided. The uterus is separated from the vaginal cuff and excised. The vaginal cuff is then closed. The floor of the peritoneal cavity is closed and the abdominal wall is closed.

PROCEDURE

1. *Opening Abdomen.* This is accomplished through a lower abdominal midline incision. (See Introduction.)

2. *Exploration.* The entire pelvis and upper abdomen can usually be explored through a midline lower abdominal incision.

3. The mesenteries to the tubes and ovaries, namely, the mesosalpinx and mesovarium, are clamped, divided, and ligated, care being taken to avoid damage to the nearby ureters.

4. The ligaments supporting the uterus, namely, the broad ligament, the uterosacral ligaments, and the cardinal ligaments, in turn must be clamped, divided, and ligated. Particular attention must be paid when dividing the broad and uterosacral ligaments to avoid injury to the nearby ureters.

5. The uterine artery and its branches pass through the broad ligament to the body of the uterus and its cervix. These must be carefully clamped, divided, and ligated.

6. The peritoneal layer overlying the bladder is separated from the superior aspect of the cervix and vagina to expose the superior wall of the vagina. An incision is made in the vagina just below the cervix and then the entire vagina is circumcised so that the uterus, including the cervix, is completely removed.

7. The vaginal cuff is then closed with interrupted 0 chromic catgut sutures.

8. The round ligaments which previously had been divided are now sutured over the vaginal cuff to act as a supporting mechanism for the retained vagina.

9. The peritoneum overlying the bladder and found in the lateral walls of the pelvis is now brought together to completely "reperitonealize" or cover the floor of the pelvis.

10. No drains are used.

11. The abdominal incision is closed in the usual manner.

SURGICAL HAZARDS

1. *Injury to Either of the Ureters.* The ureters pass dangerously close to the ligaments supporting the uterus and must be carefully observed during division of the ligaments.

2. *Massive Hemorrhage.* Bleeding from the uterine vessels is an extremely hazardous condition which must be carefully guarded against during division of the broad ligaments and incision into the vagina.

3. *Injury to the Bladder Wall.* The bladder is adjacent to and superior to the vagina and cervix, and must be properly mobilized and freed from the underlying vagina and cervix before division into the vagina. Otherwise, injury to the bladder may result, and this in turn can lead to the formation of a vaginal or cystovaginal fistula postoperatively.

4. *Injury to Bowel.* This could result in peritonitis or formation of a fecal fistula.

POSTOPERATIVE MANAGEMENT

1. The patient may be started on a liquid diet as soon as she is alert.

2. Vital signs are watched carefully. Any change in blood pressure or pulse may signify the development of pelvic bleeding.

3. A sponge is often left in the vagina postoperatively and will be removed by the surgeon 24 hours after the operation.

4. A Foley catheter, which had been inserted preoperatively, is connected to dependent drainage and observed for any signs of bright red bleeding. The surgeon should be notified if any blood is found in the drainage bag.

5. The patient is ambulated the day after surgery, and the diet is advanced to solids in 2 to 3 days.

6. The patient may be discharged 7 to 8 days after surgery.

STUDY QUESTIONS

1. What is the purpose of introducing a Foley catheter preoperatively in a patient about to undergo a hysterectomy?

2. Do you think that all women of the patient's age whose bleeding is attributable to fibroids of the uterus require hysterectomy? Explain your answer.

3. What are some of the endocrine or metabolic effects of total hysterectomy (which includes both ovaries) in the premenopausal and postmenopausal female?

4. What are some of the factors which lead a surgeon to decide whether or not to remove the ovaries at the time of hysterectomy?

5. What are some of the conditions which might be diagnosed by D and C?

6. Name the five major ligaments to the uterus. What are their functions?

7. Ten hours following a hysterectomy, the patient's blood pressure begins to fall and the pulse rises. The blood pressure is now 70/40 and the pulse 140 per minute. The patient is pale and restless. What conditions may have brought this about and what role does the nurse play in the management of this patient?

8. What is the significance of bright red blood in the Foley catheter following a hysterectomy?

9. Discuss some of the psychological factors which have to be considered by the physician and nurse in preparing a patient for hysterectomy.

49

Operation: Repair of Cystocele

TYPICAL HISTORY

A 58-year-old mother of four children noticed the onset of stress incontinence approximately 1 year prior to admission. This has increased during the year to such a degree that whenever she strains, laughs, or even walks she is incontinent of urine. She is in excellent health otherwise and denies any other symptoms.

PHYSICAL EXAMINATION

The patient is a well-developed, somewhat obese female in no acute distress.

Significant Findings

1. Pelvic examination reveals a large prolapse of the bladder and a redundant anterior vaginal wall. The urethra is normal.
2. The remainder of the physical examination is normal.

DIAGNOSTIC STUDIES

There are no particular laboratory or x-ray studies used in the evaluation of a cystocele, diagnosis being made by clinical evaluation.

PROBABLE HOSPITAL COURSE

As soon as the patient's general condition permits, she will be taken to the operating room for repair of her cystocele.

PREPARATION FOR SURGERY

1. *Levin Tube.* Not necessary.
2. The patient is typed and cross-matched for one unit of whole blood.
3. *Skin Prep.* This includes the pubic area, the perineum, and the perianal area. (See "Abdominoperineal Resection.")

4. *Enema.* A Fleet or soapsuds enema is given on the evening prior to surgery.

5. *Premedications.* Routine.

6. *Special Medications.* None.

7. *Operating Room Skin Prep.* This includes the pubis, the perineum, and the perianal region. (See "Abdominoperineal Resection.")

8. *Position.* Lithotomy position.

9. A Foley catheter is inserted either preoperatively or at the beginning of the operation.

PATHOLOGY

A cystocele represents herniation of the urinary bladder against a redundant, weakened vaginal floor. This often occurs as a result of multiple deliveries in which the stress against the perineal floor results in a weakening of the structures which support the bladder.

Under normal conditions, the pubic muscles supporting the urethral outlet of the bladder prevent any involuntary loss of urine. When these muscles are stretched and dilated they become weakened and the bladder becomes patent involuntarily. Consequently, any abdominal stress, such as occurs in straining, laughing, or walking, can result in contraction of the bladder against a patent urethral outlet causing loss of urine.

GENERAL RATIONALE AND SCHEME

Minimal stress incontinence can often be treated by muscular exercises in which the perineum is strengthened. When a cystocele becomes moderate to severe in degree, no amount of exercise can prevent loss of urine. Consequently, the bladder outlet musculature and the perineal floor must be repaired to prevent loss of urine.

Scheme

1. The anterior wall of the vagina is opened.
2. The bladder is dissected free from its attachment to the vaginal septum.
3. The pubic muscles are sutured below the urethral outlet.
4. The vaginal wall is sutured closed.

PROCEDURE

1. The patient is placed in the lithotomy position.

2. The vagina, perianal, and perineal areas are prepped with Septisol and tincture of Zephiran.

3. A Foley catheter is inserted, decompressing the bladder.

4. The anterior vaginal wall is incised and flaps are formed laterally.

5. The herniated bladder is returned to the normal position by suturing of the lateral fascial bands of the perineum, which are found below the vaginal flaps. This is usually accomplished with interrupted chromic catgut sutures of heavy caliber.

6. Any redundant vaginal tissue is excised.

7. The vaginal flaps are now sutured in the midline with interrupted chromic sutures.

8. The Foley catheter is left in place.

SURGICAL HAZARDS

1. Damage to the urethra.
2. Entrance into the bladder.
3. Bleeding may occur in the angles of the bladder near the urethra. This may be difficult to control.
4. Damage to the perianal musculature resulting in fecal incontinence.

POSTOPERATIVE MANAGEMENT

The patient is returned to the recovery room until sufficiently reactive from the anesthetic. The usual postanesthesia management is carried out. In addition:

1. The perianal region should be inspected every 2 hours to be certain significant bleeding is not occurring. If the dressing soaks through, the surgeon should be notified at once.
2. The Foley catheter is connected to dependent drainage. Any blood noted in the drainage bag should be reported to the surgeon.
3. The patient is allowed liquids to solid diet when reactive from the anesthetic.
4. If a vaginal pack has been left in place, it should be removed 24 hours following surgery. It is well to tag the chart as a reminder that a vaginal pack exists.

STUDY QUESTIONS

1. Define cystocele, rectocele, and enterocele.

2. Discuss the etiology of these perineal herniae.

3. What are some of the muscular exercises which can be carried out to control the mild cystocele with minimal stress incontinence?

4. Discuss the essential steps in the operative repair of a cystocele.

5. List three indications for vaginal hysterectomy as opposed to abdominal hysterectomy.

6. Following repair of a cystocele in a 43-year-old female, you notice a good deal of blood in the Foley catheter. What are some of the possible causes of this condition? How would you manage it?

7. Describe a nursing plan for the early care of a patient who has undergone a cystocele repair.

GENITOURINARY SURGERY

INTRODUCTION

50

BOUNDARIES, ANATOMY, AND CONTENTS

The genitourinary system consists of the paired kidneys and ureters, the bladder, urethra, prostate, seminal vesicles, and testes. Somewhat arbitrarily, the female genital structures are more properly the province of the gynecologist and will not be considered in this chapter.

The rather diffuse location of the genitourinary system does not lend itself well to a discussion of boundaries as such. Nevertheless, several points should be emphasized. The paired kidneys and ureters constitute the *upper urinary system* and are located retroperitoneally, adjacent to the vertebral column and in close juxtaposition to the aorta, vena cava, and iliac vessels. The kidneys are housed in a dense layer of tissue called Gerota's fascia. A surrounding zone of perirenal fat serves as a buffer for the kidneys. They are also protected by the diaphragm and lower rib cage posteriorly, laterally, and anteriorly.

The ureters descend almost parallel to the vertebral column, hugging the vena cava on the right and the aorta on the left. They then cross over the iliac vessels and, passing through the pelvis, enter the bladder somewhat posteriorly.

The bladder is a retroperitoneal structure also and is partly protected by the symphysis pubis, below which the urethra courses.

The prostate and seminal vesicles surround the proximal urethra in the male just before the urethra passes through the penis.

Inadvertent injury during surgery is always a result of the anatomical proximity of vital structures to the surgical area under consideration. The following list, while hardly complete, may serve as a useful reminder of some of the organs and structures situated close to the genitourinary system:

Kidneys:
  Right: biliary system, adrenal gland, renal vessels, duodenum.
  Left: spleen, pancreas, adrenal gland, renal vessels.
Ureters:
  Right: vena cava, iliac vessels.
  Left: aorta, iliac vessels.
Bladder: ureters, seminal vesicles, rectum.
Prostate: bladder, rectum.

SURGICAL APPROACHES

The kidneys are usually approached posteriorly, often through the bed of the eleventh or twelfth rib, which is removed and not replaced. They may also be approached anteriorly through the peritoneal cavity; this is often the approach for operations on the renal artery when good control of the aorta is mandatory.

The ureters are approached through muscle-splitting flank incisions. The peritoneum and its contents are reflected medially. The three muscles which must be split to reach the ureters are the external oblique, the internal oblique, and the transversus abdominus.

The bladder is approached through a midline lower abdominal incision. The peritoneum and its contents are reflected superiorly.

The prostate and urethra may be approached suprapubically, perineally, or transurethrally, depending on the nature of the problem and the experience of the surgeon.

SPECIAL FEATURES OF GENITOURINARY SURGERY

Hemorrhage. The kidneys and prostatic bed are extremely vascular structures. Renal tissue generally holds sutures well, but the high head of pressure and large vascular spaces dispose the kidney toward occasional postoperative hemorrhage. This may manifest itself as bleeding into the dressing or as hematuria, depending on whether the caliceal system has been entered or not. Periprostatic venous and arterial plexuses are not easily visualized during suprapubic and perineal surgery. Hemostatic measures other than direct suturing must be relied upon, including the use of Surgicel or Gelfoam and the use of tamponade with a balloon catheter. Postoperative bleeding is an ever-present threat whenever the prostate has been enucleated.

Fistulae. The collecting and drainage system for urine includes the renal pelvis, ureters, bladder, and urethra. Once this system has been surgically transgressed, no closure is water-tight, and postoperative urinary fistulae are the rule rather than the exception. Fortunately, most such fistulae will close, but their postoperative management becomes an important part of urological nursing.

Infection. The urinary system does not tolerate infection well, and surgery always disposes the urinary tract to infection. Proper attention to catheter management is an essential prerequisite of good urological nursing if serious infection is to be avoided or minimized.

Catheters and Drains. Almost no other form of surgery depends so much on proper drainage. This dependence is a result of the high volume of excretion from the kidneys and the potential disaster when drains and catheters become occluded or fail to function for one reason or another. Adequate drainage of extravasating urine and efficient decompression of the urinary collecting system are the hallmarks of success in this field of surgery. The urological nurse must understand the rationale behind the use of each catheter and drain. She should recognize the complications involved in achieving and maintaining proper drainage, and she should appreciate the need to prevent dislodgement of any drain or catheter.

Intake and Output Measurement. Since a substantial amount of urological surgery is performed on already compromised urinary systems — and since the occasional sacrifice of renal tissue is involved as well — extremely accurate intake and output balance sheets must be maintained until the patient is safely recuperating from the operative procedure. When fistulae are present, every effort and every "stretch of the imagination" must be made to gauge, as accurately as possible, the amount of urine that is being secreted from normal as well as abnormal exit ports. The use of external collecting bags, carefully cemented to the skin, the careful appraisal of urine-impregnated sponges, and the use of other measuring procedures must preoccupy the urological nurse intent on presenting to the surgeon an accurate tally of daily urine flow.

Operation: Nephrectomy

TYPICAL HISTORY

A 65-year-old male has noted the onset of intermittent painless hematuria for the preceding 4 months. He denies any recent trauma or past history of blood in the urine. He has noted chronic back pain for several weeks.

PHYSICAL EXAMINATION

A well-developed, well-nourished male is admitted in no acute distress. There are usually no positive abnormal findings on physical examination. Occasionally, a hard mass is palpable in the flank.

DIAGNOSTIC STUDIES

1. The urine is loaded with red blood cells.
2. The urine grossly appears to be somewhat rust colored, suggesting the presence of a good deal of blood in the urine.
3. Intravenous pyelogram confirms the presence of a mass occupying lesions in the upper pole of the left kidney.
4. A renal scan may also yield evidence suggestive of a space-occupying lesion, but the scan is usually not diagnostic of tumor.

PROBABLE HOSPITAL COURSE

The patient who demonstrates hematuria will undergo a complete evaluation of his genitourinary tract, as well as his hematologic system, to determine the location and cause of this bleeding. The following procedures are used in the evaluation of hematuria:
1. *Urinalysis.* This may or may not show a good many red blood cells in the urine. The fact that the patient has complained of blood in the urine must be taken as first evidence that there is blood in the urine, in spite of a negative urinalysis which may have been done during a time when the lesion was not bleeding.
2. *Intravenous Pyelogram.* This has been described previously. A lesion of the kidney may well show itself on intravenous pyelography.

3. *Cystoscopy and Retrograde Pyelography.*   In this examination, the surgeon passes a tube through the urethra into the urinary bladder and is able to directly visualize the inner wall of the urinary bladder. In this way, such lesions as polyps, tumors, fissures, and cystitis may be diagnosed. Following evaluation of the inner lining of the bladder, the surgeon will pass long catheters through the cystoscope into the bladder where he will catheterize the ureters as they enter the bladder. The catheters will pass up a good distance into the ureters, through which dye will be introduced into the ureteral system retrogradely. The dye will pass up into the pelves of both kidneys so that these areas can be evaluated for possible tumors or stones.

4. *Hematologic Studies.* Occasionally a blood dyscrasia, such as leukemia, may first manifest itself as hematuria. Consequently, hematologic studies should be carried out when there is any difficulty in determining the cause of hematuria.

5. *Special studies.*

Renal scanning may be done when there is some doubt as to the presence or absence of a tumor mass.

Selective renal arteriography may help to distinguish a renal cyst from a solid tumor.

Once a mass is demonstrated in the kidney, surgery will be planned, provided the patient's general condition warrants this.

PREPARATION FOR SURGERY

1. A Levin tube is not necessary.
2. The patient is typed and cross-matched for six units of whole blood.
3. A Fleet enema is given the night before or the day of surgery.
4. Anemia, when present, should be corrected preoperatively.
5. Premedications are routine.
6. There are no special medications.
7. A Foley catheter is introduced into the bladder on the morning of surgery.
8. The appropriate side is prepped, including the axilla, the anterior chest, and the appropriate side of the anterior abdomen. Also, the entire back on the side of proposed surgery is prepped. (See Introduction.)
9. *Position.*   Kidney position. (See Introduction.)

PATHOLOGY

The hypernephroma or renal cell carcinoma is the most common malignancy of the kidney in an adult. This tumor forms a rounded mass, usually in the upper or lower pole of the kidney, and it may attain an extremely large size. The tumor tends to spread into nearby veins. Consequently it may be found growing directly into the renal vein and even into the inferior vena cava with widespread metastases. Distant metastases are most likely to be found in the lungs and bones, as well as the liver.

GENERAL RATIONALE AND SCHEME

The surgeon must remove the entire kidney in order to effect a cure. Removing only a part of the kidney would not be adequate in the case of a carcinoma of the kidney.

Scheme

    1. The incision is usually made in the left or right flank below the twelfth rib.
    2. This is carried to the *perirenal fascia of Gerota* which is incised, exposing the kidney.
    3. The renal pedicle containing the artery and veins is clamped and divided, as is the ureter. The kidney is then removed.
    4. The incision is closed.

PROCEDURE

    1. The *incision* is made parallel to and 2 cm. below the twelfth rib, extending from the costovertebral angle downward to a point about 4 cm. below the crest of the ilium. This incision is extended through the latissimus dorsi, oblique muscles, and lumbodorsal fascia to expose the retroperitoneal fat.
    2. After opening the perirenal fascia, the kidney is freed and delivered into the wound.
    3. The ureter is identified, clamped, divided, and tied with ligatures at its insertion into the bladder.
    4. The renal pedicle is next isolated. Surrounding tissue is carefully cleansed. This pedicle must be carefully clamped and triply ligated to avoid massive hemorrhage. Transfixing ligatures are used, in addition to free ties, to assure adequate security of these pedicles.
    5. The wound is closed in layers using 0 chromic catgut or interrupted silk. A Penrose drain may or may not be used.

SURGICAL HAZARDS

    1. The most important surgical hazard is massive hemorrhage caused by the pedicle slipping away from the surgeon's grasp or instruments. Meticulous dissection to remove tissue surrounding the artery and veins is imperative, so that the sutures will hold without slipping.
    2. *Injury to the Duodenum.*   The second part of the duodenum is very close to the pelvis of the right kidney and can be injured during dissection of the kidney, particularly if hemorrhage occurs.
    3. *Injury to the Spleen.*   The upper pole of the left kidney is close to the spleen. The spleen may be injured during nephrectomy.

POSTOPERATIVE MANAGEMENT

    The patient is returned to the recovery room until sufficiently reactive from the anesthetic. The usual course of the postnephrectomy patient is smooth, and few problems are to be anticipated.
    1. *Urinary Output.*   The urinary output should be measured carefully, the nurse bearing in mind that the remaining kidney is now fully responsible for excretion of urine. If the patient's urinary output tends to be low, this should be reported to the surgeon.
    2. *Care of Wound.*   If a drain is used, the wound dressing may become soaked. This should be called to the surgeon's attention. However, if no drain is used, the wound is usually dry, and no problems develop in the first 24 hours.
    3. The patient is ambulated within 24 hours after surgery.
    4. The drain is removed 5 or 6 days after surgery.
    5. The patient is usually discharged 7 to 10 days after the nephrectomy.

STUDY QUESTIONS

1. What is Wilms' tumor of the kidney?

2. *Define:* intravenous pyelogram, cystoscopy, retrograde pyelography, renogram.

3. List as many causes of painless hematuria as you can.

4. Describe the positioning on the operating room table for a patient undergoing nephrectomy. What is the advantage of this position to the surgeon?

5. Differentiate between nephrostomy and nephrectomy.

6. Describe the structure and function of a renal pedicle clamp.

7. Discuss in class the essential steps in the performance of a nephrectomy. What are some of the problems or surgical hazards which should be anticipated by the scrub nurse?

8. Following an uneventful nephrectomy, there is a small amount of blood in the Foley catheter bag. What may be one of the causes of this situation? Is it sufficiently alarming to require that the surgeon be notified?

9. In the immediate postoperative period, what should the hourly urine output be? What steps are taken if the amount is too little or too much? What are the nursing implications in each situation?

10. Following a nephrectomy, a certain amount of bloody drainage is to be expected from the drain site. Describe how you would determine whether bleeding is excessive in the early postoperative period.

11. A 40-year-old male has had one episode of painless hematuria 2 weeks before being seen by his physician. What type of study do you think will be carried out on this patient if he is hospitalized?

12. Describe a nursing care plan for a patient who has had a nephrectomy. (Cover, particularly, the first 24 hours.)

13. What is selective renal arteriography? Describe its technique, uses, and risks.

THE PATIENT WITH A URETERAL STONE

52

Operation: **Ureterolithotomy (Removal of a Stone From the Ureter)**

TYPICAL HISTORY

A 43-year-old male, in good health previously, noted the sudden onset of acute left groin pain, followed by nausea and vomiting and the passage of a small amount of bright red blood in the urine. He has had no previous episodes of this kind and states that the bleeding was accompanied by a low-grade, dull backache on the left side. He denies any other difficulty with urination or defecation.

PHYSICAL EXAMINATION

The patient is a well-developed, well-nourished male in acute abdominal pain, lying restlessly in bed.

Significant Findings

1. Pallor, cold clammy skin, and an agonized expression are noted.
2. There is mild to moderate left costovertebral angle (CVA) tenderness.
3. There is some left lower quadrant tenderness in the abdomen, but no spasm of the abdominal wall.

DIAGNOSTIC STUDIES

1. Flat and upright films of the abdomen may reveal the presence of distended loops of large and small intestine which are consistent with ileus. Occasionally, a radiopaque urinary calculus may be seen lodged in the ureter.
2. WBC is 17,000 per cu. mm.
3. Hematocrit reading is 41 per cent.
4. Urinalysis reveals moderate to large numbers of red blood cells in the urine.

PROBABLE HOSPITAL COURSE

If the diagnosis appears to be consistent with the presence of a ureteral stone, the surgeon may do emergency intravenous pyelography to determine to what extent the ureter is blocked by the

339

stone. Twenty to 30 cc. of radiopaque dye is injected intravenously and several films are taken over the abdomen. The dye is excreted by the kidney and passes down the ureters. As the dye reaches the obstructing stone, blockage will be evident. The ureter proximal to the stone may be dilated (hydroureter) and the kidney pelvis on this side may also be dilated (hydronephrosis).

With the diagnosis of obstructed ureter proven by intravenous pyelogram, the surgeon must now choose the appropriate form of therapy. Very frequently, narcotics and antispasmodics relax the patient and relax the ureter, so allowing the stone to pass into the bladder, whence it will be passed in the urine. If this form of therapy is elected on a trial basis, the surgeon will ask the nurse to strain all specimens of urine in the hope of finding and recovering the stone.

If the stone appears to be too large for passage, or if a reasonable trial of conservative therapy does not succeed in bringing about spontaneous passage of the stone, the patient may undergo spinal anesthesia and cystoscopic examination. The surgeon is able to pass stone-grasping instruments up the ureter in an attempt to remove the stone by nonsurgical means. This is only feasible when the stone is lodged in the lower third of the ureter.

Should the stone fail to pass spontaneously or should it be unretrievable by cystoscopic means, the patient will undergo surgery on the ureter for removal of the stone. This operation may be done days, weeks, or months after the disease onset, depending on such factors as pain, location of stone, development of hydroureter and hydronephrosis, and a host of other factors deemed important by the urologist.

PREPARATION FOR SURGERY

1. A Levin tube is introduced into the stomach because of the unusual amount of ileus which is often associated with this painful abdominal crisis.

2. The patient is typed and cross-matched for two units of blood.

3. The skin prep extends from the nipple line out laterally over the axillary region of the chest and down across the abdomen to the iliac crest. (See Introduction.)

4. A Fleet enema is given the morning of surgery.

5. *Premedications.* Routine.

6. *Special Medications.* None.

7. *Operating Room Skin Prep.* Extends from the axilla laterally to the anterior iliac crest, anteriorly to the umbilicus, posteriorly to the dorsal vertebral line. (See Introduction.)

8. *Position.* The patient is placed in the kidney position with his right side down. (See Introduction.)

PATHOLOGY

When the ureter is exposed at the time of surgery, it will be seen to be greatly dilated proximal to the stone, and it will be completely collapsed distal to the stone. Thus, the surgeon knows precisely where to make his incision in the ureter.

GENERAL RATIONALE AND SCHEME

Acute ureteral obstruction becomes a surgical emergency when the stagnating urine causing hydroureter and hydronephrosis results in the development of infection of the kidney tract. This is usually manifested by high fevers, chills, and shakes.

Scheme

1. The lateral flank is opened.
2. The intestinal contents and peritoneum are reflected medially, exposing the ureter over the psoas muscle.
3. A small incision is made in the ureter.
4. The stone is removed.
5. A drain is placed near the ureter and brought out through the flank.
6. The wound is closed.

PROCEDURE

1. *Skin Incision.* This extends from a posterior to anterior direction, obliquely one finger below the twelfth rib. It is carried down into the groin on the appropriate side. (See Introduction.)
2. *Draping Skin.* This should be done, as often the urine is infected.
3. The oblique musculature of the abdominal wall is divided. The peritoneum is recognized and, along with the intestines, is reflected medially toward the umbilicus.
4. The obstructed ureter is identified as it passes near the vertebral column over the psoas muscle.
5. The ureter is palpated to determine the exact location of the stone.
6. A small incision, appropriate to the size of the stone, is made in the ureter directly over the stone (Fig. 52–1).
7. The entire stone is extracted.

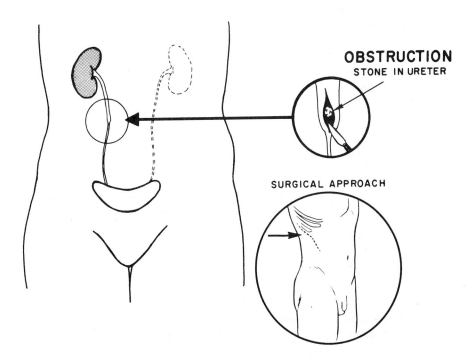

OBSTRUCTION
STONE IN URETER

SURGICAL APPROACH

FIGURE 52–1 Right hydroureter due to obstructing calculus. Inset shows incision in ureter for removal of stone.

8. Some surgeons prefer to close the ureter using a stent or t-tube placed in the ureter and brought out through the flank. Others do not close the opening in the ureter, but merely place a Penrose drain near the incision and bring it out through the flank. In their judgment, this offers the least likelihood of any stricture of the ureter developing and the urine flow through the flank incision will cease within a week.

9. The oblique muscles are closed with running or interrupted chromic stitches.

10. The skin is closed in the usual fashion and a dressing is applied.

SURGICAL HAZARDS

1. The most common hazard is uncontrolled bleeding from the lumbar veins which is avoided by very careful and meticulous dissection.

2. The peritoneum may inadvertently be opened during reflection of the peritoneum medially. This offers no difficulty provided it is recognized and the peritoneum is sutured immediately. Otherwise, incisional hernia may occur postoperatively.

3. *Inadvertent Damage to the Lumbar Sympathetic Chain.* This occurs if the lumbar sympathetic chain is confused with the ureter. Proper knowledge of the anatomy should obviate this difficulty.

POSTOPERATIVE MANAGEMENT

The patient is taken to the recovery room until sufficiently reactive from the anesthetic. The usual general postoperative care is given to the patient undergoing kidney surgery. Particular attention is given to the following:

1. If there has been no ileus and a Levin tube has not been used, fluids should be forced in the early postoperative period to prevent sludging of blood clots in the ureters and bladder.

2. A careful record of intake and output should be kept, since reflex renal failure may occur occasionally following ureterolithotomy.

3. A Foley catheter is usually kept in place for several days postoperatively. This should be connected to dependent drainage and irrigated only on the instruction of the surgeon. Abrupt cessation of urine flow suggests a malfunction in the catheter that could result in back pressure of urine on the ureter. The catheter should be gently and aseptically irrigated and the surgeon notified if prompt urine flow is not observed.

4. The wound offers no particular difficulties in the early postoperative period, although it should be reinforced if urine leaks through. Provided there is no distal obstruction beyond the incision in the ureter, the fistula should close in 7 to 10 days. Good skin care is maintained by changing the dressings frequently and by applying a plastic collecting bag to the incision (if so ordered by the surgeon).

STUDY QUESTIONS

1. Describe the procedure *retrograde pyelography* in the diagnosis of ureteral obstruction. How is this procedure performed?

2. Describe some of the illnesses which may become confused with an acute ureteral stone.

3. What are the major signs and symptoms of an obstructing calculus in the ureter?

4. What are some of the common indications for cystoscopic manipulation of a urinary calculus?

5. What preparation of the patient is necessary prior to this procedure?

6. Name some of the antispasmodics commonly used in the medical treatment of a ureteral calculus.

7. Describe some of the instruments used in an attempt to retrieve a stone through the cystoscope.

8. Why does the surgeon place a drain near the opening in the ureter following ureterolithotomy?

9. Describe a nursing plan for the postoperative care of the patient who has undergone ureterolithotomy.

THE PATIENT WITH BENIGN PROSTATIC HYPERTROPHY

53

Operation: Suprapubic Prostatectomy

TYPICAL HISTORY

A 65-year-old male has noticed increasing frequency, nocturia, and weakness of his urinary stream for several months, but he has noticed no blood in his urine and no flank pain. His general health has been excellent otherwise. He has no complaints referable to the cardiorespiratory or gastrointestinal tract.

PHYSICAL EXAMINATION

The patient is an elderly, well-developed, well-nourished male in no acute distress.

Significant Findings

The findings are limited to the rectal examination, which reveals an enlarged, smooth, symmetrical, nontender prostate gland.

DIAGNOSTIC STUDIES

1. The routine studies are unremarkable except that the urinalysis may reveal several white cells and red cells due to mild chronic cystitis associated with the obstruction from the prostate gland.

2. BUN is slightly elevated at 30 mg. per cent.

3. X-rays are described in the section following.

PROBABLE HOSPITAL COURSE

It is important that the surgeon determine whether or not any back pressure on the kidneys or bladder has resulted from the chronically obstructing prostate gland. Several studies that will be done include the following:

1. *A Postvoiding Catheter Residual Study.* In this test, the patient is asked to void and empty his bladder as completely as possible. The moment this has been done a catheter is inserted into the bladder and the amount of residual urine is noted. A significant amount of residual urine, such as 150 to 200 cc., is indicative of the obstructing tendency of the enlarged prostate gland. If less than 30 cc. of urine is found on residual catheterization, it suggests that the prostate gland is not responsible for the symptomatology.

2. *An Intravenous Pyelogram, or IVP.* In this test, 20 to 30 cc. of radiopaque dye is injected intravenously, and the time when excretion from the kidneys begins is noted. Any delay in excretion of the dye or any tendency of one kidney to excrete more dye than the other is suggestive of renal disease. Also, the size of the renal pelvis and the ureters may suggest prostatic obstruction with reflux of urine into the ureters if these or the renal pelves appear to be enlarged. These conditions are known, respectively, as *hydroureter* and *hydronephrosis.* If hydroureter or hydronephrosis is found, the patient will be placed on Foley catheter drainage for several days until the kidneys and ureters return to normal size before the prostate surgery is done.

3. The surgeon may elect also to perform cystourethroscopy in order to determine whether or not the bladder is obstructed and to what degree this has resulted in chronic thickening of the bladder wall. This will also permit the surgeon to evaluate the type of obstruction being caused by the prostate gland and how best to remove this gland.

4. Assuming that there is no hydroureter or hydronephrosis, and that the patient has no urinary tract infection, the suprapubic prostatectomy, if indicated, will be performed shortly after these tests are completed.

PREPARATION FOR SURGERY

1. Levin tube is not necessary.

2. The patient is typed and cross-matched for two units of whole blood.

3. The abdomen is prepped from the costal margins as far as and including the pubic and scrotal areas. (See Introduction.)

4. A Fleet enema is given the night before or the day of surgery.

5. No special medications are given.

6. Routine medications only are necessary.

7. The surgeon may wish to have a Foley catheter inserted preoperatively. Often, however, he may insert the catheter with a large 25 cc. balloon at the time of surgery.

8. *Position.* Horizontal supine. (See Introduction.)

PATHOLOGY

Enlargement of the several lobes of the prostate gland is an extremely common occurrence in the elderly male. It seems almost to be a normal part of the process of aging and frequently gives rise to urinary symptoms, particularly those of frequency, nocturia, dribbling, diminished force of urinary stream, and hesitancy in starting to void. If minimal in development, this hypertrophy does not cause extensive symptomatic obstruction and the patient may defer surgery indefinitely. Some patients, however, because of a rapidly progressing enlargement of the prostate gland, go on to complete urinary obstruction requiring emergency surgery. The prostate gland is divided into several lobes, and it is usually the median lobe or the lateral lobes which hypertrophy and obstruct the bladder. Occasionally, carcinoma of the prostate gland may mimic benign hypertrophy and cause obstruction.

GENERAL RATIONALE AND SCHEME

The goal of prostatectomy for benign hypertrophy is to remove the cause of obstruction to urinary flow. In time, this will allow complete or nearly complete emptying of the bladder without loss of continence. If allowed to progress untreated, benign prostatic hypertrophy can go on to complete urinary obstruction which will require immediate decompression of the bladder or cystostomy.

Scheme

There are four methods of approach to prostatectomy, the one described herein being referred to as suprapubic. Other approaches include perineal, retropubic, and transurethral. At the present time, most small glands are removed by the transurethral approach. Suprapubic prostatectomy is reserved for large glands.

1. A midline vertical incision is made in the lower part of the abdomen. The bladder is opened. The mucosa over the urethra is incised and the offending prostatic lobes are enucleated with the finger.

2. A large suprapubic catheter and a standard Foley catheter are left for adequate drainage. A small Penrose drain is placed in the suprapubic space.

3. The incision is closed.

PROCEDURE

1. A No. 18 or No. 20 catheter is introduced into the bladder through the urethra. The bladder is distended with 200 to 300 cc. of water.

2. *Skin Incision.* This is a vertical midline, lower abdominal incision in the suprapubic region. (See Introduction.)

3. The incision is carried down to the presacral space and the bladder exposed underneath the transversalis fascia.

4. The bladder is grasped with two Babcock clamps and opened.

5. The Foley catheter is now removed.

6. The surgeon introduces his left hand doubly-gloved below the drapes into the rectum to stabilize and push the prostate gland into a position that is more accessible to his operating hand. (This is optional.)

7. A small opening is made in the urethral mucosa, and the surgeon inserts his finger through the urethral mucosa to enucleate the gland with his finger.

8. The offending lateral and medial lobes are enucleated and brought out through the bladder incision.

9. The Foley catheter is reinserted and inflated with 25 cc. of water in the balloon and then placed on tension against the vesicle outlet to obtain hemostasis.

10. When hemostasis has been obtained, a large suprapubic catheter is placed in the opening through the bladder and brought out through the suprapubic incision.

11. The bladder incision is closed with interrupted chromic sutures.

12. A small Penrose drain is placed in the suprapubic space of Retzius, and both it and the suprapubic catheter are brought out through the incision.

13. The incision is closed in the usual fashion.

SURGICAL HAZARDS

1. *Uncontrollable Hemorrhage.* The prostatic bed is extremely vascular, inaccessible, and difficult to visualize. Bleeding from this area cannot be controlled by fulguration or sutures. Consequently, hemostasis must depend primarily on pressure from the Foley balloon as well as Surgicel or other hemostatic agents which are inserted into the prostatic bed. At times, bleeding may be extremely uncontrollable and difficult to manage postoperatively.

2. *Embolism.* The periprostatic venous plexus may often contain many clots, particularly when there has been chronic or acute infection of the prostate gland. Enucleating the prostatic lobes can lead to fatal pulmonary embolism.

3. *Damage to the Sphincter of the Vesicle.* Improper handling of the tissues in this area may lead to damage of the muscle which controls the continence of urine in the bladder. This may lead to permanent or incapacitating incontinence postoperatively.

4. *Acute Epididymitis.* This can be prevented by performing bilateral *vasectomy* prior to prostatectomy.

POSTOPERATIVE COURSE

1. The suprapubic tube is connected to dependent drainage, as is the Foley catheter (Fig. 53–1). The surgeon may order these to be irrigated to prevent excessive clots from forming in the bladder. If at any time the Foley catheter *does not drain,* check for unseen bleeding. This is confirmed by:

   a. Clot formation in the bladder and impaired flow through the Foley catheter.

   b. Distention of the bladder.

   c. Leakage of the anastomoses and drainage out through the wound, wetting the dressing and bedclothes.

   d. Bladder spasms, as evidenced by the patient's subjective complaint and by objective signs.
A three-way Foley catheter may be irrigated with sterile solution (normal saline).

2. Traction via the Foley catheter may be maintained for 2 to 3 hours after the operation. The catheter is taped to the inner thigh. The nurse should expect the patient to experience painful bladder spasms as traction is exerted.

3. Bright red or continuous bleeding in either tube should be brought to the surgeon's attention immediately. Failure to recognize and evacuate blood clots as they form may lead to blockage of the drainage tube with resulting distention of bladder by urine.

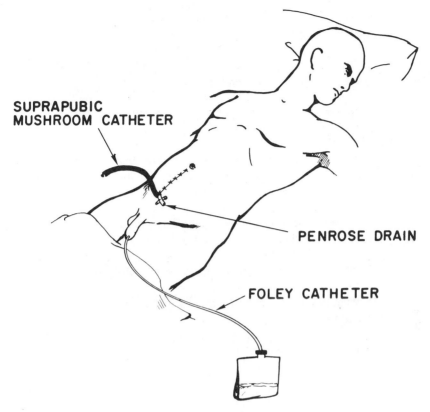

FIGURE 53–1 Postoperative positions of drainage tubes following suprapubic prostatectomy.

4. The incisional area may have to be reinforced because of the small Penrose drain which may allow a good deal of blood and serous fluid to escape. Should this dressing soak through, the surgeon should be notified.

5. Because this procedure is usually performed in the elderly patient, careful attention to vital signs and cardiorespiratory function as in other major operations is extremely important.

6. After traction is removed from the Foley catheter, the patient is kept in the recovery room for about an hour so that the status of his bleeding and the patency of the Foley catheter may be checked. An increase in the amount of bleeding should be expected for a short period of time after the traction on the Foley catheter has been removed by the house officer or surgeon in charge.

7. No rectal temperature should be taken after surgery because of the proximity of the rectum to the operative area.

8. Proper charting of urinary output is imperative when irrigating solutions are utilized. Notation must be made on the intake and output sheet as to whether the irrigating solution *has* or *has not* been subtracted from the total hourly output.

STUDY QUESTIONS

1. List all the possible symptoms of prostatic hypertrophy in the elderly male.

2. What is the significance of hydroureter and hydronephrosis in the male undergoing prostate surgery?

3. What other approaches to the prostate gland can be used besides the suprapubic approach?

4. Discuss the significance and the meaning of the BUN test, particularly with respect to the patient undergoing prostate surgery.

5. Describe the surgical steps in the suprapubic removal of a prostate gland. What surgical hazards are involved in this maneuver?

6. A 75-year-old male has undergone suprapubic prostatectomy. Bright red blood is seen in his Foley catheter and suprapubic tubes. What will the surgeon probably request the nurse to do and why?

7. Describe the nurse's steps in the irrigation of a suprapubic catheter. What precautions should be taken during this procedure?

8. What are the advantages and disadvantages of the suprapubic approach?

9. What are the rehabilitative aspects in the nursing care of a patient who has had a prostatectomy?

10. What psychological support may be needed in the daily care of this patient?

54
THE PATIENT WITH A MALIGNANT TUMOR OF THE TESTICLE

Operation: Excision of Testicular Tumor

TYPICAL HISTORY

A 31-year-old male, in previous excellent health, enters the hospital for evaluation of a relatively painless swelling of his right testicle that has been evident for about two months. The patient first noted this swelling while bathing. At first he attributed it to a mild strain that had occurred while he was playing basketball. Although generally painless, the swelling did feel "like a hardness" of the testicle, sometimes causing a mild aching sensation. He sought medical attention because the swelling seemed to be increasing.

PHYSICAL EXAMINATION

The patient is a well-nourished male in no acute distress and appearing in excellent health.

Significant Findings

1. The right testis is distinctly harder and larger than the left. It is not particularly tender and not irregular in shape. There is no fixation of the testis to the surrounding scrotum, and the epididymis is separate and normal.
2. The spermatic cord, palpable in the inguinal canal, is normal.
3. There are no palpable masses in the abdomen; the supraclavicular spaces are also normal.
4. There is no gynecomastia.

DIAGNOSTIC STUDIES

1. Chest x-ray reveals no evidence of pulmonary or mediastinal masses.
2. An intravenous pyelogram shows no evidence of ureteral displacement.
3. An assay of urine for chorionic gonadotropin-like acitvity is negative.
4. Lymphangiography and inferior vena cavography show no lymph node replacement and no vena caval displacement or obstruction.

PROBABLE HOSPITAL COURSE

1. All tumors of the testicle are presumed to be malignant until proven otherwise. Prior to surgery, the surgeon will wish to exclude regional or distant metastases in an effort to *stage the disease* and to determine the correct course of therapy.
2. Chest x-ray and IVP are standard diagnostic tests in the evaluation of a testicular mass. Less clear is the value of lymphangiography and inferior vena cavography. Some physicians feel that these tests are very sensitive means of determining retroperitoneal extension of testicular neoplasms. Others feel that too often the tests yield false negative results, and that time is lost in searching for retroperitoneal spread instead of proceeding to the surgery.

PREPARATION FOR SURGERY

1. Psychological preparation is very important. The patient should understand that the dangers associated with testicular tumor require that unilateral castration be performed, but that this will not demasculinize or sterilize him. He should be informed that prostheses are available to replace the removed testis.
2. Levin tube is not necessary.
3. *Blood.* The patient is typed and cross-matched for two units of whole blood.
4. *Skin Prep.* The entire lower abdomen and the pubic and scrotal areas are shaven while the patient is on the ward.
5. *Enema.* A Fleet enema is given the evening prior to surgery.
6. *Premedications.* Routine.
7. *Special Medications.* None.
8. *Operating Room Skin Prep.* The lower abdomen, pubis, and scrotum are prepped.
9. *Position.* Horizontal supine.

PATHOLOGY

1. Most tumors that are discovered early are confined to the testis and are surrounded by a dense testicular capsule referred to as the *tunica albuginea.* The tumor is usually separate from the scrotum, epididymis, and spermatic cord.

2. There are a wide variety of malignant tumors of the testicle. Standard textbooks of urology or oncology should be consulted for a full description of this interesting group of tumors. Some of these tumors are radiosensitive, others radioresistant. It is this distinction that will ultimately determine the full course of treatment recommended by the surgeon.

3. Tumors that are discovered late may already have spread beyond the tunica albuginea into the retroperitoneal lymph nodes. From these nodes, deposits spread by way of the thoracic duct into the left subclavian vein, from which they may be transported in the blood to the lungs, liver, brain, and bone.

GENERAL RATIONALE AND SCHEME

1. Confronted with a mass in the testis, the surgeon must first explore this mass to determine if it is a malignant tumor of the testicle. He may make this determination by orchiectomy and await the final pathological report before proceeding with other modalities of treatment. Alternatively, he may proceed, on the basis of a frozen section, with an immediate retroperitoneal lymph node dissection.

2. For illustrative purposes in this chapter, we will assume that no lymph nodes are clinically evident on preoperative studies and that the surgeon will adopt the "conservative" course of awaiting a definitive pathological report before proceeding with any other form of treatment.

3. Following ligation of the vas deferens and its blood supply high in the inguinal canal, a simple orchiectomy will be carried out and the procedure terminated. Further definitive surgery will depend on the radiosensitivity or radioresistance of the tumor.

PROCEDURE

1. *Skin Incision.* This is an oblique incision in the right inguinal canal extending into the upper scrotum, not unlike a hernia incision.

2. *Draping Skin.* This is carried out with wound towels or sutures in the usual manner. The inguinal-scrotal area is a relatively contaminated area, and efforts to prevent soiling of the gloved hand or instrument are advisable.

3. The subcutaneous tissue, fat, and superficial fascia are split obliquely. Bleeding is controlled with hemostats and fine catgut sutures.

4. The external oblique aponeurosis — the "roof" of the inguinal canal — is opened, exposing the vas deferens and the blood supply to the testicle.

5. To avoid lymphatic or blood-borne metastases, the cord and blood supply are immediately ligated at the internal ring, effectively trapping any tumor cells in transit to higher levels.

6. The testis is then evacuated from its scrotal location and removed by transecting the cord just below the ligatures.

7. The wound is irrigated with saline and the external oblique aponeurosis closed with interrupted sutures of silk or nylon.

8. The subcutaneous layers are closed with fine catgut.

9. The skin is closed with fine sutures of silk. No drains are used.

SURGICAL HAZARDS

1. Rarely, injury to the nearby femoral vein or artery could lead to serious hemorrhage or deep phlebitis.

POSTOPERATIVE MANAGEMENT

1. The patient is returned to his room as soon as he has recovered from the anesthesia.
2. The patient may be ambulated within 12 to 24 hours after surgery.
3. Difficulty in voiding is possible, and the patient must be checked frequently for bladder distention.

STUDY QUESTIONS

1. What is the age incidence of carcinoma of the testicle?

2. What other diseases or illnesses could produce a painless swelling in the scrotum and be confused with tumor?

3. What is the significance of gynecomastia in a patient with a tumor of the testicle?

4. Discuss lymphangiography and inferior vena cavography in terms of technique, hazards, diagnostic accuracy, and postoperative difficulties.

5. Prepare a list of tumors of the testicle by consulting a standard textbook of urology or oncology. Which tumors are radiosensitive? How does this alter the prognosis and treatment plan?

6. Thirty-six hours after a right orchiectomy for tumor of the testicle, the patient complains of a dull ache in his right calf. He is certain this pain was not present prior to surgery. You examine the patient and feel slight induration in the calf, which is also slightly tender. Which of the following is the correct course of action?
a. Reassure the patient and give him the analgesic prescribed for postoperative pain by the surgeon.
b. Reassure the patient and notify the surgeon immediately.
c. Dispense the pain medication prescribed by the surgeon and see if this gives relief.
d. Reassure the patient, relieve his pain, and be certain the morning shift of nurses is aware of the problem.

7. What are some of the possible causes of the calf pain described in question 6? How can you tell when a serious problem is developing?

8. An acute postoperative psychosis in a young male who has undergone orchiectomy suggests many precipitating factors. Discuss them with your class. How might you anticipate this problem and, hopefully, prevent its development?

55

THE PATIENT
WITH A CUTANEOUS
URINARY FISTULA

Operation: Ileal Loop for Urinary Diversion (Urostomy)

TYPICAL HISTORY

The patient is a 75-year-old man who several weeks ago underwent a radical retropubic prostatectomy for cancer of the prostate. He developed an anastomotic leak from the bladder that did not respond to re-exploration and pelvic drainage. It has been decided to proceed with a higher urinary tract diversion to permit the inflammatory disease in his pelvis to subside and his bladder to heal.

PHYSICAL EXAMINATION

A cutaneous urinary fistula has developed in the patient subsequent to radical retropubic prostatectomy for cancer of the prostate. A suprapubic examination with bilateral catheterization has since been performed and attempts were made to close the bladder leak with 0 chromic catgut sutures. There was much inflammation apparent at that time, and it was very difficult to achieve adequate closure.

Significant Findings

1. Obvious leakage of urine through a cutaneous fistulous tract, soiling and saturating the patient's skin and dressing.
2. Abdominal discomfort and pain.
3. *Peritonitis.* The signs and symptoms are:
   - diffuse abdominal tenderness
   - fever
   - intermittent vomiting
   - constipation
   - paralytic ileus
   - abdominal distention and rigidity
   - Hippocratic facies
   - tachycardia
   - leukocytosis
   - hemoconcentration; hypovolemia
   - oliguria
   - circulatory collapse
   - septic shock
4. Poor wound healing.

DIAGNOSTIC STUDIES

1. Endoscopy confirms the anastomotic breakdown.
2. Intravenous urography shows leakage of urine out through a tract to the skin.
3. Subcutaneous injection of dye into the fistulous tract establishes its location on x-ray.

PROBABLE HOSPITAL COURSE

The surgeon will elect to divert the urinary stream into an ileal loop as soon as the patient's general condition permits. However, the status of the structures to be included in the surgical site must first be determined. Thus cystoscopy is performed to evaluate the bladder and urethral orifices; intravenous urography is carried out to determine the degree of lower urinary tract obstruction; a small bowel series is performed to evaluate the function and patency of the bowel; and a retrograde pyelogram (injection of dye through a retrograde catheter) is performed to evaluate the function of the lower urinary tract. When these tests are completed — and show satisfactory results — the surgeon can schedule the operation.

PREPARATION FOR SURGERY

1. The nutritional state of the patient is evaluated. Severe loss of fluid and electrolytes will require replacement before surgery.

2. Skin prep and bowel prep are carried out. The current practice is to use mechanical preparation (enemas, and high caloric irrigations performed repeatedly until clean returns are obtained) and a 36 to 48 hour course of wide spectrum antibiotic therapy.

3. *Evaluating the Placement of the Stoma on the Patient's Abdomen.* Poor operative placement of the stoma can create severe physical and psychological problems for the patient postoperatively and can impede adjustment and rehabilitation. Before surgery, the surgeon should assess the best location for the stoma. This is best done by having the patient assume various body postures while the surgeon observes the abdomen. It is most important to keep the stoma away from bony areas (such as the hip and pelvis), the old cicatrix, any deep folds in the skin, and the umbilicus. When the best position for stomal placement has been decided, a mark should be made on the skin with indelible ink or gentian violet so that optimum and accurate placement of the stoma can be achieved at the time of surgery.

The stoma should be placed so that it will not complicate the wearing of a collection appliance under the many conditions of sitting, standing, bending, and twisting. The patient's desire to conceal the presence of the appliance under clothing postoperatively should not be underestimated.

4. Surgery in this situation requires a rearrangement of body image. The patient will be concerned about how things are going to function in the future, especially with regard to:
   a. continence problems
   b. odor control
   c. social activities

5. Arrange appropriate meetings with other patients who have undergone the same procedure successfully.

6. Type and cross-match for 4 units of blood.

7. Teach coughing, turning, and deep breathing exercises.

8. Explain recovery room procedures.

PATHOLOGY

A number of pathologic conditions can require the surgical creation of an ileal loop. Among these conditions are:

1. Bladder carcinoma
2. Cervical uterine carcinoma
3. Cancer of the urethra
4. Cancer of the vagina
5. Cancer of the prostate
6. Myelomeningocele
7. Urinary complications of paraplegia
8. Neurogenic bladder
9. Exstrophy of the bladder
10. Bladder neck contracture, causing hydronephrosis

In the case presented here, the patient developed a postoperative anastomotic suture line leak, which then progressed as a fistulous tract to the skin.

A fistula of the urinary tract may communicate with the skin, intestines, or other organs. In this patient's situation, because of an inability of the bladder sutures to heal, a tract from the bladder to the skin (cutaneous fistula) developed. In such a situation, the fistula developed as the result of:

a. Surgery in and near the urinary bladder, with resulting tissue trauma.
b. The prior presence of cancer of the prostate, and the need for a radical prostatectomy.
c. Poor wound healing potential, leading to the anastomotic suture line leak at the bladder.

Fistulae that communicate with the skin produce skin irritation and unpleasant odors.

A urinary diversion in this patient's situation is necessary to allow healing of the bladder suture line by by-passing the organ and allowing the urine to be excreted by means of an ileal conduit.

GENERAL RATIONALE AND SCHEME

Usually, patients need urinary diversion for one of 4 reasons:

1. Cancer that requires radical removal of part of the urinary tract.
2. Birth defects in which the urinary tract is absent or malfunctioning.
3. A neurogenic bladder resulting from infection, spina bifida, multiple sclerosis, paraplegia, or quadriplegia.
4. Formation of a fistula of the urinary tract to another organ or to the skin.

For an ileal conduit, the surgeon isolates a segment — usually about 7 to 8 inches — of small bowel (ileum) from the intestinal tract, making sure to keep the segment's nerve and blood supply intact. After anastomosing the remaining intestine for bowel continuity, he closes the proximal end of the ileal segment with sutures. He then implants the ureters in the ileal segment and brings the distal end of the segment through a circular hole in the abdomen. He forms a stoma by everting the bowel (Fig. 55–1).

Scheme

1. In this type of urinary diversion (Bricker's pouch, ileal loop, ileal bladder), a small section of the ileum close to the ileocecal valve is resected without being disconnected from the mesentery, which supplies its blood.

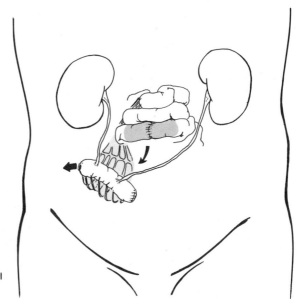

FIGURE 55–1 Ileal conduit, showing ileal segment with anastomosed ureters.

2. The proximal end of the ileal section is sutured closed, and the distal end is brought out through the abdominal wall, everted, and sutured to the skin to form an orifice.

3. The ureters are implanted in the ileal segment near its closed proximal end.

4. Peristalsis in the ileal segment propels the urine toward the stoma on the abdominal surface. The flow of urine out of the stoma will be almost continuous. The conduit does *not* become a reservoir for urine; rather it serves as a passageway for urine to flow from the ureters to the exterior.

5. During surgery, the surgeon will establish indwelling ureteral catheters throughout the area where the ureters are anastomosed to the ileal segment. These indwelling catheters are called *ureteral stents.* Their purpose is to keep the urine flowing from the kidneys even when post-operative edema occurs at the uretero-ileal anastomosis. The stents will remain in place until the postoperative edema resolves. When removing the urinary drainage appliance at any time postoperatively, the members of the staff should be careful not to disrupt or pull the stents from the ureters.

PROCEDURE

1. The patient is placed under general anesthesia. He is prepped and draped in the usual fashion.

2. The midline incision from the previous surgery is opened in its uppermost portion and extended into the patient's mid-abdomen.

3. An exploration of the abdomen is performed.

4. A segment of ileum is resected to be used for the ileal stoma.

5. A standard two-layer bowel anastomosis is carried out with interrupted silk sutures.

6. The butt of the loop is oversewn with running 3–0 chromic sutures and with interrupted 3–0 silk sutures.

7. The ureters are dissected in the retroperitoneum.

8. The left ureter is brought beneath the sigmoid mesocolon in a gentle curve.

9. The ureter on the right side is positioned to reach the butt of the loop.

10. The butt of the loop is then sewn in place in the retroperitoneum at the level of the aortic bifurcation with interrupted 3–0 silk sutures.

11. A standard uretero-ileal anastomosis is then carried out with interrupted 4–0 and 5–0 chromic sutures.

12. A stoma is fashioned in the right lower quadrant.

13. Interrupted 3–0 chromic sutures are placed in the peritoneum and fascia to secure the loop in the stomal opening.

14. 3–0 chromic sutures are used to evert the mucosa; the mucosal skin margins are reapproximated with interrupted 4–0 chromic sutures.

15. The uretero-ileal anastomosis is reperitonealized.

16. The wound is closed with various sutures: 0 nylon tension sutures are placed as necessary, running 0 chromic sutures are used for the peritoneum and posterior fascia, and interrupted 0 Dexon sutures are used for the anterior fascia.

17. The skin is closed with interrupted 4–0 silk sutures.

SURGICAL HAZARDS

1. Urinary leak can occur at one or both of the uretero-intestinal anastomotic sites; this may be caused by technical factors or by poor ureteral blood supply.

2. Gangrene of the ileal segment may occur. There may be a cyanotic stoma of questionable viability at the end of the procedure.

3. *Contamination of the Wound and Peritoneal Cavity.* Failure to apply rubber shod clamps and to drape the abdominal contents in the wound may result in massive contamination from the bowel. This can result in serious postoperative sepsis, extensive ulceration, and digestion of tissues surrounding a drain site.

4. A blind loop of ileum may be produced that can gradually enlarge and cause stasis, with resultant bacterial growth and destruction of vitamin B_{12}, followed by anemia.

IMMEDIATE POSTOPERATIVE MANAGEMENT

1. *Care of Patient with Small Bowel Resection.* A primary principle in the care of the ileal conduit patient is to make certain that the intestine remains absolutely undisturbed until the intestinal anastomosis has healed sufficiently. Accordingly, the following measures are taken:

   a. The gastrointestinal tract is decompressed with an intestinal tube.

   b. The patient receives nothing by mouth (mouth care will be required).

   c. The patient receives fluids and electrolytes intravenously.

2. *Care of the Stoma.* A bag with adhesive backing or a urinary drainage pouch may be used. The hole is centered over the stoma and the back portion of the pouch quickly smoothed so that the adhesive adheres securely to the skin surface. It is frequently recommended that in the immediate postoperative period the patient's drainage appliance should be attached to a bedside collector so that there is no opportunity for overfilling the appliance and to facilitate easy observation and measurement of drainage. The transparent tubing leading from the appliance to

this collector should be gently anchored to the thigh by strips of tape so that the tubing will not be compressed or kinked or develop dependent looping. Since this collection system is a gravity system, the end collector must always be positioned below the mattress level. The nurse will regularly check drainage of urine to make certain there is no urinary stasis caused by mucus, clots, or debris after surgery. The urinary output should be measured and recorded, and the bedside drain disconnected and properly cleansed as often as necessary.

If the patient's pouch leaks, it should be changed at once. Conversely, drainage bags and bottles should not be allowed to fill, as this interferes with continual flow of urine from the stoma. An important principle in utilizing the urinary drainage bag or pouch is that the skin must be kept free of urine while the nurse is preparing and applying the bag.

Peristomal skin usually needs no special cleansing. Plain warm water is adequate. Many physicians recommend that no soaps or detergents be used around this area because of possible irritation of the stomal mucosa. If the hair grows back on the peristomal skin, clipping or careful shaving will help to maintain a smooth surface for reapplication of the appliance. Odor will not normally be a problem for the patient who is regularly provided with disposable appliances. Malodorous urine coming directly from the stoma is an indication of a serious complication, usually bacterial infection; this should be reported promptly to the physician. One problem in using the disposable adhesive appliance is the stripping of peristomal skin, with resultant irritation and excoriation. If removal and reapplication of the temporary appliance are carried out twice daily, serious irritation of the skin may develop within 3 to 4 days. Cements and tincture of benzoin should be avoided in the immediate postoperative period. Any product capable of sensitizing the patient or requiring the use of harsh solvents should be avoided.

3. Problems to be anticipated postoperatively include:
a. *Stomal bleeding,* especially when the permanent bag is in place.
b. *Peritonitis,* due to urine leakage from the bowel anastomosis.
c. *Distention of the ileal segment by urine*, caused by:
   (1) Reflux of backed-up urine to the ureters. This is the major cause of distention after ileal surgery.
   (2) Hydronephrosis.
   (3) Dehiscence of the ileal suture line.
d. *Too large or too long a loop.* When an oversized loop is present, there is a stagnation of urine in the conduit, and this can lead to pyelonephritis and stone formation. Moreover, the blind loop syndrome may appear. The patient with too large or too long an ileal loop may present with the following:
   (1) Anorexia.
   (2) Fever.
   (3) Pyuria.
   (4) Oliguria.
   (5) Abdominal pain.
e. *Swelling of the new stoma,* causing incomplete emptying of the conduit.
f. *Stricture of the stoma at the skin level.*
g. *Abdominal distention,* which may put pressure on the ureters and prevent emptying. Causes:
   (1) Prolonged postoperative ileus.
   (2) Bowel obstruction.
h. *Trauma to the stoma,* causing ulceration (from the face plate or from slippage of the face plate). Pressure is placed on the stoma and bleeding occurs.
i. *Prolapse of the stoma.*

STUDY QUESTIONS

1. Differentiate between:
   a. ileal loop
   b. ileal conduit
   c. cystostomy
   d. ureterosigmoidostomy
   e. nephrostomy
   f. ureterostomy
   g. cutaneous urostomy

2. Specify when each of the procedures listed in question 1 would be used, or the major indication for performing each procedure.

3. Design a preoperative teaching plan for a patient who is to have an ileal conduit.

4. Review the types of pouches or collecting devices that are available for the patient with a urostomy.

5. How could you provide preoperative emotional support for the patient described in this chapter?

6. Describe the changes in body image that a patient with an ileal conduit would have to make.

7. A patient has just undergone surgery for urinary diversion through an ileal loop. Review the complications to be expected in:
   a. the early postoperative period (1 to 5 days after surgery)
   b. 6 to 10 days after surgery
   c. 11 to 30 days after surgery

8. What are the symptoms of dysfunction of the ileal loop postoperatively?

9. Develop a postoperative nursing care plan for the patient with an ileal loop. Use the patient in this chapter as the subject.

10. Be able to describe what a fistulous tract is and why it would develop in the situation described in this chapter (after radical prostatectomy).

11. Review the potential for development of fistulae in general in the surgical patient.

12. What factors are necessary for optimum wound healing after any surgical procedure?

13. Discuss the different types of access routes in prostatectomy. Review the postoperative implications of each surgical approach.

14. What adjustments in life style would a patient with an ileal loop have to make?

HEAD AND NECK SURGERY

INTRODUCTION

56

BOUNDARIES, ANATOMY, AND CONTENTS

The external boundaries of the head and neck are quite obvious. What should be kept in mind, however, is that the neck represents a bridge, so to speak, between the vital structures of the cranial cavity and the remaining vital organs of the body contained within the thorax and abdomen. Consequently, there is no internal boundary between neck and chest, but rather a continuity of structures which passes from the head, down through the neck and into the chest and abdomen.

The head and neck regions have been grouped together here for anatomical convenience, but there are several surgical principles which may be contrasted between the head and neck regions.

The simplest way of conceiving the anatomical nature of the neck is to consider it as a hollow cylinder made up of several layers of fascia which envelop various vital structures, including trachea, esophagus, large vessels passing from the chest into the head, important endocrine organs such as the thyroid and the parathyroid, and other important nerves passing from the brain into the chest and abdomen.

Surgical entrance into the neck is usually accomplished through transverse incisions which lay in the normal skin creases, thereby affording minimum cosmetic abnormalities.

SURGICAL APPROACHES

As stated, vital structures in the neck are most often approached through transverse and oblique incisions. These incisions are illustrated and labeled in Figure 56–1.

SKIN PREPS

Skin preps for the various operative procedures outlined in this section are diagrammed and labeled in Figure 56–2.

POSITIONS

Most head and neck surgery is done in a high semi-Fowler's position, with the head extended to the opposite side of the contemplated surgery. These positions are diagrammed and labeled in Figure 56–3.

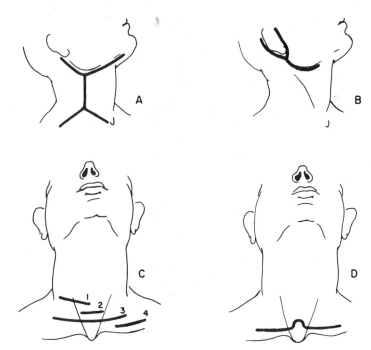

FIGURE 56-1 Standard neck incisions. *A.* Right radical neck dissection. *B.* Incision for parotid surgery. *C.* (1) Branchial cleft surgery, carotid endarterectomy; (2) tracheostomy; (3) thyroidectomy; (4) scalene node biopsy. *D.* Laryngectomy.

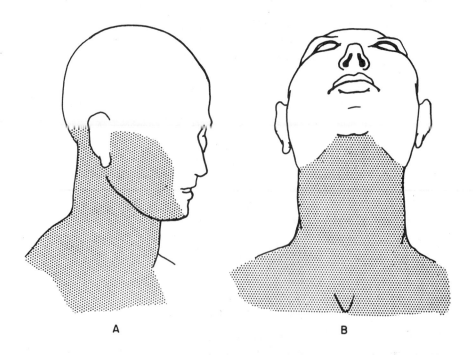

FIGURE 56-2 Skin Preps. *A.* Radical neck dissection; parotid surgery; scalene node biopsy (prep need not extend into face); carotid endarterectomy; branchial cleft surgery. *B.* Thyroidectomy; laryngectomy; tracheostomy.

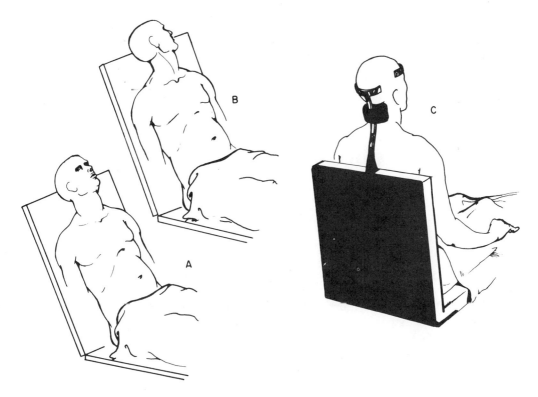

FIGURE 56–3 Positions for head and neck surgery. *A.* Thyroidectomy; tracheostomy; laryngectomy. *B.* Scalene node biopsy; branchial cleft surgery; parotid surgery; carotid endarterectomy; radical neck dissection. *C.* Craniotomy.

SPECIAL FEATURES OF HEAD AND NECK SURGERY

As stated, it is difficult to combine head and neck procedures in terms of the surgical principles involved.

Concentration of Vital Structures. Anatomically, the neck region represents the most concentrated area of vital structures in the body. Meticulous surgery and a good deal of anatomical knowledge are requisites for the performance of surgery in the neck region, as surgical error in this area can cause severe cosmetic or physiological disability.

Exposure. This is usually simple, owing to the absence of any structure — such as the small intestine — which might obscure the surgical dissection.

Wound Closure. Venous oozing in the neck usually requires the use of drains following wound closure. Heavy dressings are applied, and when drainage occurs the surgeon should be notified.

Return of Gastrointestinal Function. The patient is usually able to tolerate an unrestricted diet as soon as he is fully reactive from the anesthetic agent.

Respiratory Function. Significant edema or bleeding into the neck following neck surgery may result in tracheal compression. This, in turn, may lead to respiratory obstruction and death.

Careful observation for the sequence of events as outlined must follow every head and neck procedure.

57

Operation: Tonsillectomy and Adenoidectomy

TYPICAL HISTORY

A 7-year-old male has had repeated attacks of upper respiratory infections, sore throats, and an infected left ear. On several occasions, beta hemolytic streptococcus has been grown from the tonsillar bed and he has responded well to penicillin therapy. His mother states that he is a "mouth breather," and that he tends to speak with a nasal tone.

PHYSICAL EXAMINATION

A well-developed, thin male is admitted in no acute distress.

Significant Findings

1. The tonsils are cryptic and enlarged and almost meet in the midline of the pharynx.
2. The left eardrum is cloudy and shows residual old scarring.
3. The patient talks with a definite nasal tone.

DIAGNOSTIC STUDIES

No diagnostic studies are necessary.

PROBABLE HOSPITAL COURSE

If proper indications are present, the patient will be taken to the operating room for tonsillectomy and adenoidectomy shortly after admission to the hospital.

PREPARATION FOR SURGERY

No specific preparation is needed for this type of surgery except for routine blood studies and the usual psychological preparation of the patient. Medications are routine.

PATHOLOGY

The tonsils will be found to be enlarged and to contain several crypts from which caseous material can be easily expressed. Microscopically, the tonsils will show signs of thickening and chronic inflammation.

GENERAL RATIONALE AND SCHEME

In the past, the indications for tonsillectomy and adenoidectomy were rather liberal. It has been found, however, that many upper respiratory infections continue in spite of tonsillectomy. Consequently, recurrent attacks of respiratory infections per se, do not constitute adequate justification for removal of the tonsils.

At the present time, several strong indications persist for removal of tonsils and adenoids. These may be listed as follows:

a. When the tonsils are constantly infected with beta hemolytic streptococcus and are so enlarged as to meet in the midline of the pharynx, virtually obstructing respiration.

b. When there have been one or more attacks of otitis media, presumably secondary to acute tonsillitis and adenoiditis.

c. Chronic otitis media.

d. Chronic tonsillitis, with constant soreness of the throat unrelieved by appropriate antibiotic therapy.

Scheme

1. A self-retaining retractor is put in the mouth to maintain the mouth in an open position.
2. The capsule of the tonsil is incised.
3. Bleeders are clamped, divided, and ligated.
4. The tonsils are excised.
5. An adenomatome is inserted into the posterior pharynx and the adenoids are removed.

PROCEDURE

1. The patient is placed in the semi-Fowler's position or in a horizontal position with the neck hyperextended. (See Introduction.)

2. The base of the tongue is depressed and the tonsils are grasped with an Allis clamp.

3. The mucosa of the anterior and posterior pillars of the pharynx is incised, as is the capsule of the tonsil.

4. The vessels to the tonsils are clamped, divided, and ligated with catgut.

5. A snare is placed around the tonsil and the tonsil is removed.

6. The fossa is then carefully inspected and any bleeding vessels are clamped and tied.

7. Attention is now directed to the nasopharynx, into which the adenomatome is inserted; the adenoids are removed en bloc. Bleeding is controlled with pressure.

SURGICAL HAZARDS

1. Uncontrolled bleeding from the tonsillar bed may start and persist postoperatively. All blood vessels should be ligated and divided, and pressure should be applied until all bleeding is controlled.

2. Suture ligatures should not be placed in the tonsillar bed as the internal carotid artery may be injured. Bleeding may be very difficult to control.

3. In the performance of an adenoidectomy, the eustachian tube orifice may be injured.

POSTOPERATIVE MANAGEMENT

The patient is kept in the recovery room until fully reactive from the anesthesia. The usual general postoperative measures are carried out. In addition:

1. The patient should be kept in semi-Fowler's position or on his side horizontally to avoid aspiration of blood and venous engorgement.

2. He may be given clear liquids when reactive from anesthesia.

3. The blood pressure and pulse should be recorded every hour and the patient should be checked carefully for continued bleeding. If this is noted, the surgeon should be called immediately.

STUDY QUESTIONS

1. What is the supposed function of the tonsillar tissue?

2. What is the treatment of acute tonsillitis?

3. What is otitis media?

4. What are some of the dangers of tonsillectomy?

5. Where is the eustachian tube located and what is its use?

6. Describe the various instruments used in the performance of tonsillectomy and adenoidectomy.

7. What is the most serious postoperative complication of tonsillectomy and how is it managed?

8. What is the nurse's role in the management of postoperative tonsillar or adenoidal bleeding?

9. Describe the procedure of anterior and posterior nasal packing with particular reference to the nurse's role in this procedure.

58

Operation: Elective Tracheostomy

TYPICAL HISTORY

A 63-year-old male, who had been a heavy smoker for 30 years, has had a chronic productive cough and shortness of breath for many years. The cough and dyspnea have recently worsened to such a degree that he is constantly short of breath even at rest and is mildly cyanotic. Various bronchodilating drugs, expectorants, and postural breathing exercises have been instituted in recent months, but the patient remains extremely dyspneic, anxious, and cyanotic. He now enters for an elective tracheostomy.

PHYSICAL EXAMINATION

The patient is a well-developed, thin, cyanotic, and dyspneic male; he is sitting up in bed and using his accessory muscles of respiration.

Significant Findings

1. There is cyanosis of the nail beds and lips.
2. Clubbing of fingers is seen.
3. The patient has acute dyspnea at rest.
4. Diffuse pulmonary rales and rhonchi are noted.
5. Blood gases reveal a low pO_2 and a high pCO_2.

DIAGNOSITC STUDIES

The patient with chronic lung disease has usually had several admissions to a general hospital, where repeated x-rays and bronchographic studies have demonstrated some form of chronic lung disease for which no curative therapy can be offered. If the patient has had these studies, probably he will now have simply a repeat chest x-ray to be certain no acute infection exists prior to surgery.

PROBABLE HOSPITAL COURSE

As stated, the patient with known chronic lung disease for which no specific therapy can be offered will probably undergo his elective tracheostomy as soon as this can be scheduled. However, in the event that the patient has not been adequately studied in the past, several tests must be done to rule out a possible correctable lesion as well as to determine his pulmonary functional status. These tests include the following:

1. *Chest X-ray.* If this shows localization of disease to one or more lobes of the lung, the patient may be symptomatically improved by undergoing lobectomy.

2. *Bronchography.* The patient is given a dye through a catheter directly into the tracheobronchial tree. The tracheobronchial tree is then visualized by x-ray and obstructive disease such as bronchiectasis can be diagnosed. If the bronchiectasis is segmental, that is, localized to one or more segments of the lung, surgery can help such a patient. If, on the other hand, the bronchiectasis is diffuse or generalized, then no specific form of surgery is indicated.

3. *Bronchoscopy.* The surgeon introduces a bronchoscope into the tracheobronchial tree and visualizes the several orifices of the lung segments. Any obstruction caused by, for example, carcinoma of the bronchus, is thereby visualized and a biopsy can be taken.

4. *Functional Tests.* These are tests which attempt to determine the pulmonary functional status of a patient who is suffering from chronic lung disease.

   a. By far the simplest test to perform is an *exercise tolerance test,* in which the patient is asked to walk up one or two flights of stairs to determine how rapidly he becomes dyspneic. In the patient under discussion, who is dyspneic at rest, there is obviously no need to perform this type of test.

   b. Sophisticated quantitative tests of functional lung capacity are now available, and the student is referred to appropriate texts on pulmonary physiology for a discussion of this complex subject.

   c. Blood gas analysis is another useful set of tests for evaluating present lung function and for predicting future function. The student should consult appropriate pulmonary references for a discussion of blood gas testing.

Following these studies, the patient is prepared for elective tracheostomy.

PREPARATION FOR SURGERY

1. Complete history and physical examination.

2. *Psychological Preparation.* The patient about to undergo a tracheostomy must be carefully instructed concerning his postoperative vocal and pulmonary status. It should be carefully explained to him that his voice box will not be injured during this operation, but that, at the same time, intermittent blockage of the tracheostomy will be necessary in order for speech to be audible. Generally, the patient with severe dyspnea is willing to accept this inconvenience in order to alleviate his symptoms.

3. *Skin Prep.* The entire neck from the submental region to the supraclavicular and anterior chest regions is prepped anteriorly as well as laterally to the lateral borders of the sternomastoid muscles. (See Introduction.)

4. *Enema.* Not necessary.

5. *Levin Tube.* Not necessary.

6. *Blood.* Not necessary.

7. *Premedications.* Routine.

8. *Special Medications.* The patient may be started on expectorants, antibiotics, or various bronchodilator agents 2 to 3 days prior to surgery in order to obtain the maximum pulmonary status for tolerating the surgery.

9. *Operating Room Skin Prep.* This extends from the submental region anteriorly down to the anterior chest wall and laterally to the lateral borders of the sternomastoid muscle. (See Introduction.)

10. *Position.* The patient is placed in a high semi-Fowler's position with the neck hyperextended. (See Introduction.)

PATHOLOGY

Generally there is no local pathologic condition at the site of the tracheostomy.

GENERAL RATIONALE AND SCHEME

A tracheostomy is done either on an elective or on an emergency basis. An elective tracheostomy is often carried out in the presence of chronic lung disease. The rationale behind the tracheostomy under these circumstances is to diminish the dead space which exists from the opening of the mouth down to the supraclavicular region, where the tracheostomy is to be created. This dead space or column of air occupies a large percentage of the patient's total lung volume of air. Consequently, by creating a new vent closer to the functional areas in the lung, greater efficiency is given the patient, who already is functioning with a partly destroyed lung.

Emergency tracheostomy, on the contrary, is usually performed because of obstruction in the upper respiratory tree, in which case the opening is made below the obstruction to afford immediate relief.

Scheme

1. The skin, fascia, and *pretracheal* muscles are divided in the lower part of the neck.
2. One or two of the tracheal rings are partially removed.
3. A properly fitted tracheostomy tube is inserted.
4. The skin is closed around the tube.

PROCEDURE

1. *Skin Incision.* The vertical or transverse incision may be used, the latter being more popular and preferred. This incision is made approximately one finger breadth above the suprasternal notch parallel to it and extending from the anterior border of one sternomastoid muscle to the opposite side. (See Introduction.)

2. *Deepening the Incision.* The incision is deepened through the subcutaneous tissue and the underlying platysmal muscle fibers are divided.

3. The upper and lower flaps of skin, the subcutaneous tissue, and the platysmal muscle are retracted, and the deep cervical fascia is divided.

4. The isthmus of the thyroid gland which joins both lobes of the thyroid gland in the midline over the trachea is retracted in an upward direction, thereby exposing the underlying tracheal rings. An oval segment of tracheal tissue is excised often incorporating a segment of the second or third tracheal ring.

5. The tracheostomy tubes are examined for proper size and a tube with its obturator is inserted into the tracheal opening. In the adult, No. 5 and No. 6 tubes are the most frequently used (Fig. 58–1).

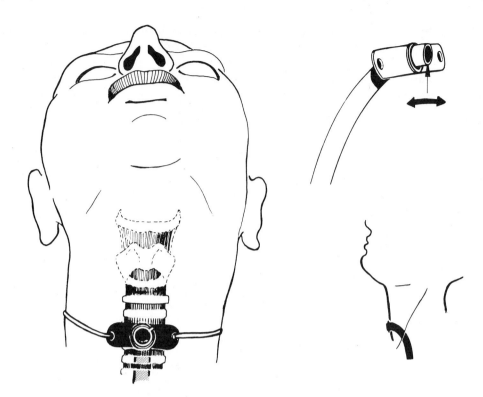

FIGURE 58-1 Tracheostomy, demonstrating position of the tracheostomy tube below the second tracheal ring.

6. *Skin Closure.* The skin is loosely closed around the tracheostomy tube and a small petroleum jelly dressing is placed between the tube and the skin to prevent excoriation. The margins of the skin should be checked for bleeding at this time. Ribbons should be placed around the tracheostomy tube and tied around the patient's neck to prevent loss of the tube during coughing.

SURGICAL HAZARDS

1. *Severe Bleeding.* This occurs most often from the thyroid bed, particularly when the operation is performed too hastily.

2. *Damage to the Jugular Veins.* This also may result in severe bleeding and, if much air is suctioned into the veins after they are opened, an air embolism may occur.

3. Damage to the larynx can occur if the incision in the trachea is made too high. The third ring is the preferable ring to incise; certainly, incision should be no higher than the second ring.

4. *Damage to the Recurrent Laryngeal Nerves.* These are lateral to the trachea and, as long as the incision is kept in the midline of the anterior wall of the trachea, this complication should not occur.

5. Damage to the cricoid cartilage.

6. Perforation of the esophagus.

7. *Subcutaneous and Mediastinal Emphysema.* These conditions can occur as a result of inadvertent laceration of the pleural domes. They may also occur after tracheostomy; an excessively tight skin closure can cause negative intrathoracic pressure to suck air into the wound.

8. Pneumothorax.

9. Injury to the carotid artery.

10. Aspiration of blood during the tracheostomy.

IMMEDIATE POSTOPERATIVE MANAGEMENT

The patient is returned to the recovery room until sufficiently reactive from the anesthetic. He is kept in a high semi-Fowler's position, and oxygen should be administered through the tracheal tube by way of a respirator or a Brigg's adaptor. Oxygen should be humidified during administration, as should be room air introduced through a tracheostomy.

1. *Respiratory Management.* The tracheostomy may need deep endotracheal suctioning in the recovery room. This should be done with use of sterile gloves, a sterile tracheal catheter, and sterile saline (to cleanse the catheter). Indeed, all suctioning of the trachea should be performed with such sterile precautions in mind. Suctioning should not be done for more than 5 to 10 seconds, since oxygen will be removed from the tracheobronchial tree and this may lead to anoxia, with resulting cardiac arrest. The patient should be allowed to rest between tracheal suctionings. Nasopharyngeal suctioning should be employed whenever the cuff of a tracheostomy tube is deflated.

2. General pulmonary measures will include:

a. Encouraging coughing and deep breathing.

b. Use of expectorants and antibiotics.

c. Use of humidification.

3. *Care of the Wound.* Moderate serosanguineous drainage around the tracheostomy tube is to be expected for 2 to 3 days. If bleeding persists, the surgeon should be notified, as a small blood vessel may occasionally begin to bleed after the patient coughs vigorously. Dressings and tapes around the patient's neck should be changed as necessary.

4. Postoperatively, careful attention must be focused on:

a. Preventing the tracheostomy tube from sliding out of place.

b. Preventing plugging of the tracheostomy tube with tenacious mucous secretions.

c. Deflating the cuffed tracheal tube as ordered, to prevent tracheal necrosis and resulting stricture.

5. Anti-infection precautions must be employed to prevent contamination of the patient's wound and respiratory tract with pathogens. All members of the staff should wear masks when they come in contact with the patient.

STUDY QUESTIONS

1. Define tracheostomy and tracheotomy.

2. List five conditions demanding an emergency tracheostomy.

3. What is the incision of choice for an emergency tracheostomy? Why?

4. What instruments should be contained in an emergency tracheostomy kit?

5. What is the nurse's role in aiding the surgeon in the performance of an emergency tracheostomy in the pateint's bed?

6. What structures are liable to be damaged during an emergency tracheostomy?

7. What is the pulmonary dead space? How is this relieved by tracheostomy?

8. Describe the proper care of a tracheostomy patient postoperatively.

9. Why should this care be carried out under sterile conditions?

10. One hour following a tracheostomy, the patient coughs vigorously and the tracheostomy tube is suddenly ejected from his trachea. How would you handle this emergency?

11. What are some of the psychological consequences of tracheostomy to a patient? How are these prevented or treated?

12. Describe the steps in an elective tracheostomy procedure to your class.

59   THE PATIENT WITH A PAROTID GLAND TUMOR

Operation: Superficial Parotid Gland Resection

TYPICAL HISTORY

A 48-year-old male has noted a painless swelling over his right jaw near the ear. The swelling has been present for about 5 months and has been slowly increasing in size. He does not develop any discomfort on eating or drinking and the mass causes no pain whatsoever. He has noted no facial droop, excess salivation, or other related symptoms.

PHYSICAL EXAMINATION

The patient is a well-developed, well-nourished male in no acute distress.

Significant Findings

1. There is a firm, nonmoveable mass over the angle of the mandible on the right side in the region of the parotid gland.
2. Stensen's duct is milked intraorally and no purulent material is expressed.
3. The remainder of the physical examination is unremarkable.

DIAGNOSTIC STUDIES

1. X-rays of the face, particularly of the mandible and maxilla, are taken to rule out the presence of any radiopaque calculi in the duct of the parotid gland. A sialogram may be obtained to visualize the parotid ductal system.

PROBABLE HOSPITAL COURSE

The most likely diagnosis is a tumor of the parotid gland and, by far, the most common tumor is the *mixed tumor.*

The surgeon will wish to rule out the presence of an obstructing calculus in the duct of the parotid gland with resultant parotitis. The absence of tenderness and swelling and of purulent material from Stensen's duct militates against this diagnosis in the present case.

PREPARATION FOR SURGERY

1. A careful neurological examination with particular regard to the facial and mandibular nerves should be done prior to the operation to determine any preoperative weakness of these nerves which could be misinterpreted postoperatively as damage to the nerves.
2. The face and neck region on the right side including the hair line anterior to the ear is shaven preoperatively. (See Introduction.)
3. Typing and cross-matching for blood is not necessary.
4. *Enema.* Not necessary.
5. *Premedications.* Routine.
6. *Special Medications.* None.
7. *Operating Room Skin Prep.* The ear, face, neck, and jaw regions on the appropriate side are prepped. (See Introduction.)
8. *Position.* This will vary with the surgeon but, generally, a high semi-Fowler's position is used, the neck being turned laterally to the opposite side of surgery and hyperextended. The head should be stabilized with tape and sandbags to prevent motion during the operation. (See Introduction.)

PATHOLOGY

The majority of tumors of the parotid gland are benign, *mixed* tumors; however, 30 to 40 per cent are malignant. The tumor usually appears grossly as a small, firm, and painless swelling in any part of the parotid gland tissue. If a benign mixed tumor of the parotid gland is found in the superficial lobe, only this lobe will be removed, as removal of the deep part of the gland involves danger of injury to the facial nerve which passes through the gland (Fig. 59–1).

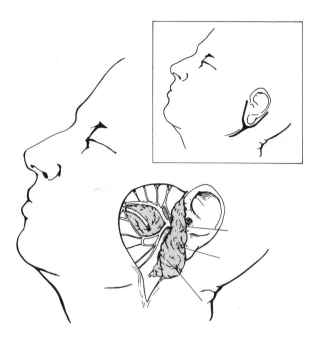

FIGURE 59-1 Considerable skill must be used in surgery on the parotid gland because of its proximal relationship to the facial nerve, as shown in the larger drawing. One type of incision used to approach the parotid gland is shown in the inset.

GENERAL RATIONALE AND SCHEME

It is impossible to distinguish clinically a benign from a malignant tumor of the parotid gland. Consequently, every painless swelling thought to be a tumor must be explored and removed.

Benign mixed tumors of the parotid gland usually occupy the superficial lobe of the gland and are therefore more easily removed without undue danger of injury to the underlying facial nerve. However, careful and complete dissection of this tissue must be done because of the high incidence of local recurrence even of the benign mixed tumor.

Should a malignant tumor of the parotid gland be proven at the time of surgery, then a total parotid resection will be required. This involves a very extensive and dangerous resection due to the involvement of the facial nerve.

Scheme

1. A proper Y-type skin incision is made on both sides of the ear and below the angle of the mandible, and skin flaps are raised and reflected. (See Introduction.)
2. The facial nerve is identified, as well as all its branches.
3. The superficial lobe of the parotid gland containing the tumor is excised.
4. The skin incision is drained and closed, and a heavy dressing is applied.

PROCEDURE

1. *Skin Incision.* A pre- and postauricular incision is made with a curved cervical extension below the angle of the mandible. (See Introduction.)
2. Anterior and posterior skin flaps are raised. Biopsies are carried out to determine the nature of the tumor.

3. The mastoid process is palpated and the facial nerve is identified as it exits from the stylomastoid foramen. Identification may require a long, tedious exploration.

4. The tail of the parotid gland is reflected from the underlying sternocleidomastoid muscle.

5. After the main facial nerve trunk is visualized, dissection is carried between the superficial and deep lobes of the parotid gland, totally dissecting free and preserving the branches of the facial nerve.

6. Stensen's duct is transected and ligated at the anterior margin of the incision.

7. The wound is closed and a small drain is placed in the dependent aspect of the wound.

8. A firm pressure dressing is applied.

SURGICAL HAZARD

By far, the most common surgical hazard is injury to the facial nerve or one of its branches. This can be avoided only by performance of meticulous and bloodless surgical dissection. Some surgeons prefer to use an electric nerve stimulator to identify various fibers of the facial nerve. Whatever the method, the procedure can be done only by neat, careful, and time-consuming surgery.

POSTOPERATIVE MANAGEMENT

The patient is returned to the recovery room until sufficiently reactive from anesthesia. The general principles of postoperative management are applied. In particular:

1. The patient should be kept in high semi-Fowler's position to avoid venous oozing from the incision.

2. The dressing is changed p.r.n. if it soaks through. This should be done under aseptic conditions, the first dressing preferably being changed by the surgeon.

3. A tracheostomy kit is kept by the bedside, although it is rare for this type of surgery to result in any significant respiratory difficulty.

4. The patient is allowed clear liquids by mouth as soon as he is awakened from the anesthetic.

5. As soon as he is able to cooperate, he should be asked to smile, show his teeth, and purse his lips so it can be determined as early as possible whether any damage has been done to the facial nerve. If one delays in this examination for 48 to 72 hours, operative edema will have developed around the facial nerve and palsy will ensue. It will be difficult to know whether this palsy is due to edema or permanent injury unless an examination is done right after surgery.

STUDY QUESTIONS

1. List several causes for a lump in the parotid gland. What is a *mixed tumor* of the parotid gland?

2. What is Stensen's duct and where is its opening?

3. Describe the location of the facial nerve and its five main branches. Explain the function of these nerves.

4. Describe the clinical condition resulting from total transection of one facial nerve at its main trunk.

5. What is the treatment of a stone in Stensen's duct?

6. Describe the make-up and function of an electric nerve stimulator. What is the nurse's role in preparing this machine for use in parotid surgery?

7. Describe the surgical steps involved in the removal of the superficial lobe of the parotid gland.

8. Which is more hazardous in terms of facial nerve injury — a superficial lobectomy or a parotidectomy?

9. What are some of the theoretical hazards associated with frozen section of a parotid tumor at the time of surgery?

10. What is a sialogram? How does it aid in the evaluation of parotid gland disease?

11. What is Frey's syndrome?

60

THE PATIENT WITH CANCER OF THE LARYNX

Operation: Laryngectomy

TYPICAL HISTORY

A 59-year-old male, who was a heavy cigarette smoker, had been treated with irradiation of his larynx 5 months earlier for a small, noninvasive carcinoma of the larynx.

Two months before admission he noted recurrent hoarseness which has progressively worsened. He now enters for evaluation and further therapy.

PHYSICAL EXAMINATION

A well-developed, well-nourished male is admitted in no particular distress.

Significant Findings

1. There is obvious hoarseness.
2. Laryngoscopic examination reveals a small carcinoma in the left vocal cord which appears to have fixed this cord, thus producing malfunction and resulting hoarseness of the voice.
3. Examination of the neck reveals no evidence of metastatic disease. (A radical neck dissection would be indicated if the patient had palpable metastases, usually on the same side as the tumor.)
4. The remainder of the examination is unremarkable.

DIAGNOSTIC STUDIES

1. A chest x-ray is done usually to rule out distant metastatic disease.
2. Apart from direct visualization of the lesion through a laryngoscope, there are no other particular studies used. If the diagnosis has not been confirmed previously, a biopsy can be taken of the lesion through the laryngoscope.

PROBABLE HOSPITAL COURSE

If surgery is planned for the treatment of the lesion, the patient's general status is evaluated and, when feasible, total laryngectomy is carried out.

PREPARATION FOR SURGERY

1. *Levin Tube.* Unnecessary.
2. The patient is typed and cross-matched for two units of whole blood.
3. The skin prep extends from the submental region to the clavicles and laterally out to the angles of the mandibles. (See Introduction.)
4. *Enema.* Not necessary.
5. *Premedications.* Routine.
6. *Special Medications.* None.
7. *Psychological Preparation.* The loss of voice which follows total laryngectomy is, of course, a most tragic psychological event for the patient. This requires a great deal of preparation and all members of the surgical team must lend moral support to the patient. It is usually explained to the patient that several electronic devices are available to aid him in vocal communication with his fellow human beings. If possible, it is even worthwhile to present to the patient another person who has undergone laryngectomy and who has adapted to the use of electronic vocalizing devices. This is often of greater value to the patient than any other preparation which he can be given.
8. Operating room skin prep extends from the submental region to the clavicles and laterally to both mandibular angles. (See Introduction.)
9. *Position.* The patient is placed in the semi-Fowler's position with the head hyper-extended. (See Introduction.)

PATHOLOGY

Usually the pathologic condition is limited to the intrinsic anatomy of the larynx and will not be visualized during the dissection.

Should any lymph nodes be involved in the cervical area, a combined laryngectomy and radical neck dissection will be performed by the surgeon.

GENERAL RATIONALE AND SCHEME

There is considerable controversy concerning the proper treatment of cancer of the larynx. In the early stage the lesion is amenable to x-ray therapy and this will preserve the voice box. Consequently, early lesions or those localized to one vocal cord are often treated with x-ray therapy first.

Some of the commonly accepted indications for surgery for cancer of the vocal cords include the following:

1. Fixation of a vocal cord.
2. Recurrence of cancer after radiation therapy.
3. Extensive cancers growing out of the larynx, and
4. Cancer involving the hypopharynx.

Removal of the entire larynx and associated nodal structures offers the best hope for a radical cure of this condition. Should there be any nodal involvement in the neck region where this disease commonly metastasizes, a radical neck dissection is often added to the laryngectomy.

Scheme

1. *Skin Incision.* This consists of raising large flaps and exposing the entire anterior surface of the neck.
2. The muscles attaching the larynx to the trachea are divided.
3. The trachea is opened and the larynx is removed.
4. The gastrointestinal tract in the area of the pharynx is reconstituted.
5. Tracheostomy is performed.
6. The skin incision is closed.

PROCEDURE

1. *Skin Incision.* There are many types of skin incisions employed. The one used in the present case is an upright T-shaped incision overlying the larynx and thyroid. (See Introduction.)
2. The flaps created by the incision are dissected and reflected inferiorly and superiorly, exposing all the structures of the anterior neck region.
3. The hyoid bone, which is attached to the larynx and is to be removed during this dissection, is separated from its suprahyoid muscular attachments.
4. The lower attachment of the larynx to the clavicle via the strap muscles of the neck is now divided.
5. The final attachment of the larynx is to the pharynx. The pharynx must, therefore, be entered so that laryngectomy may be completed. The pharynx is opened and the trachea is divided below the larynx.
6. The specimen is now removed en bloc and given to the circulating nurse.

7. A Levin tube is now passed by the anesthetist through the nose. It will be visualized in the pharynx and fed through into the distal esophagus.

8. The pharynx is now closed with running sutures and with interrrupted silk suture.

9. The lower end of the trachea is sutured to the skin as a permanent tracheostomy.

10. Penrose drains or suction catheters are used to drain the subcutaneous space.

11. The skin is closed with interrupted silk sutures.

12. A No. 10 or No. 12 tracheal cannula is inserted snugly into the tracheostomy and tied behind the patient's neck to avoid slipping.

SURGICAL HAZARDS

1. There are numerous vital structures in the neck which must be avoided. These include large blood vessels such as the carotid artery, from which there may be uncontrollable massive hemorrhage. Bleeding may also occur without evidence, because blood may be swallowed.

2. The vagus nerves and phrenic nerve must be preserved.

3. Dissection too close to the clavicle may injure the apex of the pleura, resulting in pneumothorax.

POSTOPERATIVE MANAGEMENT

The patient is returned to the recovery room and kept in a high semi-Fowler's position to minimize postoperative bleeding.

1. Constant suction is applied to catheters in the neck wound.

2. Humidified air is introduced into the tracheostomy.

3. Routine aseptic tracheostomy care is carried out.

4. The patient is kept n.p.o. for the first 24 hours.

5. The surgeon should be notified if the dressing soaks through.

STUDY QUESTIONS

1. Describe the anatomy of the larynx to your class.

2. How do electronic devices aid in vocalization after a laryngectomy?

3. State some of the indications for laryngectomy for carcinoma of the vocal cords.

4. Describe a nursing plan for the postoperative care of a patient who has undergone total laryngectomy.

5. Why is the semi-Fowler's position utilized in the postoperative period?

61

THE PATIENT
WITH METASTATIC
CARCINOMA
TO THE NECK

Operation: **Radical Neck Dissection**

TYPICAL HISTORY

A 68-year-old male underwent resection of a carcinoma of the lip approximately 6 months prior to this admission. He now enters with a nontender firm mass in the right side of the neck overlying the sternocleidomastoid muscle. He denies any pain, local tenderness or other symptoms and appears to be in good health otherwise.

PHYSICAL EXAMINATION

The patient is a well-developed, well-nourished male in no acute distress.

Significant Findings

1. There is a well-healed scar at the angle of the mouth near the lower lip at the site of the previous excision of a carcinoma. There is no evidence of local recurrence in this area.
2. In the right side of the neck overlying the sternocleidomastoid muscle is a firm, nontender, moveable mass, 3 by 3 cm.
3. Remainder of the physical examination is unremarkable.

DIAGNOSTIC STUDIES

1. WBC is normal.
2. Chest x-ray shows no evidence of primary or metastatic disease in the chest.
3. Thyroid scan is normal.
4. Laryngoscopy reveals no abnormality.
5. Sinus studies are unremarkable.

PROBABLE HOSPITAL COURSE

The patient appears to have developed a metastatic node in the right side of the neck secondary to the previous lip cancer. The surgeon is usually able to determine this by clinical examination of the mass, which appears to be extremely hard and nontender, but somewhat

378

moveable. The absence of this mass 6 months previously and the fact that the patient has had a carcinoma of the lip removed constitute ample evidence of metastatic disease.

The surgeon is hesitant to do a biopsy of this mass because, should it be cancerous, the overlying lymphatics would be disrupted at the biopsy site and the cancer might be spread. However, he must be reasonably certain of the diagnosis prior to submitting the patient to radical neck dissection.

Assuming that carcinoma metastatic to the neck has been diagnosed and that there is no evidence of metastases below the clavicle or on the opposite side, the patient will undergo radical neck dissection.

PREPARATION FOR SURGERY

1. Levin tube unnecessary.
2. A large-bore intravenous needle or intracatheter should be inserted for possible massive blood transfusions during the operative procedure.
3. The patient should be typed and cross-matched for four units of whole blood.
4. *Skin Preparation.* This should include the entire right side of the face and neck from the level of the upper pole of the ear to the nipple line. Behind the ear, the hairline should be shaven cleanly over the entire mastoid process and down toward the prominence of the trapezius muscle. (See Introduction.)
5. Enema is not necessary.
6. *Premedications.* Routine.
7. *Special Medications.* None.
8. *Psychological Preparation.* Operations on the head and neck are usually associated with greater anxiety than operations anywhere else in the body because the patient is worried primarily about the cosmetic effect of the operation. He also has an instinctive awareness of the vital structures contained within the neck.

It should be explained to the patient that the cosmetic results of radical neck dissection are not particularly disturbing, nor will he have any significant limitation of function of the neck following this operation.

It should also be explained to the patient that he may have to undergo temporary tracheostomy and that during this period he will be unable to talk.

9. *Operating Room Skin Prep.* This also extends from the superior pole of the ear down to the nipple line and the entire side of the neck on the appropriate side. The retroauricular hairline down to the suboccipital area and trapezius should also be prepped. (See Introduction.)
10. *Position.* The patient is placed in a semi-Fowler's position with the neck hyperextended and turned to the extreme left side, exposing the entire right side of the neck. (See Introduction.)

PATHOLOGY

In addition to the obvious clinical node which has been palpated, other metastatic nodes may be found in the course of the dissection. To the extent that these nodes are confined to the field of dissection, a reasonably good cure rate is to be expected from this type of operation.

GENERAL RATIONALE AND SCHEME

A peculiarity of carcinoma of the head and neck region, in general, is its pattern of slow growth and slow spread. Disease of the oral cavity and lips and even of the thyroid tends to spread to the neck in a slow fashion prior to any further spread to the chest region. Consequently, metastatic disease from the lip to the neck does not constitute an incurable situation. The entire lymphatic chain and nodal system of the neck is removed on the involved side. There is a good possibility of permanent cure. A radical neck dissection has been devised to remove all nonvital structures of the neck including all lymphatics and nodes which may contain the tumor.

Scheme

1. The neck is widely opened by large superior, inferior, lateral, and medical flaps.
2. All nonvital structures of the neck region are removed in one continuous mass of tissue.
3. Suction catheters are put in place.
4. The incision is closed.
5. A compression dressing is applied.
6. If necessary, a tracheostomy is done.

PROCEDURE

1. *Skin Incision.* An H-shaped incision is made on the appropriate side of the neck. The four large flaps are reflected to their full extent, exposing the entire side of the neck. (See Introduction.)

2. Michel clips are used to clip skin towels to the surrounding skin flaps after they have been fully dissected.

3. The sternocleidomastoid muscle is exposed and transected at its lower attachment to the clavicle.

4. The external jugular vein is ligated and transected, following which the internal jugular vein is clamped, ligated, and divided.

5. Care should be taken to avoid injury to the carotid artery and vagus nerve, which are retracted medially during the dissection. All the lymphatic tissue, including nodes overlying the carotid sheath, the brachial plexus, and the vagus nerves, is swept superiorly along with the sternomastoid muscle and the jugular veins.

6. When the superior aspect of the incision is reached, the submandibular space is also dissected cleanly, avoiding injury to branches of the facial nerve.

7. At the superior aspect of the incision, the internal jugular vein is again clamped, ligated, and divided.

8. After removal of all nonvital tissue in the neck, the entire wound must be well irrigated with saline and all small bleeding vessels clamped and ligated. The operative field must be as dry as possible prior to closure. An electrocautery may be used at this point.

9. Large Penrose drains or suction catheters are placed under the flaps and brought out through the lower poles of the incision.

10. A heavy compression dressing is placed around the incision to minimize postoperative oozing. If suction catheters are used, a light dressing is sufficient.

11. If the surgeon feels there will be any postoperative respiratory distress, a tracheostomy should now be done.

SURGICAL HAZARDS

1. *Massive Hemorrhage.* There are several large vessels in the neck, including the external and internal carotid arteries, the internal and external jugular veins, and several other smaller

tributaries. Any one of these may be lacerated inadvertently or a suture ligature torn, resulting in massive hemorrhage in the neck.

2. Injury to the thoracic duct on the left side of the neck in a left radical neck dissection may occur. If a laceration is noted at surgery, simple ligatures are placed around it and there is no difficulty postoperatively. Failure to treat a laceration of the thoracic duct may result in formation of a lymph fistula postoperatively, which can be very difficult to manage.

3. Injury to vital structures, such as the vagus nerve, the carotid artery, the recurrent laryngeal nerve, or the phrenic nerve, may cause one or more postoperative problems depending on the structure injured. Thorough knowledge of the local anatomy must be kept in mind and meticulous dissection must be carried out in a bloodless field.

4. *Hypotension.* This can be caused by a hypersensitive carotid sinus, which is affected by minimal surgical manipulation; arterial blood pressure may decrease to 50 to 60 mm Hg for a few minutes during surgery.

5. A pneumothorax can be produced as a result of trauma to the apex of the pleural cavity at the root of the neck. Its presence may be manifested by a flow of air through the wound and by the usual pulmonary symptoms of pneumothorax.

6. Intracranial pressure may be increased as a result of a rise in cerebral venous pressure during surgery (due to unilateral ligation of the jugular vein). The increase in intracranial pressure is usually slight but can persist for several days postoperatively.

7. *Complications Resulting from the Sacrifice of Various Nerves.* The sacrifice of:

a. The *spinal accessory nerve,* that is, the motor nerve to the trapezius muscle, will cause atrophy of the muscle, drooping of the shoulder, difficulty in lifting the arm laterally or over the head, and discomfort and lameness of the shoulder.

b. The *lingual nerve* will cause the ipsilateral side of the tongue to become numb.

c. The *hypoglossal nerve* will result in paralysis in that side of the tongue; the protruded tongue will then deviate to the side of the trauma.

d. The *vagus nerve on one side* will cause paralysis in the same side of the vocal cord.

e. The *glossopharyngeal nerve* will result in dysphagia on that side of the throat.

f. The *phrenic nerve* will leave the patient with a hemidiaphragm.

g. The *sympathetic nerves* will cause Horner's syndrome.

h. The *brachial plexus* will cause sensory and/or motor dysfunction in the upper extremity.

POSTOPERATIVE MANAGEMENT

1. The patient is returned to the recovery room in semi-Fowler's position to discourage venous oozing from the wound.

2. If a tracheostomy has been performed, routine postoperative management should be undertaken.

3. If the dressing soaks through with blood, the surgeon should be notified at once.

4. The operative wound may be drained by means of a Penrose drain or by catheters attached to negative pressure and a collecting drainage system. Optimum drainage is accomplished by the use of negative pressure; adequate drainage is facilitated when suction is employed. Suction catheters should be connected at once to suction to prevent clotting of blood within the tubing. These suction catheters should not be irrigated except by specific order of the surgeon.

5. The external suture line may be cleansed with sterile mineral oil or hydrogen peroxide every 2 hours; sterile technique must be used. (In some cases the surgeon may not elect any special wound care postoperatively.)

6. A bulky dressing is applied with some firmness to prevent oozing from the wound and to keep the skin flaps intact and firmly in contact with underlying tissues. If the dressing is too tight,

the patient may develop bradycardia, cyanosis, and restlessness. The surgeon should be notified of these events and the dressing should be loosened.

7. A nasogastric tube will be in place, and the patient will receive nothing by mouth. He will require mouth care frequently (at least every 2 hours) and periodic suctioning of his mouth and throat. Suctioning must be done very gently to prevent any undue trauma to the internal suture lines. The patient may drool, since the swallowing reflex may be absent or the act of swallowing may be too difficult for the patient to accomplish. Edema of the recurrent laryngeal nerve and of the nerves to the pharynx may cause difficulty in swallowing and in expectorating secretions.

8. Edema of the lower part of the face on the same side as the surgery is to be expected.

9. Insufficient replacement of blood lost during surgery may manifest itself as tachycardia and hypotension in the early postoperative period. Vital signs must be checked frequently and carefully so that any changes that indicate hypovolemia may be evaluated by the surgeon; appropriate replacement must be made in order to relieve this situation.

10. The nurse must check for signs and symptoms of increased intracranial pressure. She must note especially the patient's complaint of headache, which may be indicative of the increase.

STUDY QUESTIONS

1. Why is tracheostomy sometimes performed during the course of a radical neck dissection?

2. Why is a pressure dressing indicated postoperatively for a patient who has had radical neck dissection?

3. Describe the nursing care concerned in the management of suction catheters in the neck.

4. Name five anatomic structures that are removed in the course of a radical neck dissection.

5. Name five anatomic structures that must be preserved in the course of a radical neck dissection.

6. While performing a radical neck dissection, the surgeon inadvertently severs the phrenic nerve to the diaphragm. What postoperative complications might be expected?

7. What postoperative complication might be expected from severance of the recurrent laryngeal nerve?

8. Draw up a nursing plan describing the postoperative nursing management of a patient who has undergone a radical neck dissection.

THE PATIENT WITH A THYROID TUMOR

62

Operation: Thyroidectomy

TYPICAL HISTORY

A 38-year-old female, in excellent health previously, accidentally noticed a lump in the left side of her neck approximately 1 month prior to admission. This lump has not been tender nor has it caused any other symptoms.

PHYSICAL EXAMINATION

The patient is a well-developed, well-nourished female in no acute distress.

Significant Findings

1. There is an enlarged thyroid gland with a distinct tumor mass or nodule on the left side of the thyroid. This mass is firm, freely moveable, and nontender; it moves up and down when the patient swallows.
2. The remainder of the physical examination is unremarkable.

DIAGNOSTIC STUDIES

Although clinically the mass does not appear to be causing any symptoms of hyperthyroidism — that is, it does not appear to be a *functioning nodule* — the surgeon generally will perform several studies to determine whether or not the thyroid is chemically hyperactive. The decision to operate or to observe this tumor mass may well be altered pending the results of studies. Some of the studies include:

1. *Basal Metabolic Rate (BMR).* This is not the most accurate means of determining hyperfunction of the thyroid gland, inasmuch as an apprehensive, anxious patient may show hypermetabolism. However, a normal metabolic rate, as determined by the BMR test, certainly argues against the gland's being hyperactive. This study is done with the patient under mild sedation. Description of the exact technique is beyond the scope of this book.

2. *Protein Bound Iodine (PBI).* This indicates the iodine binding capacity of the thyroid gland; consequently, elevated levels suggest hyperthyroidism, whereas low levels suggest hypoactivity or normal thyroid function.

3. *Radioactive Iodine Test (RAI).* This is a study made directly over the thyroid gland. The patient swallows a radioactive iodine solution which is concentrated in the thyroid gland and measured with a counter. The test also helps to determine overactivity or underactivity of the thyroid gland and is an extremely valuable one.

4. Other studies that are used for evaluating the thyroid include:

a. Serum cholesterol.

b. X-rays of the neck and chest to determine the possible presence of a substernal thyroid gland.

c. If there is any question of injury or impingement on the recurrent laryngeal nerves by the thyroid mass, the vocal cords will be directly visualized with the laryngoscope and their degree of function determined.

d. Thyroid scanning may detect the "hot" or "cold" nodule.

e. Resin T_3 uptake usually is high in thyrotoxicosis and low in hypothyroid states.

PROBABLE HOSPITAL COURSE

There are several indications for surgery on patients suffering from thyroid disease. The indications are determined by the type of thyroid disease found. Basically, there are four types of thyroid illnesses:

1. *Nodules, Either Discrete or Multiple.* These may obviously be benign or malignant. Often the surgeon must explore the patient simply because he cannot otherwise rule out a malignant nodule of the thyroid gland.

2. *Hyperactivity of the Thyroid Gland.* Here, the surgeon is removing thyroid tissue because he is unable to control the hyperactivity with medication.

3. *Inflammation of the Thyroid or Thyroiditis.* In this case, surgery is justified only if the condition cannot be distinguished from carcinoma.

4. *Diffuse Goiter.* In this case surgery, if indicated at all, is only for cosmetic purposes should the gland become extremely large. Tracheal compression, with symptoms of wheezing and shortness of breath, may also require surgery.

The hospital course will be determined by the type of disease process occurring in the thyroid gland. If, for example, the patient is suffering from a hyperactive thyroid gland, he may be treated medically to determine how well the thyroid gland responds to medication. If, on the other hand, the patient is found to have a nodule in the thyroid gland, the surgeon will immediately proceed to surgery if he cannot rule out malignancy in this nodule. A thyroid scan that indicates a "cold" nodule is often a strong impetus to surgery.

PREPARATION FOR SURGERY

In addition to the general measures outlined in Part I, the particular approach to the patient undergoing thyroid surgery is as follows:

1. A complete history and physical examination is obtained, as this is of great importance in thyroid disease, particularly with respect to certain endemic conditions which can occur in certain parts of the country. Nutritional deficiencies, history of previous nodules excised, as well as a history of symptoms suggesting toxicity of the thyroid gland should also be considered.

2. *Psychological Preparation.* The patient undergoing thyroidectomy is quite anxious concerning the incision in the neck. There is a certain amount of anxiety related to the cosmetic results, particularly in women, and it should be explained to the patient that the *collar incision* is barely perceptible 6 months after the operation. Another source of anxiety is simply that the neck is being operated upon — there is an instinctive fear of any surgery in the head, neck, or face region. Again, it should be explained that the vital structures in the neck will be avoided and that there is very little danger of any damage to these structures.

The patient with a lump in the thyroid gland is also quite anxious over the possibility of cancer. While this cannot be ruled out with any certainty preoperatively, a frank discussion with the patient concerning the improbability of the lump being a malignant tumor should be carried out.

3. *Skin Prep.* The entire neck, supraclavicular regions, clavicular regions, and anterior chest should be widely shaven on the evening prior to surgery. (See Introduction.)

4. *Enema.* Not necessary.

5. *Levin Tube.* Not necessary.

6. *Blood.* The patient should be typed and cross-matched for two units of whole blood as significant hemorrhage may occur if a large blood vessel is inadvertently damaged during the operation.

7. *Premedications.* Routine.

8. *Special Medications.* In the case of a patient undergoing surgery of the thyroid for tumors or nonfunctioning adenomata, there are no special medications used. However, when a patient with hyperthyroidism is to undergo surgery in order to cure this type of thyroid disease, it is imperative that the toxicity of the gland be reduced preoperatively. If this is not done, the highly vascular toxic gland, once mobilized during surgery, may release an immense quantity of thyroxin into the circulation, thereby causing postoperative thyroid storm. The physician uses Lugol's solution and propylthiouracil to control the thyroid gland for 4 to 6 weeks prior to surgical extirpation.

9. *Operation Room Skin Prep.* This includes the entire neck, supraclavicular, infra-clavicular, and anterior chest regions. (See Introduction.)

10. *Position.* High semi-Fowler's position with the neck hyperextended. (See Introduction.)

PATHOLOGY

The pathologic condition of the thyroid gland at the time of surgery is quite varied. Four basic conditions are usually found:

1. One or more nodules in one or both major thyroid lobes. These nodules may be benign or malignant.

2. *Inflammation of the Thyroid Gland.* This usually presents as a firm, diffusely swollen gland adherent to surrounding structures.

3. Diffuse enlargement of the thyroid gland — *diffuse goiter.* This is usually a very nodular, irregular thyroid gland of varying size and containing many colloid cysts.

GENERAL RATIONALE AND SCHEME

The surgeon attempts to cure or palliate the disease by removing part or all of the diseased glandular tissue.

1. *For Nodules:*

a. *For benign nodules,* mere excision of the nodule is all that is required.

b. *For malignant nodules,* the entire thyroid lobe involved or, at times, the entire thyroid gland must be sacrificed.

2. *For a hyperactive gland,* subtotal thyroidectomy to reduce the amount of functioning tissue is necessary.

3. *For inflammation of the gland or thyroiditis,* a biopsy only is performed to rule out carcinoma. If the gland is impinging upon the trachea, the isthmus may be removed to relieve tracheal compression.

4. *For diffuse thyroid goiter,* sufficient tissue is removed for cosmetic results or for decompression of the trachea.

Scheme

1. The gland is exposed in the neck by incising the skin and overlying fascia and muscle.
2. The blood supply of the segment of thyroid gland to be removed is divided.
3. The nerves to the vocal cords are carefully identified and preserved.
4. Resection of the desired portion of the gland is carried out.
5. The incision is closed.

PROCEDURE

1. *Skin Incision.* The proposed area of the skin incision is outlined by pressure with a fine silk thread to ensure an even, cosmetic incision. This incision is a curvilinear incision, one finger-breadth above the supraclavicular notch parallel to the lower crease in the neck, and it extends lateral to the clavicular insertions of the sternocleidomastoid muscles. (See Introduction.)

2. *Deepening Incision.* The incision is deepened through the underlying platysma down to the cervical fascia, which is also incised.

3. *Exposing the Thyroid Gland.* Once the fascia and infrahyoid muscles are divided and retracted, the fascia overlying the thyroid gland is found and also incised, thereby exposing the gland.

4. *Mobilizing Skin Flaps.* The superior and inferior skin flaps are sufficiently mobilized and retracted to expose the entire thyroid gland.

5. *Ligating the Blood Supply.* The three main blood vessels which must be ligated are:

  a. *Superior Thyroid Artery.* Care must be taken to avoid injury to the superior laryngeal nerve.
  b. *Middle Thyroid Artery.*
  c. *Inferior Thyroid Artery.* Care must be taken to prevent damage to the recurrent laryngeal nerve.

After complete division of blood supply to the thyroid gland has been accomplished, the surgeon estimates the amount of gland which must be sacrificed.

6. Serial clamping and ligating of the tissue to be removed is next accomplished.

7. The remaining stubs of thyroid tissue are sutured to the pretracheal fascia to accomplish adequate hemostasis.

8. *Closure.* One or more drains are left in place deep to the infrahyoid muscles and brought out through the lateral aspect of the incision.

SURGICAL HAZARDS

1. *Damage to One or Both Recurrent Laryngeal Nerves.* During the course of ligation of the inferior thyroid vessels, the recurrent laryngeal nerves which pass very close to these vessels may be damaged or divided, resulting in hoarseness or total loss of voice.

2. *Damage to the Parathyroid Glands.* The parathyroid glands are adjacent to the thyroid substance and may be damaged during the removal of the thyroid. If no parathyroid tissue is left in situ, acute tetany will develop postoperatively.

3. *Severe Uncontrollable Hemorrhage.* The superior thyroid arteries may retract into inaccessible areas in the neck during the course of dissection. These must be carefully isolated and ligated prior to division to prevent this complication.

4. *Damage to the Trachea.* The trachea may be punctured while the surgeon is clamping off small vessels in the thyroid substance. This can result in aspiration of blood through the trachea or the formation of a tracheocutaneous fistula postoperatively.

5. *Perforation of the Esophagus.* This can occur if a goiter is wedged between the trachea and the esophagus or if cancer of the thyroid has invaded the esophagus.

POSTOPERATIVE MANAGEMENT

The patient is returned to the recovery room until sufficiently reactive from the anesthetic. She should be kept in a high semi-Fowler's position to encourage easy venous return of blood from the head and the neck, thereby diminishing any venous oozing into the incision. Several complications are prone to occur in the post-thyroidectomy patient in the immediate postoperative period and may be hazardous or fatal if not appreciated early.

1. *Tracheal Compression.* A significant amount of venous oozing may occur in the early postoperative period. If this blood does not drain through the drains onto the dressing, it may cause compression of the trachea.

Early tracheal compression is usually heralded by the onset of restlessness, crowing respirations, tachycardia, and, finally, cyanosis. Symptomatic tracheal compression can often be prevented or minimized by placing the patient in a semi-Fowler's position directly after the surgical procedure to encourage venous drainage from the neck. Administration of adequate sedation, which minimizes the possibility of the sutures being disengaged from the small vessels due to coughing and restlessness, is also used. Should early tracheal compression be suspected by the nurse, the surgeon should be notified immediately, oxygen therapy started at once, and a tracheotomy set obtained and made ready at the bedside. It is wise to have a tracheotomy set at the bedside routinely. Hemorrhage in the wound can occur during the first 48 hours after thyroidectomy and can cause respiratory obstruction through compression.

If a surgeon is not immediately available and the patient's condition is deteriorating, the neck skin sutures or clips should be removed immediately and the skin edges separated with a Kelly clamp, thereby allowing accumulated blood to escape.

2. When the patient develops the signs and symptoms of *laryngeal edema* and *stridor* postoperatively, treatment includes:
   a. Placing the patient in a high Fowler's position.
   b. Initiating steam inhalation.
   c. Administering humidified oxygen by mask.
   d. Rapidly inserting an endotracheal tube (the nasal route is preferred).
   e. **Acting quickly to prevent anoxia and resulting cardiac arrest.**

It is a safe policy to call the responsible surgeon immediatley whenever his patient has respiratory difficulty after thyroidectomy.

3. *Hypocalcemic Tetany.* This may last for 2 to 3 days after surgery.
   a. *Cause.* Removal of parathyroid glands incidental to thyroidectomy.
   b. *Diagnosis.* Hypocalcemic tetany is often heralded by nervousness, muscular twitching, muscle cramps, and paresthesias of the hands and feet. These signs usually develop within the first 24 to 48 hours after a thyroidectomy, but may be delayed for 6 to 7 days. The surgeon will perform two tests in an effort to confirm the diagnosis:
      (1) *Chvostek's sign.* Tapping the facial nerve near the mastoid process will result in twitching of the upper lip. This indicates neuromuscular irritability, which occurs in impending tetany. (This sign may also be found in an individual not affected by tetany.)

   (2) *Trousseau's sign.* A blood pressure cuff is inflated around the arm. If the hand takes on a characteristic claw-like position, this again indicates neuromuscular irritability. If one or both of these signs are positive, a blood specimen should be examined for serum calcium and intravenous calcium given before the laboratory report is returned.

c. *Preventive Measures.* Early recognition of impending tetany by close observation for above signs and symptoms.

d. *Treatment.* The principle of treatment is concerned with avoiding the serious respiratory distress threatened by the patient's poor muscle coordination or muscle dysfunction in the wake of the tetany. An intravenous line should be available.

   (1) Serum calcium and phosphorus levels should be assessed as soon as feasible.

   (2) Calcium gluconate in a dose of one gram is administered intravenously (a 10 per cent solution of the drug is used). Prompt improvement in the patient's condition is indicative of hypoparathyroidism. Calcium per os is then administered, where feasible, in the next 24 hours.

   (3) If calcium therapy proves ineffective, parathyroid hormone may have to be given intramuscularly in repeated doses until long-acting massive doses of vitamin D (50,000 to 100,000 units 3 times a day) become effective.

4. *Loss of Voice*

a. *Cause.* Injury, edema, or severance of both recurrent laryngeal nerves results in loss of voice.

b. *Diagnosis.* If the voice is present immediately after surgery, but then becomes hoarse or absent several hours postoperatively, this usually implies edema of the nerves and the condition is temporary. If the voice loss is total and follows immediately after the procedure, this may indicate total severance of nerves which will be permanent. Also, if the vocal cords are paralyzed, the glottis will be closed and respiratory obstruction may result. Consequently, the condition may be fatal.

c. *Preventive Measures.* There are none postoperatively. However, if respiratory obstruction is suspected, a tracheotomy set should be immediately available for possible use. The condition can also be temporarily abated by the introduction of an endotracheal tube through the paralyzed glottis and positive pressure breathing maintained through the endotracheal tube by the anesthetist.

d. *Treatment.* For voice loss — expectant; for respiratory obstruction — oxygen, tracheotomy, or endotracheal intubation.

5. *Thyroid Storm or Crisis.* This complication, which can prove fatal, is rare nowadays.

a. *Cause.* Sudden excretion into the circulation of excess thyroid hormone due to manipulation of a toxic gland during surgery.

b. *Diagnosis.* Extreme restlessness, high fever, and extreme tachycardia.

c. *Prevention.* In the preoperative course, if there is any suspicion of an overactive thyroid gland, antithyroid drugs should be given to decrease glandular activity and to make the patient euthyroid.

d. *Treatment.* This condition is very serious and must be treated aggressively. Intravenous sodium iodide, steroids, sedatives, and oxygen are administered. On suspicion, the surgeon is notified and these drugs are secured for possible emergency use.

   6. *Pneumothorax* may follow injury to apical pleura during removal of a large substernal goiter. Chest x-ray will confirm the diagnosis.

   Most of these complications are unusual and the patient's postoperative course is generally unremarkable. If the dressing soaks through, the surgeon should be notified for first dressing change. The presence of drains may encourage some soiling of dressings but this is usually of no significance.

STUDY QUESTIONS

1. What is Graves' disease and what medications are used for its treatment?

2. What is Hashimoto's disease?

3. Describe the various types of carcinoma of the thyroid, paying particular attention to the prognosis of each type.

4. What syndrome occurs if the entire thyroid gland is removed?

5. What syndrome occurs if the parathyroid glands are removed?

6. Why must an overactive thyroid gland be made *less active* prior to surgery?

7. How is an overactive gland suspected clinically and proven chemically?

8. Explain the significance of the positioning in the operating room.

9. Describe the location and function of the superior and inferior laryngeal nerves. Based on their locations, when are they most apt to be injured during thyroid surgery?

10. What are the infrahyoid muscles and what function do they serve?

11. Describe the blood supply to the thyroid gland.

12. Why does the surgeon drain the thyroid bed prior to closure?

13. Describe the syndrome of thyroid storm. What type of thyroid disease is likely to predispose the patient to this condition? Why is thyroid storm such a rare complication at present?

14. Is tetany ever fatal? Must all the parathyroid glands be removed before tetany occurs? Can a person live without any parathyroid tissue?

15. Is cancer of the thyroid gland curable by surgery or by any other means?

16. Make a list of things to do and problems to anticipate in the postoperative management of the thyroidectomized patient.

17. Define the purpose and technique of thyroid scanning. What is a "hot" thyroid nodule?

BREAST SURGERY

63   INTRODUCTION

This section, devoted to surgery of the breast, will discuss two procedures that are performed directly on the breast and a third, adrenalectomy, used in connection with the management of advanced breast cancer.

BOUNDARIES, ANATOMY, AND CONTENTS

The breast is a modified skin appendage consisting of functioning glands (alveoli) encased, in varying degree, in areolar and fibrous tissue, surrounded by a loose "capsule" or superficial fascia, and supported by dense connective tissue cords called Cooper's ligaments. The alveoli secrete their products into ducts that converge like branches of a tree and exit from the nipple through a dozen or more larger ducts.

The breast is variable in shape, tending to be hemispherical, with a "tail" or enlongated segment which extends up into the corresponding axilla. The breast is closely approximated to the underlying pectoralis major and minor muscles, to which it is attached by loose areolar tissue and through which lymphatics and blood vessels migrate to nourish the breast tissue. Superficial lymphatics also extend to the subdermal lymphatic plexus along with appropriate arteries and veins.

The lymphatic drainage system of the breast merits special attention because it is through these channels, primarily, that malignant cells migrate. Indeed, radical surgery for cancer of the breast is tailored to a thorough knowledge of the anatomy of the lymphatic system. There are three main lymphatic channels exiting from the breast. These channels in turn connect to an extensive network of smaller lymphatics that completely surround the breast and converge at the nipple. Because of this rich lymphatic network surrounding the breast, a malignancy beginning in one part of the breast has ready access to any other part of the breast. The rationale for total mastectomy whenever any part of the breast is involved in malignancy is thus readily apparent.

The three main lymphatic channels pass toward the *axilla* and *mediastinum* and directly through the pectoralis muscles via the *interpectoral group* of nodes. A fourth group of lymphatic channels passes through the upper rectus sheath and into the liver (this group is not as important as the three others).

Radical mastectomy, in its classical form, eradicates the entire breast, the axillary lymphatics, the pectoral muscles, and the upper segment of the rectus sheath, all in an effort to incorporate most of the lymphatic channels exiting from the breast. Super-radical mastectomy adds to this eradication the removal of the upper internal mammary lymph nodes which form the mediastinal group of nodes. Defenders of the super-radical mastectomy argue that a significant number of malignancies enter this internal mammary chain early in the development of cancer; failure to remove these nodes, as in any less radical procedure, defeats the entire rationale for mastectomy. Those who argue for the traditional radical mastectomy believe that the vast majority of tumors first embolize through the axillary and interpectoral group of nodes; the less accessible internal mammary nodes can thus be spared. The latter, it is argued, should be treated with x-ray for any medial quadrant tumor.

Recently, some physicians have argued for less radical approaches to surgery for cancer of the breast. Some would treat the disease by performing a simple mastectomy followed by x-ray treatment. Others, who question the necessity for breast mutilation, recommend simple extirpation of the malignancy itself, followed by appropriate x-ray treatment.

These controversies, while important to the surgeon, cannot be settled in an introductory text. Nevertheless, the surgical nurse should be aware of the continuing debate in surgical circles in regard to the appropriate therapy for breast cancer. The debate does have substantive anatomical grounds, for it centers on (1) the possibility or impossibility of total lymph node extirpation for breast cancer, (2) the efficacy or inefficacy of x-ray sterilization of malignant lymph nodes, and (3) the probability or improbability of early blood-borne metastases rendering lymph node extirpation somewhat futile.

SURGICAL APPROACHES

Breast masses are approached by curvilinear incisions that follow the normal concentrically disposed skin lines overlying the breast. When feasible, the mass is totally excised. Larger masses may be biopsied with a small wedge excision, followed by local excision if benign, or radical surgery if malignant.

Mastectomy, with or without a radical dissection, is carried out with an elliptical incision that removes the entire breast. The lines of incision are determined partly by the surgeon but must *not* pass through the axilla, as this could create disabling contractures.

Diseases of the nipple are generally approached by passing a small probe into the offending duct and opening the duct to uncover the disease (usually an intraductal papilloma or carcinoma).

SPECIAL FEATURES OF BREAST SURGERY

Psychological and Legal Problems. The potentially grave psychological problems attendant upon removal of a woman's breast can be readily appreciated. There are sexual connotations to the breast and strong associations with body image as well, and these must be taken fully into account both by the physician and the nurse. Often, the nurse is privy to the patient's anxieties to a far greater extent than is the doctor, and she must take advantage of her special position with the patient. Not the least of these anxieties is concern over the husband's acceptance of mastectomy; clearly, exceptional tact and discretion, along with a genuine sense of empathy, are needed here. As for legal entanglements, these can be avoided by arranging a careful preoperative discussion of the possibility of mastectomy with the patient.

Postmastectomy Pneumothorax. The possibility of surgical entry into the thoracic cavity, which can lead to postoperative pulmonary distress, must be recognized by the surgical nurse. Any dyspnea, restlessness, or cyanosis should alert the nurse to pulmonary complications, and appropriate physical examination and x-ray studies should follow.

Suction Catheters. Mastectomy leads to extravasation of blood and serum below the skin flaps, particularly if a radical dissection has been performed along with the procedure. The extravasation can lead to hematoma and seroma formation, with resultant wound infection and necrosis of skin flaps. Suction catheters are usually placed below the skin flaps to minimize these complications. The catheters are placed on continuous negative pressure, and the nurse must see to it that they are functioning properly.

64

THE PATIENT WITH A BREAST LUMP

Operation: Breast Biopsy

TYPICAL HISTORY

A 28-year-old female enters the hospital for evaluation of a painless lump in the left breast. She discovered the lump quite by accident while bathing one month ago. The patient reports no local pain associated with this lump, no nipple discharge, nor any breast trauma. There is no family history of breast disease.

PHYSICAL EXAMINATION

The patient is a well-developed, well-nourished female in no distress but appearing quite apprehensive about her impending surgery.

Significant Findings

There is a moveable, smooth, firm, and nontender mass in the upper outer quadrant of the left breast. The mass is about 2 cm X 2 cm and has well-defined margins. It is not fixed to the skin or to the underlying tissue.

DIAGNOSTIC STUDIES

1. Mammography is consistent with a benign lesion of the breast.
2. Chest x-ray is normal.

PROBABLE HOSPITAL COURSE

All true breast masses must be excised in order to rule out malignancy. Mammography and xeroradiography are helpful in ruling out malignancy but are not absolutely determinative.

Following routine laboratory testing and physical examination, the patient will be scheduled for biopsy, usually on the day after admission, unless routine studies reveal some other disease requiring further evaluation.

PREPARATION FOR SURGERY

1. A complete history is obtained and a physical examination carried out.
2. *Skin Prep.* The entire breast, axilla, and chest wall are shaven in anticipation of a radical mastectomy, should this be necessary.
3. *Enema.* Not necessary.
4. *Levin Tube.* Not necessary.
5. *Blood.* The patient is typed and cross-matched for 2 units of blood.
6. *Premedications.* Routine.
7. *Special Medications.* None.
8. *Psychological Preparation.* A careful and discrete discussion of the possibility of radical mastectomy should be carried out by the surgeon with his patient. The patient may wish to discuss the matter with the nurse. It therefore behooves the nurse to discuss the possibilities with the surgeon in order to get some idea of his estimates about the nature of the breast mass.
9. *Operating Room Skin Prep.* The entire breast, chest wall, axilla, and upper abdomen on the appropriate side are prepped according to the particular hospital routine.
10. *Position.* Horizontal supine, with the arm extended on an arm board.

PATHOLOGY

Breast masses in young females are usually benign. They include fibroadenomas, cysts, fat necrosis, and galactocoeles. A fibroadenoma is usually a discrete, moveable, firm mass occurring in young women. Fibroadenomas seem to be causally related to excessive estrogen levels or, perhaps, to an unusual sensitivity of certain segments of the breast to normal estrogen levels.

GENERAL RATIONALE AND SCHEME

Breast masses are considered malignant until otherwise is proven. *Nothing short of biopsy can assure the surgeon and his patient that a mass is benign.*

Scheme

1. A small incision is made over the breast mass.
2. The mass is removed en toto.
3. Frozen section analysis is performed to determine whether the mass is benign.
4. If the mass is benign, the skin incision is closed over a drain and a dressing is applied.

PROCEDURE

1. A curvilinear incision is made in a natural skin line in the breast overlying the mass.
2. Small subcutaneous bleeders are clamped and ligated with fine plain catgut sutures.

3. An incision is made through normal breast tissue until the mass is exposed. The incision is extended around the entire mass to include it *in its entirety* in the biopsy specimen.

4. The mass is taken for frozen section analysis and the surgeon awaits the findings from the pathologist before proceeding.

5. If the mass is benign, the breast tissue is approximated with catgut sutures on a cutting needle.

6. A small Penrose drain is left in the subcutaneous tissue and is sutured to the skin edge.

7. The skin is closed with interrupted fine nylon or silk sutures.

8. A small compression dressing is applied.

SURGICAL HAZARDS

There are no specific hazards associated with this procedure.

POSTOPERATIVE MANAGEMENT

The patient is returned to her room after a short period of time in the recovery room. An intravenous fluid may be administered for the next 12 to 24 hours but is discontinued as soon as the patient's vital signs are stable and she can tolerate fluids orally. She may be ambulated whenever awake, and can be given a house diet the following morning.

There is usually minimal discomfort associated with this procedure, and narcotics should be used moderately.

The patient will probably be discharged from the hospital the day after surgery, after the dressing has been changed and the drain removed.

The patient is liable to be very apprehensive the moment she awakens, for she will be wondering if radical surgery has been performed. The surgical nurse should anticipate this problem and obtain permission from the surgeon to assure the patient that the lesion was benign. Not infrequently, a patient waits hours in dread of the worst until her surgeon returns in his postoperative visit to reassure her. The nurse can play a very important role here by discussing the biopsy with the patient. It is absolutely necessary, however, that the surgical nurse be *certain* that the lesion was benign and that she *make no assumptions about it.* This is possible only if she discusses the matter directly with the surgeon before talking with the patient.

STUDY QUESTIONS

1. What is a galactocoele?

2. Discuss mammography and xeroradiography as diagnostic tools for breast masses.

3. When is needle aspiration of a breast mass safe and useful?

4. Discuss *incisional* and *excisional* breast biopsy.

5. What postoperative problems should the surgical nurse anticipate in any patient undergoing breast biopsy?

Operation: Radical Mastectomy

TYPICAL HISTORY

A 54-year-old female accidentally noticed a painless lump in her right breast while bathing 2 months prior to admission. At first she paid little attention to it, thinking it to be insignificant "since it caused no pain." As the lump gradually enlarged, she consulted her physician, who suggested immediate hospitalization for evaluation and treatment.

The patient has been in excellent health otherwise, denying any previous breast lumps or other breast symptoms.

PHYSICAL EXAMINATION

A well-developed, well-nourished female is admitted and is in no acute distress.

Significant Findings

1. There is a nontender, firm, irregular but discrete mass in the upper outer quadrant of the right breast. The axilla is free of masses, as is the other breast.
2. The remainder of the physical examination is essentially negative.

DIAGNOSTIC STUDIES

1. If there is any suggestion of widespread disease, a metastatic x-ray series and a total-body bone scan may be ordered (see below).
2. There are no other studies, short of biopsy, that can reveal the true nature of a breast lump. However, mammography may be done in search of other lesions in either breast.

PROBABLE HOSPITAL COURSE

1. Following a general examination, the patient will be taken to the operating room for breast biopsy. If necessary, radical mastectomy will be done during the same operation.
2. Occasionally, if the surgeon suspects advanced cancer, he will order a metastatic series and a total-body bone scan. The metastatic series includes x-rays of the skull, chest, ribs, pelvis, arms, and legs. Metastatic disease to one of these areas represents a contraindication to radical mastectomy.
3. The lesion is carefully marked off on a diagram used for staging (Fig. 65–1).

DATE _____

T_____ N_____ M _____

STAGE _____

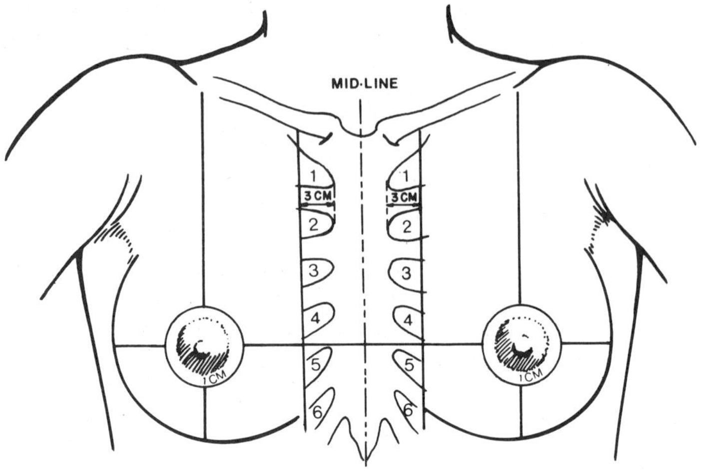

FIGURE 65-1 Diagram used for charting the stages of breast cancer. The lesion is sketched into the appropriate quadrant of the breast and its staging determined by use of the applicable indices. (Modified from Sabiston, David C., ed., *Davis-Christopher Textbook of Surgery,* Tenth Edition, Philadelphia: W. B. Saunders Company, 1972.)

T	**N**	**M**
(Local Tumor)	*(Regional Lymph Nodes)*	*(Distant Metastasis)*
T_1 Tumor of 2 cm. or less in its greatest dimension; Skin not involved, or involved locally with Paget's disease.	N_0 No clinically palpable axillary lymph node(s) (no metastasis suspected).	M_0 No distant metastasis.
T_2 Tumor over 2 cm.; or with skin attachment (dimpling); or nipple retraction (subareolar tumors). No pectoral muscle or chest wall attachment.	N_1 Clinically palpable axillary lymph nodes that are not fixed (metastasis suspected).	M_1 Clinical and radiographic evidence of metastasis except those to homolateral axillary or infraclavicular lymph nodes.
T_3 Tumor of any size with any of the following: skin infiltration, ulceration, peau d'orange, skin edema, pectoral muscle or chest wall attachment.	N_2 Clinically palpable homolateral axillary or infraclavicular lymph node(s) that are fixed to one another or to other structures (metastasis suspected).	

PREPARATION FOR SURGERY

1. *Psychological Preparation.* It is extremely important for the surgeon to adequately prepare his patient for the possible loss of her breast. Failure to do so may result in grave psychological as well as legal problems. It is also obvious that the patient who does lose her breast will realize the true nature of her disease. The surgeon must therefore speak with utter frankness to his patient. This is done, needless to say, with great tact and as gently as possible. It is explained to the patient that the cure rate for cancer of the breast is quite high and that the breast is sacrificed only because the surgeon is optimistic for a cure.

The cosmetic effects of mastectomy are often grossly exaggerated by the patient who attaches strong psychosexual connotation to the breast. The various types of prosthetic devices available should be briefly described to the patient. It is often helpful to present a patient who has undergone mastectomy to the prospective patient.

The fear of sexual change causes anxiety in the premastectomy patient. It should be explained to the patient that the breast carries no hormonal entities capable, for example, of "defeminizing" a patient when once removed.

2. Levin tube not necessary.

3. Type and cross-match for three units of whole blood.

4. *Skin Prep.* This includes the entire chest and axilla on the involved side, as well as the upper abdomen. If skin grafting is anticipated, the anterior and lateral thigh should be prepared.

5. *Enema.* A Fleet or soapsuds enema is given on the evening prior to surgery.

6. *Premedications.* Routine.

7. *Special Medications.* None.

8. *Operating Room Skin Prep.* Same as skin prep.

9. *Position.* Horizontal prone, with arm hyperextended.

PATHOLOGY

Many lesions may mimic breast cancer. The common breast lesions include:

a. *Fibroadenoma.* A firm, discrete, nontender, benign breast tumor, occurring particularly in young females.

b. *Cyst.* A benign, often tender, and sometimes discrete mass containing a small amount of cloudy or serous fluid.

c. *Hematoma.* Injury to the breast may result in the development of a calcified mass containing old blood; it may be firm, moveable, discrete, and nontender.

GENERAL RATIONALE AND SCHEME

Every breast lump must be assumed to be malignant until pathological evaluation proves otherwise. It does not matter what the patient's age is, how long she has had the lump, or whether it pains or is painless.

Certain characteristics of a breast lump may make the surgeon suspect that it is benign rather than malignant. These include:

a. The fact that the lump is tender.

b. The fact that the lump compresses like a cyst.

c. The fact that the patient has noted premenstrual breast pains.

d. The young age of the patient.

But in spite of the presence of all these characteristics in a given lump, cancer cannot be ruled out with certainty. Two further studies, somewhat more sophisticated, are sometimes used by the surgeon:

a. *Mammography.* Breast lumps have certain x-ray characteristics, and the benignancy or malignancy of a breast lump can be determined with a high degree of accuracy (but not certainty) by the radiologist.

b. *Needle Biopsy.* This may help determine whether the lump is cystic or solid. While helpful in arriving at a probable diagnosis, this procedure has many pitfalls.

Radical mastectomy means removal of the entire breast along with its lymphatics. A small breast cancer and any possible metastases to the axilla are theoretically encompassed by this radical extirpation of breast and lymphatics.

Scheme (Assuming Positive Report on Breast Biopsy)

   1. Large skin flaps are raised, encompassing the desired area of surgical dissection.
   2. The entire breast and all the muscles of the chest wall on the involved side, along with the lymphatic tissue in the axilla, are removed.
   3. Drains are left in place. Suction catheters may also be used.
   4. A compression dressing is applied.

PROCEDURE

   1. *Skin Incision.* There are many standard skin incisions for radical mastectomy and the incision will depend on the surgeon's preference. In general, the incision will extend from the clavicle, proceeding in a downward direction and passing widely around the tumor area and the breast. This incision is carried around the breast on both sides, forming a long vertical ellipse, the distal end of the incision being in the epigastrium. (See Introduction.)
   2. Very thin skin flaps must be raised so that all tumor-bearing lymphatics in the subcutaneous tissue will be included in the specimen. These flaps are extended laterally to the latissimus dorsi muscle, medially to the midsternal region, superiorly to include the entrance of the subclavian vessels into the thorax, and inferiorly to include the region over the upper rectus muscle.
   3. The skin flaps are carefully covered with moist saline pads to prevent injury to them.
   4. The surgeon now begins his dissection in the upper aspect of the incision near the axillary vein and axillary artery. The lymphatic, areolar, and connective tissue surrounding the axillary vein is carefully cleared away in a downward direction, all vessels being clamped, divided, and ligated in the process. The dissection is carried laterally into the axilla, where the brachial plexus is carefully cleansed of all lymphatic, areolar, and connective tissue. The specimen is removed inferiorly, all bleeding being controlled with fine catgut or silk sutures. Some surgeons prefer the electric cautery for small bleeders.
   5. The dissection includes the pectoralis major and pectoralis minor muscles, both of which are removed with the specimen.
   6. The most important nerves to protect are the (a) lateral thoracic nerve to the latissimus dorsi muscle and (b) the long thoracic nerve to the serratus anterior muscle.
   7. At the conclusion of the dissection, the tumor and surrounding breast tissue are removed en bloc. The operative area is now visualized as a perfectly clean chest wall and axilla, with all external chest muscles removed, as well as the entire breast.
   8. The chest wall and axilla are thoroughly irrigated with warm sterile saline to remove debris and clots of blood.
   9. Large multiholed suction catheters are placed in the axilla and overlying the anterior chest and brought out through stab incisions below the main incision.
   10. The surgeon must now decide whether a graft will be needed or whether the skin incision can be closed by first intention. If, on attempting to close the skin flaps, he finds that there is too much tension, the skin will be loosely approximated and a graft will be placed on the defect remaining, with use of a split thickness graft from the thigh. If, on the other hand, the tissues come together without significant tension, then the incision will be loosely closed with interrupted silk or wire sutures.
   11. A large compression dressing is applied.
   12. The catheters are immediately connected to suction.
   13. The patient is returned to the recovery room.

SURGICAL HAZARDS

1. Excessive loss of blood may occur due to injury to major vessels in the axilla.

2. Pneumothorax may occur when the bleeding vessels are clamped on the chest wall. This occurs if the clamp penetrates the intercostal muscles between the ribs and damages the pleura.

3. Injury to the long thoracic nerve or the lateral thoracic nerve will result in a certain degree of disability. (See "Review Questions.")

4. Injury to the brachial plexus or axillary artery may result in disability to the arm involved.

POSTOPERATIVE MANAGEMENT

The patient is returned to the recovery room. General postanesthetic measures are carried out. In addition:

1. The patient is kept in the semi-Fowler's position to minimize venous oozing.

2. The suction catheters from the chest wall are immediately connected to suction. Failure to begin suction on these catheters at once may result in blood clotting in the tubes. This may cause accumulation of considerable blood and serum underneath the skin flaps which may hinder healing. At no time should these tubes be disconnected or irrigated without the surgeon's permission or order.

3. As soon as the patient is alert, she may be given liquids by mouth.

4. Hematocrit value should be checked several hours after surgery to be certain that under-replacement of blood has not occurred.

CONTROVERSIAL ASPECTS

Recent evidence has suggested to some investigators that radical mastectomy may not be necessary to effect a cure of breast cancer. Opinions vary greatly, ranging from advocacy of simple mastectomy with radiation therapy to support for simple enucleation of the tumor ("lumpectomy") followed by radiation therapy. The majority of surgeons still favor radical mastectomy, but it is fair to say that not all the evidence is in at this time.

STUDY QUESTIONS

1. What is the most common cause of a painless lump in the breast in a 25-year-old female?

2. What advice should this woman be given about such a painless lump?

3. What are some of the dangers of needle biopsy of a painless lump?

4. Discuss mammography with your class, listing some of the indications and reliability of the test.

5. Describe the essential steps in the performance of a radical mastectomy.

6. Why are suction catheters used in the early postoperative period? Discuss their management from a nurse's point of view.

7. What muscles are supplied by the long thoracic nerve of Bell and the lateral thoracic nerve? What disability results if these are severed during the course of radical mastectomy?

8. Describe some of the early postoperative problems in a postmastectomy patient.

9. Are there any forms of therapy for cancer of the breast other than surgical excision? Discuss the nature of these forms of therapy, indications for them, and their rationale.

10. Prepare a plan for self-examination of the breasts for your patient. Discuss the value of this procedure.

66

THE PATIENT WITH ADVANCED BREAST CANCER

Operation: Bilateral Adrenalectomy

TYPICAL HISTORY

A 50-year-old female enters the hospital with weight loss, bone pain, anorexia, and lassitude of several months' duration. She underwent left radical mastectomy 6 years ago for stage II carcinoma of the breast, and several weeks later had cobalt therapy for the ipsilateral chest wall, axilla, and mediastinum. Following an asymptomatic 4½ years, diffuse bone pain, weight loss, and dyspnea occurred, and diagnostic studies confirmed widespread osseous, soft tissue, and liver metastases. A bilateral oophorectomy was performed, with remarkable relief of symptoms and objective evidence of regression of the disease for over 1 year. However, in the past 6 months, she has noted return of anorexia, lassitude, dyspnea, and diffuse bone pain. She now enters the hospital for further evaluation and bilateral adrenalectomy.

PHYSICAL EXAMINATION

The patient is a well-developed, emaciated female, short of breath and complaining of back, pelvic, and rib pain.

Significant Findings

1. Dyspnea, emaciation, and pain are obvious.
2. There are no signs of local tumor recurrence in the incision used for the removal of the left breast.
3. There is tenderness to percussion over the lower spine and pelvis.
4. The liver is enlarged, slightly tender, and nodular.

DIAGNOSTIC STUDIES

1. Chest x-rays and metastatic series confirm the presence of diffuse mottling in both lungs consistent with pulmonary lymphatic spread of carcinoma. Osteolytic and osteoblastic lesions in the ribs, lower spine, pelvis, and right femur are also evident.
2. A liver scan reveals multiple filling defects in both lobes consistent with diffuse liver metastases.
3. Liver function studies reveal elevated lactic dehydrogenase, as well as hypoproteinemia.

PROBABLE HOSPITAL COURSE

The work-up has confirmed the presence of widespread metastatic breast disease. There was excellent symptomatic as well as objective evidence of remission of past disease in this patient following oophorectomy 1½ years ago, and the healthy status appeared to last over a year. Removal of her ovaries reduced the hormonal environment which supports growth of breast cancer; hence, disease regression occurred. The adrenal glands also are a rich source of estrogens, and it is postulated that stimulation of breast cancer can occur from this source. With this in mind, and because of the excellent results from oophorectomy, the surgeon will consider either ablating the adrenal glands or performing a hypophysectomy, an equally effective procedure which shuts off adrenal gland function.

As soon as the patient has been fully evaluated and any deficiencies corrected, adrenalectomy will be performed.

PREPARATION FOR SURGERY

Adrenalectomy is an extensive procedure that at times can cause great shock to the patient's system. Therefore a careful preoperative evaluation is always necessary:

1. Any pre-existing anemia is corrected with transfusions of whole or packed cells.
2. Hypoproteinemia, reflected by a low serum albumin level, should be corrected if possible. If the patient is markedly emaciated, a short course of intracaval hyperalimentation may be beneficial.
3. Fluid and electrolyte deficiencies must be corrected, in view of the potential severe alterations following adrenalectomy.
4. If the liver disease is severe, hypoprothrombinemia will exist and will predispose the patient to bleed excessively during the operation. The hypoprothrombinemia may or may not be correctable with vitamin K, but every effort must be made to return the prothrombin time to normal preoperatively.
5. Pulmonary function and blood gas studies should be carried out to assess the base-line condition of the patient so that any postoperative changes can be more easily understood. Pleural effusions that impair the mechanics of respiration should be removed prior to surgery.

6. A Levin tube is inserted preoperatively.

7. A Foley catheter is inserted preoperatively.

8. *Enema.* A Fleet or soapsuds enema is given the evening prior to surgery.

9. The patient is cross-matched for 6 units of whole blood.

10. A large-bore intracatheter is inserted while the patient is on the ward and is checked for proper functioning.

11. *Skin Prep.* The entire abdomen from the nipples to and including the pubis is cleanly shaven while the patient is on the ward.

12. *Operating Room Skin Prep.* Same as skin prep on the ward.

13. *Position.* Horizontal supine.

14. *Special Medications.* Preoperative intravenous or intramuscular doses of cortisone are given to prevent intraoperative shock following adrenalectomy.

PATHOLOGY

In a significant number of cases, the adrenal glands will contain metastatic deposits of disease. As can be anticipated from the liver scan, the liver will show variable deposits in both lobes.

GENERAL RATIONALE AND SCHEME

As has been mentioned, bilateral adrenalectomy is performed because of the past indications that a reduction in the hormonal environment that favors cancerous growth can apparently yield remission of the disease.

Scheme

Note: This chapter discusses the anterior approach, favored by the senior author. More popular, at present, is the bilateral posterior approach, which is made through the beds of the eleventh ribs and remains outside the peritoneal cavity. The reader is referred to any standard atlas of surgical technique for a discussion of the posterior approach.

1. The abdomen is opened through a transverse, upper abdominal bilateral incision.

2. A general exploration is carried out to evaluate the extent of disease and to check for other, unassociated problems.

3. Each adrenal gland is approached by an appropriate dissection on each side in proximity to the superior pole of each kidney.

4. Drains are brought out through stab incisions.

5. The incision is closed in the usual fashion.

PROCEDURE

1. A long, curvilinear incision made with the convex side facing the patient's head is extended in the upper abdomen from one flank to the other. This incision will require division of the anterior rectus sheath and rectus muscles on both sides followed by opening of the posterior rectus sheaths and peritoneum.

2. Wound towels are applied in the usual fashion and a general exploration of the abdominal cavity is carried out. The extent of liver involvement is noted.

3. The hepatic flexure of the colon is mobilized and reflected downward, and the duodenal loop is observed. The posterior peritoneum lateral to the duodenal loop is incised, and the duodenum and the pancreatic head are reflected medially.

4. The right kidney is retracted downward, exposing the adrenal gland at the upper pole of the kidney. Multiple adrenal veins and arteries are clipped with a hemoclip and divided, and the right adrenal gland is removed. A drain is placed in the adrenal fossa and is brought out through a stab incision in the right flank.

5. The splenic flexure of the colon is mobilized and retracted medially, exposing the left kidney. The latter organ is retracted inferiorly and the left adrenal gland devascularized and removed as it was on the right side. A drain is placed in the adrenal fossa and brought out through a stab incision.

6. The incision is closed in standard fashion and a dressing is applied.

SURGICAL HAZARDS

1. *Hemorrhage.* Profuse hemorrhage from injury to the vena cava, aorta, or renal vessels may occur during bilateral adrenalectomy. In addition, steady bleeding often occurs during ligation of the multitude of small vessels surrounding the adrenal gland.

2. *Common Duct Injury.* Removal of the right adrenal gland requires dissection in an area very close to the common hepatic duct. Bleeding can result in blind attempts to control the bleeding points, with subsequent damage to the common duct.

3. *Injury to the Duodenum.* The duodenum is retracted medially during excision of the right adrenal gland and can be injured as a consequence. Unrecognized damage can lead to a postoperative duodenal fistula.

4. *Injury to the Spleen.* Resection of the left adrenal gland can result in injury to the spleen, accompanied by profuse hemorrhage. If the injury is not recognized during surgery, postoperative hemorrhage from a lacerated spleen can result in shock.

POSTOPERATIVE MANAGEMENT

The patient is kept in the recovery room after the procedure until fully reactive from the anesthesia. Because of the length of the procedure and the potential for postoperative shock, the patient should then be placed in the intensive care unit for careful observation until her condition appears stable.

In addition to the usual complications following any major abdominal procedure, acute postoperative adrenal insufficiency poses the most significant problem after adrenalectomy. The loss of adrenal hormones predisposes the organism to a very precarious state, and postoperative intravenous, intramuscular, and, eventually, oral administration of replacement cortisone is necessary. Failure to titrate the appropriate levels of cortisone postoperatively can lead to hypovolemic and hyponatremic shock, resembling an Addisonian crisis.

The early changes of acute adrenal insufficiency may be extremely subtle, with early signs of dehydration, restlessness, and tachycardia preceding overt shock. Postoperative monitoring of central venous pressure, of hourly urine outputs, of serum electrolytes, and (especially) of sodium levels in serum and urine, together with the evaluation of vital signs, level of consciousness, and so forth, will prevent unrecognized adrenal insufficiency. If shock should supervene, the treatment involves increased cortisone dosage, hypertonic saline infusions, and, rarely, the careful use of peripheral vasoconstrictors.

When intestinal activity resumes (2 to 3 days after surgery), the Levin tube is removed and fluids are started by mouth. Cortisone tablets will now be used to supplement parenteral cortisone; the latter is gradually tapered off, and is stopped as soon as normal intestinal activity has been established.

Barring any untoward problems such as postoperative sepsis, the patient usually is discharged from the hospital 7 to 10 days after surgery and is maintained on oral cortisone. The patient should be advised of the necessity of taking her cortisone daily and should carry a Med-Alert tag stating that she has undergone adrenalectomy.

STUDY QUESTIONS

1. What is the physiological rationale for adrenalectomy in patients with advanced breast cancer?

2. What are the indications for adrenalectomy in patients with advanced breast cancer?

3. Discuss the types of hormones produced by the adrenal glands, their functions, and the symptoms resulting from inadequate levels of these hormones.

4. What is Addison's disease? Cushing's disease? What is an acute Addisonian crisis? What are its symptoms?

5. What medications are used preoperatively and postoperatively in patients undergoing adrenalectomy? Why are these medications important? How would you recognize acute postoperative adrenal insufficiency?

6. Two days after an adrenalectomy, the patient goes into shock, accompanied by a rapid, feeble pulse, dehydration, and oliguria. Her hematocrit is 48, serum sodium 112 mEq/L. Which of the following is the most common cause of this state?
   a. acute adrenal insufficiency
   b. intra-abdominal hemorrhage
   c. acute coronary thrombosis
   d. pulmonary embolism

7. In shock due to acute adrenal insufficiency, you would expect the central venous pressure to be:
   a. very low
   b. very high
   c. unchanged

8. The treatment of acute adrenal insufficiency includes:
   a. Isuprel; sodium bicarbonate; blood; calcium
   b. hypertonic saline; blood; calcium; antibiotics
   c. hypertonic saline; fluids; occasional vasopressors
   d. none of these

9. Discuss how you would educate your patient about the dangers of adrenalectomy in terms of long-term management, use of cortisone, and unrecognized illnesses in the future. Discuss also the patient's need to wear Med-Alert identification.

CARDIOTHORACIC SURGERY

INTRODUCTION

67

BOUNDARIES, ANATOMY, AND CONTENTS

The chest cage may be looked upon as a firm but somewhat elastic bellows mechanism whose two major functions are the protection of the heart and great vessels and the creation of a vacuum system for expansion of the lungs.

It is axiomatic that the dynamic bellows action of the chest cage and diaphragm requires an intact pleural surface. Any opening in this pleural lining results in the entrance of air (pneumothorax) and collapse of the lung. The lung becomes totally inefficient in the presence of massive pneumothorax. Of necessity, operative procedures in the chest result in the creation of a pneumothorax. As long as this pneumothorax occurs *under controlled circumstances,* that is, in the operating room under endotracheal anesthesia, the situation is compatible with life.

Anatomically, the chest consists of ribs, attached muscles, and an attached diaphragm within which are the heart, the great vessels, the lungs, the esophagus, and the nerves passing from the neck through to the abdomen.

Surgical entrance into the chest cage may be obtained through a median incision in the sternum or variously placed lateral thoracic incisions. These incisions require entrance through the bed of a rib or between two ribs (intercostal) and incision into the parietal pleura where the lung is seen immediately.

SURGICAL APPROACHES

The surgeon will plan the level of incision to correspond with the anticipated pathologic condition. For example, if the surgeon plans an apical lobectomy, the incision may be made in the second or third interspace. On the other hand, repair of a hiatus hernia may be done through the seventh or eighth interspace incision. Should wide exposure be necessary, the surgeon may elect to resect one or more ribs. This usually causes very little postoperative difficulty as far as stability of the chest or cosmetic result is concerned; however, if a smaller exposure is necessary, the surgeon may merely split the ribs at their posterior attachments, and repair them later. At times, separation of the ribs with a retractor is all that is necessary.

The great danger in making intercostal incisions is that injury to the intercostal neurovascular bundle may occur. This can result in postoperative pain if the intercostal nerve has inadvertently been ligated, or in severe hemorrhage either during operation or postoperatively due to injury to an intercostal artery. Consequently, many surgeons elect to divide and tie the neurovascular bundle in the course of opening the chest wall. The most commonly used incision is a lateral posterothoracic one, which is depicted in Figure 67–1.

The incision is started posteriorly below the scapula and extended in an oblique direction anteriorly over or between two ribs. The anterior rim of the incision does not usually enter the abdominal wall. Following incision of the skin and subcutaneous tissue, the surgeon may insert his hand up along the rib cage, counting the ribs, in order to determine the exact space which he wishes to enter.

SKIN PREPS

These must encompass a wide area posteriorly as well as anteriorly. The most commonly used incision and its skin prep is depicted in Figure 67–1.

POSITION

The patient is placed on his side. A pillow is inserted between the knees to prevent any compression injury of nerves in the legs. The upper arm is extended over a pillow and stand to support it and to prevent any axillary, vascular, or neurologic complications from developing. Some thoracic surgeons prefer to operate with the patient in a head-down position in order to prevent blood from spilling into the bronchi.

SPECIAL FEATURES OF THORACIC SURGERY

WOUND SEPSIS

For reasons not clearly understood, wound sepsis occurs rather rarely in chest surgery. In spite of this, however, the same type of aseptic precautions and skin preparations must be used in preparing the patient for thoracotomy.

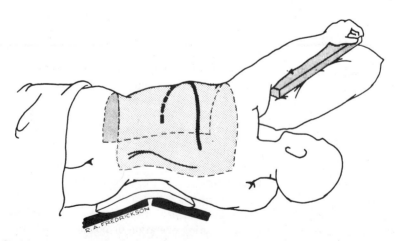

FIGURE 67–1 Position for a left thoracotomy, a standard thoracotomy incision, and extent of the prep.

ALTERATION IN THORACIC DYNAMICS

As mentioned previously, the creation of a pneumothorax during thoracotomy immediately results in poor functioning of the lung involved. As a result, thoracic surgery must be done under endotracheal anesthesia in which the anesthetist controls inspiration and expiration.

CHEST DRAINAGE

Following most thoracotomies, the surgeon drains the chest postoperatively with large, firm, rubber or plastic chest tubes. The total drainage set-up is sterile, and internal sterility is maintained during the length of time it takes to evacuate the thoracic cavity of its foreign contents. The chest tube or tubes are placed in the intrapleural space. The use of chest tubes accomplishes:

    a. The removal or drainage of blood and air from the intrapleural space.

    b. Expansion of the lung on the operative side.

    c. Restoration of subatmospheric pressure in the thoracic cavity.

It must be remembered that when drainage collects in this pleural space, heavier fluids will collect in the lower area, and air will rise to the top. For these reasons, chest tubes are placed in strategic positions to accomplish certain ends.

Placement of the Chest Tubes

Chest tubes are placed in the pleural space; they are positioned just anterior to the posterior axillary line at the site of the 8th or 9th intercostal space. If two tubes are used in this area, they are placed approximately 4 centimeters apart in the same interspace. This is done to minimize patient discomfort and decrease intercostal trauma. A third chest tube may be used in the event that alveolar leakage is excessive; it may be the only chest tube employed if the patient has experienced a traumatic pneumothorax. This tube is placed in the second thoracic interspace anteriorly. If air escaping from the functioning lung tissue is not evacuated from the pleural space, it will cause:

    a. Incomplete expansion of the lung on the operative side.

    b. Pneumothorax; occasionally tension pneumothorax.

    c. Mediastinal shift from the tension pneumothorax.

    d. Impaired function of the structures located within the mediastinum due to a shift of contents as the result of increased pressure on one side of the thorax.

It can be expected that posterior chest tubes will drain *blood and some air* and that an anterior chest tube will drain *air* only. Each chest tube will be connected to a drainage set-up with a one-way seal valve system in operation (Fig. 67-2).

One-Way Valve System

The uniqueness of chest drainage lies in the fact that a one-way valve system must be established so that fluid and air can be evacuated from the chest cavity but prevented from returning to this same cavity. Every thoracic drainage set-up must be equipped with a one-way valve system in order to protect the patient from aspiration or gravity return of his own thoracic drainage. This valve or seal is most often accomplished by the use of *water*. The chest tube is submerged in water in the collecting drainage bottle to a certain level, usually about 1 to 1½ inches below the fluid level. Thus, air and serosanguineous drainage will travel out of the chest only.

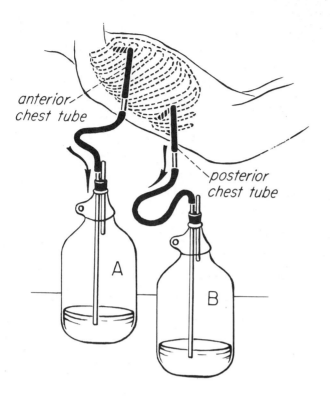

anterior
chest tube

posterior
chest tube

A

B

FIGURE 67-2 Placement of chest tubes (water-seal drainage — gravity type).

Types of Closed Chest Drainage

There are two basic types of thoracic water-seal drainage currently used. They are (1) gravity and (2) suction drainage. Their basic similarities and differences follow:

<u>Gravity Drainage</u>   <u>Suction Drainage</u>

Similarities

1. All equipment in the set-up is sterile and maintained as such until the procedure is discontinued.

2. All bottles and tubing are kept below the level of the patient's chest.

3. On inspiration, the fluid in the submerged chest tube will noticeably rise to a height of about 6 centimeters; upon expiration, the water level will drop and drainage will pass out into the water in the collecting bottle. This is called *fluctuation.*

4. The tip of the water-seal chest tube must be kept below the level of fluid in the collecting bottle (or in the second bottle, if a 2-bottle set-up is used).

5. Fluctuation of the water in the drainage tube indicates proper functioning of the apparatus, that is, the water seal is intact.

6. All connections must be air tight on the tubing; they can be sealed in such a way with adhesive.

Gravity Drainage

Suction Drainage

Differences

1. The gravity method of closed chest drainage allows gradual withdrawal of fluid and air.

1. The suction method of chest drainage will evacuate the intrapleural fluid and air faster than the simpler gravity set-up.

2. Anterior and posterior drainage tubes are usually connected to separate drainage bottles.

2. The suction control bottle has a glass tube inserted into water; the depth to which this tube is inserted will control the amount of suction reaching the pleural space. The doctor will determine and set the level of fluid in this bottle.

3. The level to which the chest drainage tube is immersed in the one-bottle set-up must be adjusted as the level of collected chest drainage rises. This necessitates raising the level of this tube so that it is only in the fluid 1 to 1½ inches at any one time.

3. There is no air vent in this system. It is attached to a suction outlet and in no way connects with the atmosphere.

4. An air vent to the atmosphere must be provided in the one-bottle set-up. The two-bottle set-up will have its air vent in the water-seal bottle.

4. A water-seal bottle is employed in addition to the suction regulating bottle.

5. Negative pressure is used; wall suction or a Gomco thoracic pump can be employed.

6. Continuous "sucking" in of outside air in the suction regulating bottle will result in constant bubbling in this bottle.

7. Constant bubbling in the suction regulating bottle indicates proper functioning of the system. If there are no bubbles in this bottle (#2 or #3) there is faulty suction due to a leak somewhere in the set-up.

Numbers of Chest Bottles or Other Types of Thoracic Drainage Apparatus Used

1 bottle	1 bottle (Gomco)
2 bottles	2 bottles
	3 bottles
Heimlich valve	Heimlich valve — with suction attached
Pleur-evac	Pleur-evac — with suction attached.

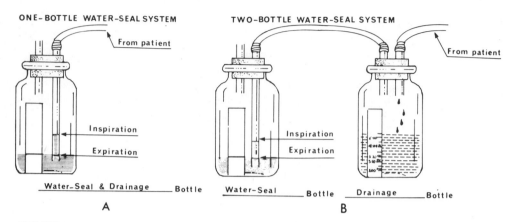

FIGURE 67-3, A and B Closed thoracic drainage of the gravity type. *A.* An underwater-seal bottle. The level of water or saline in the indicator tube rises and falls in direct response to expansions and contractions of the chest muscles and inflation and deflation of the lungs. *B.* Drainage of air and fluid from the chest without suction. Fluid from the chest drips into the empty bottle on the right. (Courtesy U.S. Dept. Health, Education and Welfare: Closed Drainage of the Chest — A Programmed Course for Nurses. Public Health Service, Division of Nursing, Washington, D.C., May, 1965.)

1. *Thoracic Thermotic Pump (Gomco).* This apparatus, powered by electricity, operates on the principle of expansion of heated air, which is then discharged through an outlet. This causes the current to go off, and the cylinder (which contains a filament) cools. A partial vacuum is created. This vacuum creates a suction, which then pulls on the contents of the pleural space. This is capable of removing air and fluid from this intrapleural space. A relatively constant suction is maintained by repeating this cycle eight times per minute. There is a switch on the machine which can be set for high (300 liters of air or fluid removed per hour) or low (160 liters) suction. (The manometer (bubble tube) serves the same purpose as the suction control bottle of the two- or three-bottle suction set-up. The height of the water in the manometer tube indicates the amount of suction exerted. Bubbling in the fluid in the manometer tube indicates that air is being removed from the pleural cavity.

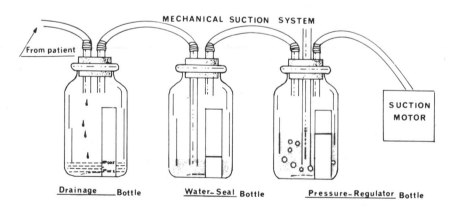

FIGURE 67-4 Closed thoracic drainage of the mechanical suction type, showing the drainage of air and fluid. The depth of the tube under the water level regulates the suction vacuum. (Courtesy U.S. Dept. Health, Education and Welfare: Closed Drainage of the Chest — A Programmed Course for Nurses. Public Health Service, Division of Nursing, Washington, D.C., May, 1965.)

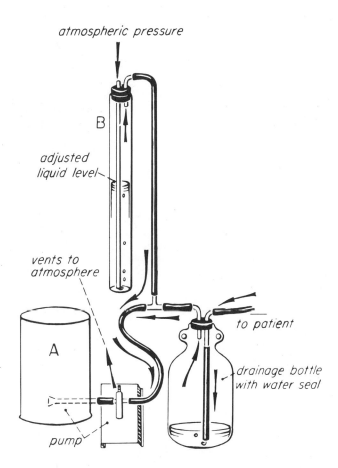

atmospheric pressure

B

adjusted
liquid level

vents to
atmosphere

A

to patient

drainage bottle
with water seal

pump

FIGURE 67-5 Movement of air in thoracic thermotic pump.

2. Some institutions are currently using the B-P Heimlich chest-drainage valve. This plastic, disposable, sterile valve is attached between the chest tube and the drainage bottle. It allows the patient more mobility to function in any position. Suction can be attached to this valve, also. No water seal is employed; the valve has a rubber diaphragm that acts as a one-way valve.

3. Another plastic, sterile, disposable unit is the Pleur-evac; this system duplicates the three-bottle set-up by its three-chamber arrangement. An underwater seal is employed. Suction can also be attached at one end of this unit for more rapid evacuation of the pleural cavity.

IMPORTANT PRECAUTIONS AND NURSING MANAGEMENT

1. Know what type of chest drainage set-up is being employed and why.

2. Maintain sterility of the chest drainage set-up. Strict asepsis and clamping of the chest tube must be employed while this change is taking place.

3. Do not allow the water seal to be broken by tilting the drainage bottles at any time.

4. Use stationary chest bottle stands or boxes, or the apparatus that is indicated to be used with disposable units.

5. Avoid accidental pneumothorax. Always *clamp* chest tubes if they become disconnected from the drainage bottle. Each chest tube is clamped with 2 clamps; put them on the tubing close to the patient's chest.

6. Keep the chest tubing straight from the bed of the patient to the collecting bottle. Avoid kinks.

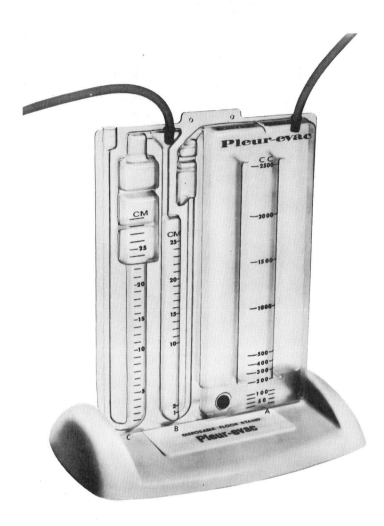

FIGURE 67-6   Disposable Pleur-evac unit. *A.* Collection trap. *B.* Water seal. *C.* Suction. All chambers are connected within the unit so that there is no exposed glass and rubber tubing. (Courtesy of Krale Laboratories, Division of Deknatel, Inc., New York.)

7. Do not allow the chest tubes to become occluded by either the patient lying on them or having clots or fragments obliterate them; milk the tubes when necessary. Check patency often.

8. Reinforce all connecting areas and stoppers. Make sure these areas are sealed tightly and that there are no "leaks" in the closed set-up.

9. Keep the chest-drainage bottles well *below* the patient's chest; this prevents the flow of water back into his chest; this does not apply when the chest tubes have been clamped and are not functioning.

10. If there is no "bubbling" in the suction control bottle, check all connections to make sure they are airtight.

11. Measure and record chest drainage either hourly or every 2 hours as ordered by the doctor. Get down to the level of the chest bottle so that you will clearly see the ascent of the drainage on the side of the bottle. Mark the bottle when you observe the level of drainage at the appointed time.

12. If the drainage collecting bottle fills quickly, *call the doctor.* Do not empty the drainage bottle yourself. When a drainage bottle overfills, it will not operate correctly or adequately.

13. When the chest tube is to be removed, instruct the patient to perform the Valsalva maneuver. Have him breathe in deeply, blow half of the inspired air out, and then hold the remaining air and bear down, as he would when having a stool.

14. When the chest tube is pulled out by the doctor, be ready to apply either a vaseline or alcohol impregnated pressure dressing to the site.

15. Have the patient deep-breathe and cough frequently even though chest tubes are in place. When the tubes have been removed, he will be instructed to perform breathing exercises that he has been taught to do prior to his chest surgery.

THE PATIENT WITH CARCINOMA OF THE LUNG

68

Operation: Pulmonary Lobectomy

TYPICAL HISTORY

A 56-year-old male, who is a heavy smoker, has had a hacking "smoker's cough" for several months which has been increasing in recent weeks. He has also noted the onset of hemoptysis and some pain in the left lower chest. This pain occurs on deep breathing and is a sharp stabbing pain relieved by his breathing lightly. He denies any weight loss, anorexia, nausea, or vomiting.

PHYSICAL EXAMINATION

A thin male is admitted in no acute distress.

Significant Findings

1. A pleuritic friction rub is heard over the left chest and, in addition, inspiratory wheezing can be heard over the left chest posteriorly.
2. The remainder of the physical examination is unremarkable.

DIAGNOSTIC STUDIES

1. A chest x-ray shows a round coin lesion, 2 cm. in diameter, in the outer aspect of the left lower lung field.

2. A "Pap." smear of deep sputum is examined on three occasions and each time is reported to be negative.

3. Pulmonary function and blood gases are found to be within normal limits.

4. Liver scan and liver function studies are normal.

PROBABLE HOSPITAL COURSE

A heavy smoker of middle age is suspected of having cancer until this can be ruled out. The diagnostic study includes chest x-ray and sputum analysis for cancer.

The surgeon may also wish to perform *bronchoscopy,* although the presence of a nodule in the periphery of the lung field makes it unlikely that anything will be visualized. Nevertheless, the lesion may be a metastasis from a central bronchogenic carcinoma which may be visualized on bronchoscopic examination. At the time of bronchoscopy, a scalene node biopsy may also be performed.

Though all studies are unremarkable, the patient will undergo exploratory thoracotomy to rule out the presence of carcinoma of the lung.

PREPARATION FOR SURGERY

1. *Levin Tube.* Not necessary.
2. The patient is typed and cross-matched for three units of whole blood.
3. Skin preparation includes the entire left chest posteriorly as well as anteriorly and the left side of the abdomen. (See Introduction.)
4. *Enema.* A Fleet or soapsuds enema is given the night prior to surgery.
5. *Premedications.* Routine.
6. *Special Medications.* None.
7. *Operating Room Skin Prep.* This includes the entire left chest posteriorly as well as anteriorly and the left upper abdomen. (See Introduction.)
8. *Position.* Thoracotomy position with the right side down. (See Introduction.) Some surgeons prefer the prone position.

PATHOLOGY

There are many lesions which can appear on x-ray as carcinoma. These include:
1. Hamartoma.
2. Tuberculoma.
3. A fungal-like lesion.
4. Benign cyst.

Often the lesion, if carcinomatous, will cause puckering and stenosis on the lung surface and, if it extends to the pleura, there will be some pleuritic chest pain. The surgeon will wish to examine the hilar lymph node area to determine whether any metastases from this lesion have occurred. If there is any doubt about the diagnosis, the segment of diseased tissue will be removed and frozen section examination will be done prior to further surgery.

GENERAL RATIONALE AND SCHEME

A nodular lesion of the lungs must be considered to represent carcinoma until proven otherwise. Consequently, as long as the patient's general condition permits, he will be submitted to exploratory thoracotomy and the surgical procedure of choice as determined by the exploration will be undertaken.

Scheme

1. The chest is opened through a left posterolateral intercostal incision.
2. The lower lobe of the lung is mobilized.
3. The vessels and bronchus to this lobe are divided and ligated.
4. The involved lobe is removed.
5. The chest is closed over a chest tube which is connected to underwater-seal drainage.

PROCEDURE

1. *Skin Incision.* This incision is made overlying the sixth intercostal space and it extends from below the left scapula, running obliquely and anteriorly between the sixth and seventh ribs. (See Introduction.) This is a posterolateral thoracotomy incision.

2. *Draping Skin.* This is important, since an opening into the bronchus is potentially contaminating to the area and could result in a wound infection.

3. The left pleural cavity is entered and the visceral pleura is incised between the left upper lobe and left lower lobe to expose the pulmonary artery and its branches.

4. The arteries to the lower lobe are clamped, divided, and ligated with silk suture.

5. The pulmonary veins supplying the lower lobe are clamped, divided, and ligated with silk suture.

6. The main bronchus of the lower lobe is clamped, divided, and closed with interrupted silk sutures.

7. The suture line of the main bronchus is covered with a segment of pleura to prevent leakage.

8. The lung segment is removed.

9. Two chest tubes are placed in the anterior and posterior chest and brought out through separate stab incisions.

10. The chest is closed in the usual fashion and the chest tubes are connected to underwater-seal drainage.

SURGICAL HAZARDS

1. Uncontrollable bleeding may occur from one of the main veins or arteries. These should be doubly ligated with strong suture material.

2. Aspiration of blood and serous fluid into the bronchus may occur and cause postoperative pneumonia. A dry field must be maintained during the opening and suturing of the bronchus.

POSTOPERATIVE MANAGEMENT

The patient is taken to the recovery room until sufficiently reactive from the anesthetic. The usual postanesthesia management is carried out. In addition:

1. The vital signs are taken and recorded every 20 minutes.
2. The head of the bed is elevated 45 degrees.

3. The patient is turned from side to side and to his back alternately every hour. The patient should not be left on his unoperated side for longer than ½ hour in the immediate postoperative period. Otherwise, the quality of respirations will be diminished and the amount of chest drainage from the operative side reduced, owing to the fact that the operative side will have to overcome gravity while turned up.

4. Coughing and deep breathing are encouraged every hour as soon as the patient is awake.

a. Routine nasotracheal suctioning may promote voluntary coughing.

b. Intermittent positive pressure breathing with mucolytic agents or saline may help to loosen tenacious secretions.

c. Deep endotracheal suctioning to remove thickened secretions mechanically may be necessary, if:

(1) Fever is present the evening of surgery.

(2) Rhonchi are heard on auscultation.

(3) Coughing is ineffective or unproductive.

Removal of respiratory secretions is mandatory if atelectasis and pneumonia are to be prevented postoperatively.

d. If nasotracheal suctioning fails to expand an atelectatic area of lung tissue, a bronchoscopy may be indicated.

e. If secretions remain a difficult problem for the surgeon from a management standpoint, and if numerous bronchoscopies have to be undertaken to remove tenacious plugs of mucus, then tracheostomy may be indicated to establish more efficient pulmonary care.

5. As soon as the patient is awake, fluids may be given by mouth.

6. The chest tubes are immediately connected to underwater-seal drainage.

7. Administration of nasal oxygen is begun at 7 liters per minute. The catheter is changed every 8 hours. The oxygen must be humidified — that is, passed through distilled water to prevent the nasal and bronchial mucosa from becoming crusted and dry. The patient's nose and mouth need meticulous attention at least every 2 hours while oxygen therapy is being used. If oxygen is administered by face mask, the flow rate is set at 10 liters per minute and a heated nebulizer is utilized for delivery. The patient may be kept intubated after surgery; in such a case the endotracheal tube is attached either to a respirator or to a Brigg's adaptor.

8. Analgesics are given in small doses every 3 to 4 hours. The respiratory rate must be checked carefully before each administration. Morphine sulfate is the drug of choice, administered intramuscularly or intravenously in doses of 4 to 8 mg at a time.

9. A chest x-ray (portable) is usually done in the recovery room immediately postoperatively *and* the morning after surgery to check the lungs for re-expansion and aeration.

10. Two chest tubes are inserted at the completion of the surgical procedure to promote drainage of the pleural space and to facilitate re-expansion of the lung. The first chest tube is placed at the apex of the pleural space. The second chest tube is placed posteriorly at the base of the pleural space. (If the surgeon chooses, both chest tubes can be placed in the base of the pleural space to make drainage of the space a certainty.) The two tubes are then connected to water-seal drainage and to suction in the form of negative pressure, usually set at −15 cm of water (alternatively, the first tube can be connected to suction and the second to gravity drainage). The tubes should be checked for patency and "milked" vigorously every hour while they are in place in the pleural space. There are certain important observations that must be made with regard to the chest drainage system:

a. *Failure of the Column of Water within the Tubing to Fluctuate on Inspiration.* This often suggests obstruction of the tubing, either by blood clots or by kinking of the tubing under the patient's body. Failure to fluctuate must be called to the surgeon's attention immediately.

b. *Inordinate Amount of Bloody Drainage.* Certain amounts of serum and serosanguineous fluid normally drain into the drainage bottle for 24 to 36 hours following thoracotomy. Frank passage of large amounts of blood within the chest tube signifies persistent thoracic bleeding and must be called to the surgeon's attention immediately.

c. *Early Postoperative Development of Subcutaneous Emphysema.* This is usually indicative of inadequate drainage of the pleural space. It may also occur if the patient has only one chest tube in place postoperatively. The treatment in this situation would be for the surgeon to insert additional chest tubes and attach them to water-seal drainage and suction for more efficient drainage of the pleural space.

STUDY QUESTIONS

1. What is a coin lesion of the lung? List five disease entities which may cause a coin lesion to develop.

2. Describe the collection of sputum for "Pap." smear in the preoperative pulmonary patient.

3. List some of the preoperative pulmonary measures which can be carried out at the bedside to increase pulmonary function in a patient with chronic lung disease. What role does the nurse play in the preoperative preparation of the patient for thoracotomy?

4. Discuss the essential steps in the carrying out of pulmonary lobectomy.

5. Diagram a three-bottle underwater-seal drainage and suction system to your class, explaining the function of each bottle in the system.

6. What dangers exist in transporting a patient who is on underwater-seal drainage from a bed to a chair? How are these circumvented?

7. While a patient on *underwater-seal drainage is ambulating,* the chest tube slips from its glass connection to the underwater-seal drainage tube. What are the most important emergency steps which the nurse must carry out before notifying the surgeon?

8. Which of the following educational plans, if successful, would result in the greatest number of lives being saved from lung cancer deaths?
    a. Promote the idea of an annual chest x-ray
    b. An anti-smog campaign
    c. An anti-cigarette smoking campaign
Discuss reasons for your answer.

69

THE PATIENT WITH
A HIATUS HERNIA

Operation: **Repair of Hiatus Hernia
(Transthoracic Approach)**

A 56-year-old obese female has noted recurring episodes of steady, boring epigastric pains, heartburn, and belching for several years. She states that the pain is aggravated by ingestion of large meals and by lying down. For the past 2 years, she has had to sleep in an upright position, propped up on two pillows, to alleviate nocturnal heartburn and belching.

PHYSICAL EXAMINATION

The patient is a well-developed, obese female in no acute distress.

Significant Findings

1. The patient is obese.
2. Pallor is noted.
3. The stool is dark.
4. Remainder of physical examination is normal.

DIAGNOSTIC STUDIES

1. Upper G.I. series reveals a hiatus hernia with some narrowing of the distal esophagus. There is no evidence of duodenal ulcer.
2. Stool is positive for occult blood.
3. Hematocrit value is 32 per cent.
4. Esophagoscopy reveals narrowing of the distal esophagus with marked esophagitis.

PROBABLE HOSPITAL COURSE

The patient exhibits many of the indications for repair of hiatus hernia (see below). A further period of medical therapy for this condition is not warranted and the patient should be explored as soon as her general condition permits.

The surgeon will probably normalize the patient's blood with one or more transfusions. Long-standing anemia may require the use of *packed red cells* instead of whole blood.

418

PREPARATION FOR SURGERY

1. A Levin tube is carefully inserted preoperatively.
2. Type and cross-match for two units of whole blood.
3. *Skin Prep.* This includes the left axilla, the left anterior chest and left abdomen, and the left side of the back. (See Introduction.)
4. *Enema.* A Fleet or soapsuds enema is given the evening prior to surgery.
5. *Premedications.* Routine.
6. *Special Medications.* None.
7. *Operating Room Skin Prep.* This includes the left axilla, the left side of the chest and abdomen, and the left back. (See Introduction.)
8. *Position.* Right side down. (See Introduction.)

PATHOLOGY

A hiatus hernia represents protrusion of part of the stomach through a weakness in the hiatal aperture of the diaphragm. Normally, the distal esophagus passes through the diaphragm and is embraced by the muscular crura surrounding the hiatus (opening in diaphragm for passage of esophagus). When these crura are weakened, they no longer maintain the lower esophagus in position, and the stomach passes, to a greater or lesser degree, into the chest.

The loss of the *esophagogastric junction,* resulting from herniation of the stomach, allows gastric juices to pass into the esophagus, resulting in esophagitis. It is this esophagitis which is responsible for the symptoms and the bleeding.

GENERAL RATIONALE AND SCHEME

Moderate symptoms from a hiatus hernia can be relieved with medical therapy. Certain indications call for surgical intervention. These indications usually include:

1. Severe stenosing esophagitis.
2. Recurrent attacks of severe gastrointestinal bleeding or intractable chronic bleeding.
3. Intractable symptoms unrelieved by medical therapy.

The present patient has suffered from peptic esophagitis for many years. On esophagoscopy she demonstrates stenosis of the esophagus. In addition, she has apparently been bleeding silently for some time. Consequently, she fulfills many of the criteria for surgical therapy of this disease.

There is much controversy as to the proper approach for repair of a hiatus hernia, which can be done transabdominally as well as transthoracically. Proponents of the transabdominal approach offer the following advantages:

1. Other associated abdominal conditions (such as gallbladder disease and gastric lesions) can be evaluated.
2. A complementary vagotomy and pyloroplasty can be performed (some argue that these two procedures should accompany repair of a hiatus hernia).

Proponents of the thoracic approach offer the following advantages:

1. Accompanying lesions of the distal esophagus can be better evaluated.
2. A better view and better repair of the hernia can be accomplished.

Scheme

1. The chest is opened in the seventh intercostal interspace.
2. The lung is reflected out of the way.
3. The sac of the hernia is mobilized.
4. The sac and stomach are reduced into the abdomen.
5. The muscular crura are brought into apposition.
6. The chest is closed.

PROCEDURE

1. *Skin Incision.* This extends from the tip of the scapula anteriorly and in a downward direction between the seventh and eighth ribs. (See Introduction.)
2. The left pleural cavity is opened and a rib retractor is inserted to spread the ribs apart.
3. The left lung is deflated and retracted medially, exposing the sac of the hernia.
4. The mediastinal pleura, overlying the hernia, is opened and reflected.
5. The hernia is mobilized between umbilical tapes.
6. A small opening is made in the diaphragm and the hernia is reduced by traction on the umbilical tape which has been inserted through the hiatus.
7. The muscular crura are apposed with silk sutures.
8. The opening in the diaphragm is closed.
9. A large chest catheter is placed in the pleural space and brought out through a stab incision.
10. The ribs are approximated with heavy catgut sutures and the wound closed.
11. The chest tube is connected to underwater-seal drainage with or without suction.

SURGICAL HAZARDS

1. Injury to the intercostal artery may result in severe hemorrhage.
2. Injury to the phrenic nerve may result in diaphragmatic paralysis.
3. Injury to the lung or heart.
4. Injury to the subdiaphragmatic organs, particularly the spleen or the pancreas.

POSTOPERATIVE MANAGEMENT

The patient is returned to the recovery room until sufficiently reactive from the anesthetic. The usual postoperative thoracic management should be instituted. In addition:

1. The patient is kept in semi-Fowler's position to aid in drainage of blood from the pleural space.
2. Narcotics should be given in adequate dosages to alleviate pain, which may be severe following thoracotomy.
3. The surgeon should be notified if the dressing soaks through with excessive bloody drainage.
4. The chest tube is connected to underwater-seal drainage and managed in the usual fashion. Any significant bloody drainage in the chest bottle should be called to the surgeon's attention.

5. The patient receives nothing by mouth for 24 hours in order to decrease the nausea associated with general anesthesia and compounded by the side effects of narcotics given to relieve chest pain.

STUDY QUESTIONS

1. Distinguish between paraesophageal and sliding esophageal hiatus hernia. Are the symptoms, treatment, and prognosis different?

2. In your opinion, what is the most important indication for repair of a hiatus hernia? Discuss your answer in your class.

3. What is the medical therapy of hiatus hernia? Do you think that *all* patients with hiatus hernia need an operation?

4. Why are the symptoms of hiatus hernia aggravated when the patient lies down?

5. Describe the essential steps in the repair of a hiatus hernia.

6. Discuss the management of chest bottles following repair of hiatus hernia. Why are they used?

7. What problems may be experienced by the patient in whom the phrenic nerve has been inadvertently cut during repair of a hiatus hernia?

8. What abdominal conditions are sometimes associated with a hiatus hernia?

9. Discuss the relationship between anemia and hiatus hernia.

10. Outline a nursing care plan for a patient who has had transthoracic repair of a hiatus hernia.

70

Operation: Closure of a Patent Ductus Arteriosus (Closed Heart Surgery)

TYPICAL HISTORY

A 6-year-old male was noted by his physician to have a heart murmur 1 year prior to admission. Except for slight diminution in growth rate and frequent upper respiratory infections, he has been in excellent health and has taken part in all childhood events in a normal manner. He has never been cyanotic or dyspneic. Cardiac surgery had been recommended at the time the murmur was first discovered but the parents declined.

PHYSICAL EXAMINATION

The patient is a well-developed, somewhat slender male in no apparent distress.

Significant Findings

1. A characteristic "machinery" murmur is heard in the left upper chest. The exact nature of this murmur and its differentiation from other murmurs is outside the scope of this book. Suffice it to say that the pediatric cardiologist can derive a great deal of information about the exact congenital defect by the type and location of the murmur or murmurs.
2. The remainder of the examination may be entirely normal.

DIAGNOSTIC STUDIES

A complete description of a *cardiac workshop* is beyond the scope of this book. Nevertheless, a brief listing of some of the tests performed and their rationale is instructive:

Chest X-ray. The size and shape of the heart, the presence or absence of increased bronchial markings in the lungs, and the size and nature of the great vessels in the thorax as depicted by plain chest x-ray are very important considerations in the differential diagnosis of congenital heart disease.

Electrocardiogram. Enlargement (hypertrophy) of one or more heart chambers is of importance not only in differentiating various cardiac lesions but also in determining, to a certain extent, the amount of heart strain brought about by a given lesion.

Cardiac Catheterization. The degree of oxygenation and the amount of pressure in each of the chambers of the heart may be determined by passing catheters into these chambers. Blood is withdrawn from each chamber and analyzed, and the pressure is determined at the tip of the catheters. These findings also aid in the differential diagnosis of congenital heart disease.

PROBABLE HOSPITAL COURSE

The patient with congenital heart disease must be evaluated with respect to the presence or absence of infection or heart failure prior to surgery.

a. *Infection.* This may take the form of respiratory or valvular infection (bacterial endocarditis). The infection must be eradicated prior to surgery.

b. *Heart Failure.* Many cardiac lesions are characterized by the presence of heart failure. This must be brought under control prior to corrective surgery when possible.

As soon as the patient is in maximum readiness, corrective surgery will be undertaken.

PREPARATION FOR SURGERY

1. Levin tube not necessary.
2. A large-bore intravenous needle or intracatheter should be inserted for possible emergency intravenous therapy or transfusion during the operation.
3. Type and cross-match for four units of whole blood.
4. *Skin Prep.* The entire left chest, left back, and upper left abdomen are prepared (See Introduction.)
5. *Enema.* A Fleet or soapsuds enema is given on the evening prior to surgery.
6. *Premedications.* Routine.
7. *Special Medications.* None.
8. *Psychological Preparation.* It is more often the parents who must be prepared for their child's heart surgery. Surgery of the heart is new and parents often have fears far out of proportion to the known results, particularly in closure of a patent ductus in which the mortality is negligible. The parents should be carefully apprised of the necessity of this operation in spite of the fact that, at the time of surgery, their child does not appear to be particularly ill.
9. *Operating Room Skin Prep.* The entire left chest, left back, and left abdomen are prepared in the usual manner.
10. *Position.* Thoracotomy position with right side down.

PATHOLOGY

The ductus arteriosus represents a connection between the pulmonary artery and the descending aorta. It is a necessary structure for the maintenance of fetal circulation. This duct usually closes at about the time of birth. Should patency persist, it will provide an abnormal course for flow of blood from the pulmonary artery to the aorta, *by-passing the lungs.* Since the pressure is greater in the aorta than in the pulmonary artery, blood is usually shunted from the aorta retrogradely through the ductus into the lungs. This reversal of flow creates a workload on the left ventricle which results in hypertrophy and finally failure.

GENERAL RATIONALE AND SCHEME

The child with a patent ductus arteriosus may go on for years in apparent excellent health. Depending on the size of the ductus and other factors not clearly understood, the excess workload on the heart will eventually cause symptoms, heart failure, and decreased longevity. Consequently, though asymptomatic, the patient with a patent ductus arteriosus should be operated upon as soon as the diagnosis is made and the general condition permits.

Scheme

1. The chest is opened through a posterolateral incision.
2. The mediastinal pleura is opened and the pericardium retracted medially, thus exposing the patent ductus.
3. The patent ductus is ligated and divided.
4. The mediastinal pleura is closed.
5. The chest incision is closed over drainage tubes.

PROCEDURE

1. *Skin Incision.* This is a posterolateral incision in the fifth to sixth interspace.
2. A retractor is put in place and the ribs are spread apart.
3. The mediastinal pleura is opened and the flaps are retracted, exposing the vagus nerve which is also retracted laterally.
4. A small tip of pericardium overlying the region of the patent ductus is dissected free, thus exposing the patent ductus arteriosus.
5. The patent ductus is freed posteriorly and ties are placed around it for ligature.
6. The duct is divided between these silk ligatures. If it is a very wide duct, it may be sutured with interrupted silk sutures after division.
7. The mediastinal pleura is sutured loosely over the ends of the patent ductus.
8. Chest tubes are put in place and brought out through stab incisions.
9. The chest incision is closed in the usual manner and a heavy dressing applied.

SURGICAL HAZARDS

1. Injury to the vagus nerve.
2. Injury to the phrenic nerve.
3. Exsanguinating hemorrhage from slippage of the ligature of the divided patent ductus.

IMMEDIATE POSTOPERATIVE MANAGEMENT

The patient is returned to the recovery room. The usual postanesthesia management is carried out. In addition:

1. The patient is kept in the semi-Fowler's position and turned from side to side.
2. The chest tubes are connected to underwater-seal drainage and managed in the usual fashion.

3. Narcotics in moderate doses are given to control pain.

4. The patient is allowed liquids by mouth as soon as he is fully alert from the anesthesia.

STUDY QUESTIONS

1. Name four other congenital valvular lesions occurring in children and treated surgically.

2. What is the usual life span of a child, not operated upon, who has a patent ductus arteriosus?

3. What is the usual cause of death in a patient with a patent ductus?

4. Discuss the fetal circulation through the patent ductus.

5. Discuss the essential steps in the closure of a patent ductus arteriosus.

6. Name five major immediate postoperative complications in a patient who has undergone closure of a patent ductus arteriosus.

7. Discuss a complete nursing plan for the early postoperative management of a patient who has undergone closure of a patent ductus arteriosus.

THE PATIENT WITH MITRAL STENOSIS

71

Operation: **Mitral Valvuloplasty — Closed Intracardiac Surgery**

TYPICAL HISTORY

A 38-year-old woman with a history of rheumatic fever as a child, now married and the mother of four children, is admitted to the hospital with dyspnea on exertion while doing her household chores and caring for her family. She notices that she needs more frequent rest periods. At times, she may raise flecks of blood. She limits her climbing of stairs to once daily; when she does go up stairs, she has to stop once or twice "to catch my breath." She has lost about 10 pounds of body weight this past year. She has three-pillow orthopnea. Before retiring, she notes that her ankles swell up a great deal. She has been admitted to the hospital twice this year for pulmonary edema.

PHYSICAL EXAMINATION

A thin, well-developed female, sitting up in Fowler's position, is observed; she rests quietly in bed.

Significant Findings

1. The typical diastolic murmur in the form of a continuous rumble is heard at the apex of the heart. The murmurs are especially easy for the physician to auscultate if the patient is placed in the left lateral position and a bell stethoscope is utilized. Brief exercises of the patient cause the murmur to be heard more easily.
2. The patient's rhythm is one of atrial fibrillation; half the patients who have mitral stenosis are fibrillators.
3. There is right ventricular enlargement. This is reflected by a left sternal border or subxiphoid heave of the heart.
4. Pulmonary hypertension is manifested by an exaggerated, snapping pulmonic second heart sound.
5. When a systolic murmur is heard in mitral stenosis, it indicates some degree of mitral insufficiency.

DIAGNOSTIC STUDIES

The patient with mitral stenosis will have many important clinical studies performed to (1) ascertain the defect through x-rays and confirm this by significant electrocardiogram findings, (2) note if there is calcification on the valve, (3) determine an exact diagnosis, and (4) evaluate the existing pulmonary function.

Roentgenologic examination is undertaken to see the size of the heart and its position. A barium swallow will outline the left atrium of the heart. These x-rays will demonstrate a straightened left cardiac border, a large pulmonary artery, and a large atrial appendage. Enlargement of the right ventricle constitutes a shelflike image on the affected side, instead of the usually smooth image or straight border. Calcification of the mitral valve may be seen on the x-ray and an old atrial thrombus may also be visualized at this time. Calcification of the valve is best seen at fluoroscopy. The patient is asked to have a barium swallow to outline the atrium and show the existing enlargement.

The electrocardiogram will reveal atrial fibrillation and right ventricular hypertrophy in about 50 per cent of these patients. Incomplete right bundle-branch block is a rhythm pattern that is a common finding in some patients.

Cardiac catheterization may be performed to determine the size of the mitral valve and cardiac output. It will also give the doctor significant information regarding intracardiac pressures within each chamber and on each side of the cardiac valves. Angiography can also be employed at this time to determine if there is a signficant degree of insufficiency of the valves visualized. This information allows the cardiologist to detect and evaluate various forms of heart disease, determine the severity of each, and recommend a course of action for the surgeon to take.

Complications of cardiac catheterization do occur; however, the mortality in adults is less than 1 in 1000 cases. Arrhythmias occur frequently during the procedure but are rarely a problem. They can usually be controlled by the administration of appropriate drugs at the time they occur. Hypotension may occur for a variety of reasons and is usually transitory and easily corrected with vasopressors. Allergic reactions to the contrast media used at the time of catheterization may occur. Cardiac perforation by the catheter itself may happen; this is a serious complication, but happens rarely. Other complications that can occur are pyrogenic reactions, air emboli, thrombo-phlebitis, hemopericardium, and cardiac tamponade (in the wake of cardiac perforation). All of these must be taken into consideration in the nursing care of the patient who has undergone cardiac catheterization.

Nursing care following the catheterization includes:

1. Checking vital signs frequently to detect hypotension, arrhythmias, respiratory distress, and thrombophlebitis.

2. Checking cutdown sites on the arm or groin to determine if there is bleeding. The patient may complain of severe pain in the area of the cutdown due to arterial spasm or hematoma formation.

3. Maintaining bed rest until vital signs are stable.

4. Medicating for pain (at the site of the cutdown) as ordered.

5. Administering antibiotics as ordered.

6. Placing sandbags or a pressure dressing on the cutdown site; this may be the care of choice if the femoral or brachial artery was used in the catheterization procedure.

Pulmonary studies will be done to determine the amount of functioning lung tissues available and to predict what the pulmonary status of the patient will be in the postoperative period. Common tests include:

1. *Vital capacity* — the patient is told to breathe deeply and forcibly exhale. The exhaled volume of gas will be measured. Norms are:

      Male = 3500 cc.
      Female = 3000 cc.

2. *Total lung capacity* is the maximum amount of air one can inhale. Norms are:

      Male = 5500 cc.
      Female = 5000 cc.

3. *Timed vital capacity* is done to determine how much air one is able to blow out in 1, 2, and 3 seconds. The average person should blow 80 per cent of vital capacity in 3 seconds.

4. *Bronchospirometry* studies are done to determine simultaneously the part played by each lung in ventilation and gaseous exchange.

5. *Tidal volume* is the amount of air taken in upon each inspiration. Usually that amount is 500 cc. for each breath.

A detailed medical examination is given to the patient and then, through the combined effort of the medical and surgical teams, a decision to operate is made.

PROBABLE HOSPITAL COURSE

What type of patient is the best candidate for a mitral valvuloplasty? Persons who are in the early stages of their disease and have a relatively normal degree of leaflet tissue and fusion at the commissures are perhaps the best candidates.

If this patient's studies indicate that she indeed has tight mitral stenosis, she will be taken to surgery, operated on through a left thoracotomy incision, placed in the recovery room for the remainder of her surgical day, and then returned to her clinical unit that evening or the following day, barring no complications. She will remain in the hospital 10 days to two weeks after surgery.

PREPARATION FOR SURGERY

The patient with mitral stenosis and congestive heart failure is managed with digitalis, diuretics, and rest. It is very important for the nurse to convince the patient of the reality of the surgery she is about to face. The nurse will have the responsibility of interpreting what the doctor has told the patient and of explaining technicalities she may not understand. The doctor will order what limitations or restrictions are to be placed on the patient's activities. Vital signs are taken at least twice daily. Apical-radial pulses are done twice daily and recorded. Blood pressure is taken as ordered. Weight of the patient is an important consideration; preferably, it is taken at the same time every day, with the same amount of clothing on the patient and by the same staff member if possible. This insures accuracy. If the patient is relatively inactive, elastic stockings may be ordered to be worn as a prophylaxis against phlebitis.

Salt substitutes may be permitted; the diet will usually consist of 2 grams sodium restriction. Between-meal foods should not contain excess sodium and what foods are permitted at these intervals should be carefully noted. Accurate intake and output will be a dual responsibility of both patient and nurse. Fluids may be limited to 1200 to 1500 cc.'s daily. This may be adjusted to the condition of the patient or to hot weather. Instruct both patient and visitors as to the importance of accurate fluid records.

Baths with pHisoHex substance may be ordered on a daily basis from the day of admission until the tentative surgery date. Shampoos may be ordered every other day.

Drugs that may be administered to the patient during this time include: polyvitamins, penicillin (rheumatic prophylaxis), digoxin, potassium chloride supplements, and Nembutal. Test doses of other drugs may be necessary to determine whether the patient is allergic to specific agents that may be used postoperatively.

The skin preparation will be quite extensive; the patient should be told what to expect in that her anterior and posterior chest will be washed and shaved. She will be given an enema preoperatively, since she will be undergoing general anesthesia. Specific remedial breathing and arm motion exercises should be taught to the patient during this phase. They are to be conscientiously practiced and mastered prior to surgery. They will play a vital part in the prevention of complications in the postoperative period. Above all, instruct the patient to discontinue smoking (if she has not by this time) at least two weeks prior to surgery.

The patient will have need of a great deal of moral support and understanding from the doctors and nurses. How the patient conceives of her heart and its relationship to her total body will have an influence on the way she handles her anxiety during the preoperative and postoperative stages. She may focus on many different aspects of care during this period. She may be openly hostile about an aspect of care, e.g., diet. Be able to determine what the patient really wants to know about her surgery, her role in the care, and what is expected of her in the postoperative phase. Remember too that the patient will tire easily during the preoperative period and the many tests that will have to be endured may be irksome and exhausting. Pain and fear of death may cause great concern.

The type of anesthesia to be received will be thoroughly explained by the anesthesiologist. It is important to assure the patient that she will be asleep during the procedure and will awaken after the procedure is all over and she is in the recovery room or the intensive care area. Tell the patient that her family will be able to visit with her on the day of surgery and will be able to go into the I.C.U. area. Explain what tubes to expect in place postoperatively and include the rationale for these. Explain the type incision she will have and where it will be. Tell her that she can ask for pain medication if she so desires it; assure her that a competent surgical and nursing staff will be alert to her physical and emotional needs while she is in the recovery area.

PATHOLOGY

When does mitral stenosis become significant and cause the patient progressive symptoms? If the mitral valve reaches 1.5 cm.^{2} in area for a man or 1 cm.^{2} for a woman, it represents significant obstruction. This can be calculated after cardiac catheterization and substantiated at surgery.

The valve area may or may not show calcification. If there is calcium on the valve, prophylaxis at the time of surgery is advised lest a particle break off and become an embolus in the systemic circulation. This safety measure is accomplished by isolating the innominate and left common carotid arteries during surgery and occluding them both in the period immediately following the valve fracture. They are held occluded in this manner for 20 to 30 seconds so that particles of suspected calcium are swept past these vessels so that they do not present a significant danger to the brain.

There may also be a mural thrombus present on the inside of the atrial appendage and atrium. This clot will be evacuated when the surgeon first opens the auricular appendage and allows a jet of blood to mobilize the clot from the inside out.

A mitral valvuloplasty procedure may also be performed on an emergency basis. This would apply to a patient who had broken off a piece of the mural thrombus in the left atrium which then became an embolus in the systemic circulation. If such fragments or a major clot is affecting the circulation to vital areas, a procedure to rid the body of the source of these thrombi is necessary.

GENERAL RATIONALE AND SCHEME

The purpose of a mitral valvuloplasty is to fracture the mitral valve and chordae tendineae and to free up the papillary muscles in order to restore mobility to the valve leaflets. When this is accomplished successfully, the mitral valve will be able to coapt freely and this restored motion will decrease the strain on the heart.

Scheme

1. An incision to facilitate adequate exposure is obtained by a complete left hemithoracic opening over the fifth interspace.

2. The chest wall is opened; the aortic arch, the texture of the lung, and its surface lymphatics and mediastinal nodes are checked for abnormalities.

3. Usual approach to the heart: the pericardium is opened; the atrial appendage is inspected; appropriate pursestring sutures are put around it to decrease the incidence of bleeding; an opening is made to allow the index finger of the operator to penetrate the heart.

4. The mitral valve is palpated, the stenotic valve is fractured, and the chordae tendineae and papillary muscles are treated similarly if they are scarred and adherent.

5. Chest tubes are placed in the thoracic cavity on the affected side (where the thoracotomy has been performed).

6. The incision is closed.

PROCEDURE

1. The patient is placed in a lateral position, with the shoulder and hips elevated on a rolled sheet to allow expansion of the right chest, EKG monitoring, and extension of the left arm.

2. A thoracotomy incision is made through the fifth interspace. The cartilage and rib posteriorly are divided.

3. The pericardium is opened posteriorly to the phrenic bundle in the direction of the pulmonary artery; marsupializing sutures are placed in the pericardium; this affords stabilization of the heart and exposure of the left auricular appendage.

4. Pursestring sutures (a double row) are placed at the base of the auricular appendage. An atrial clamp is used to control bleeding; the appendage is opened with a scalpel.

5. The bare index finger of the operator is inserted as the auricular clamp is removed. Tension on the pursestring sutures provides hemostasis during this manipulation.

6. The valve is explored. Penrose tapes are placed about the innominate and left carotid arteries for immediate occlusion if thrombotic or calcific particles are encountered.

7. The anterior fracture of the fused commissure is accomplished with the surgeon standing at the patient's back. Correction of secondary stenosis of the chordae tendineae and fused papillary muscles is accomplished.

8. Fracture of the posteromedial commissural fusion is accomplished by the surgeon, who has now moved to the front of the patient. During this maneuver, the assistant inserts his finger into the auricular appendage while the surgeon moves to the other side. Much of the fracturing of the valve is accomplished by the cutting ability of the uncovered fingernail. If a sharper edge is necessary, a valvulotome can be used.

9. When fracture of the entire valve is accomplished, the finger is removed; opposing pursestring sutures are closed and the auricular appendage is twice oversewn to prevent the trabeculae of the appendage from shifting during contraction of the heart.

10. Pericardial sutures are released and the anesthesiologist expands the lungs.

11. Two chest tubes are inserted intercostally and placed 4 cm. apart so that the patient does not lie on them in bed. If there have been alveolar leaks relative to the dissection of the adherent lung, an anterior chest tube can be placed in the second interspace anteriorly. Chest tubes are connected to an underwater-seal apparatus and connected to (a) simple gravity drainage or (b) suction drainage, according to the preference of the surgeon.

SURGICAL HAZARDS

1. Operative hemorrhage may occur when the heart is opened.

2. Trauma to the ventricular septum. This may produce heart-block.

3. Separation of the junction between the left auricle and the pulmonary veins. Pressure from behind the left ventricle can be exerted for counterpressure in this area.

4. Particles of calcium or a thrombus can migrate to the brain or other major organ and cause embolism.

IMMEDIATE POSTOPERATIVE MANAGEMENT

1. *General Thoracic Care.* The patient should be in a bed with her head elevated 30 degrees. Nasal oxygen will be administered at a rate of approximately 7 liters per minute. This catheter is to be changed at least every 8 hours while the patient is receiving oxygen therapy. Listen for the sound of oxygen flow. Sounds are more important than the reading on the oxygen gauge, which may be not registering correctly. Encourage coughing every hour. Turn the patient from her back to the operated side every 2 hours. Maintain two chest tubes to underwater-seal drainage. Tracheal suctioning may have to be performed by a competent practitioner if the patient does not raise mucus, has audible rhonchi, or has a fever the evening of surgery.

2. *Medications.* These will include morphine for pain as often as every 2 hours, quinidine and/or digitalis (digoxin) and Nembutal for sleep the evening of surgery.

3. *Fluids.* Always discontinue nasal oxygen when giving food or water. If this is not done, gastric distention may be the result. On the first postoperative day, 30 cc.'s of water every hour may be administered. The patient will gradually proceed to surgical fluids p.o.; I.V. fluid restrictions will be enforced according to the needs of the patient.

4. *Urinary considerations.* Check voiding if there is no catheter in place; this should be done on an 8- to 10-hour basis.

5. *Vital signs.* Rectal temperatures will be taken throughout the early postoperative period. Apical and radial pulses will be taken as ordered.

6. *Central venous pressure monitoring.* This reading is useful in assessing the amount of blood returning to the heart and in determining the capability of the right and left ventricles to propel this blood out into the large blood vessels of the circulatory system. A long, large polyethylene catheter is inserted into the venous circulation, usually through a vein in the arm or neck. This tubing is attached to a manometer system, with the patient receiving constant infusion when the CVP reading is not being determined. There are important specifics in the actual reading of the CVP that must be understood by all those caring for the patient. They are:

a. The manometer system must be properly set up and the 5 cm. mark on the tape (which numbers the centimeters on the water column) must be level with the patient's sternal notch.

b. Any change in the patient's position will cause a corresponding change in the readings that are obtained when the CVP is measured. The 5 cm. point must be relocated and releveled, preferably with a carpenter's level, each time the CVP reading is taken.

c. Readings of the CVP vary, depending on whether or not the patient is on a respirator. A notation of the patient's position and his respiratory status should be made when obtaining an initial CVP reading so that this may serve as a baseline assessment for all future readings. Fluid in the manometer system will fluctuate with each respiration of the patient. If the patient is on ventilatory assistance, this must be turned off for the few seconds it takes to read the CVP.

d. If the I.V. fluid in the manometer falls very slowly — or does not fall at all — the CVP catheter may be clogged with particles or with a blood clot, in which case the catheter should be irrigated. If the fluid in the manometer falls very rapidly without fluctuating as it falls, the catheter may be improperly positioned in the venous system. *The CVP should be read when the fluid level in the manometer drops to and remains at a consistent or constant level in the tubing.* If the I.V. fluid does not fluctuate, or if it falls very slowly during a reading, a notation of this fact should be made, so as to alert the staff to possible inaccuracies. Usually, the CVP reading is taken at the same time that the other vital signs are evaluated by the staff.

e. Routine nursing care of the CVP insertion site:
   (1) Dressings are changed daily.
   (2) The insertion site is cleansed with alcohol applied under conditions of strict surgical asepsis.
   (3) The insertion site and part of the tubing in the wound itself are covered with an antibiotic ointment after the skin is cleansed.
   (4) When dry, sterile gauze is applied, the nurse must check to see that the catheter is not kinked or bent under the new dressing.
   (5) The general skin condition around the catheter and in the site where tape has been placed for security is evaluated. The nurse should check areas where pressure from an arm board might pose a threat.

f. The rate of infusion of the I.V. fluid must be constant in order to prevent clotting of the CVP catheter. If blood samples are taken from the CVP line, it must be adequately flushed with saline after the specimen is obtained; the I.V. fluid is again infused only when this flushing has been completed.

7. *Cardiac monitoring.* The patient will have EKG monitoring after closed surgery (a lead II reading being chosen for representation of the heart pattern) to assess and continually evaluate the presence of arrhythmias. If the patient has atrial fibrillation, ventricular pacing wires may have been inserted at the time of surgery to control heart block.

STUDY QUESTIONS

1. Review the historical development of heart surgery.

2. Review the anatomy and physiology of the cardiovascular system.

3. Review congestive heart failure. Discuss its mechanism, treatment, and nursing care.

4. What are the major causes of heart disease? What relationship does each have to cardiac surgery?

5. Compare the operative risks of open-heart surgery and closed heart surgery.

6. What factors play a part in the evaluation of an individual's operative risk?

7. Review the classification of patients with heart disease according to the American Heart Association.

8. What is the difference between stenosis and insufficiency of a valve?

9. Can both conditions exist in a patient at the same time? If so, how?

10. Define cardiac neurosis and cardiac cachexia.

11. Describe the preoperative care for a patient who is to have a mitral valvuloplasty.

12. What are the psychological implications for a patient who is to undergo heart surgery?

13. How should the family be treated during the hospitalization of the patient? What part do they play in the over-all rehabilitation of the patient?

14. How could you include the patient's family in the over-all preoperative teaching plan?

15. Why is a mitral valvuloplasty called "closed-heart surgery?" Is this terminology correct?

16. You are assigned to care for a patient in the recovery room who has had a mitral valvuloplasty today. What are some nursing assessments you would be required to make?

17. List the nursing actions and the scientific principles involved in the care of a patient who has thoracic drainage tubes in place and connected to underwater-seal drainage.

18. *Define:*

atrial fibrillation	embolization
ventricular fibrillation	central venous pressure
heart-block	closed heart surgery
Valsalva maneuver	mitral valve
defibrillation	cardiac catheterization
cardioversion	

THE PATIENT WITH MITRAL INSUFFICIENCY

72

Operation: Mitral Valve Replacement: Open-heart Surgery (Requiring Cardiopulmonary By-pass)

TYPICAL HISTORY

A 56-year-old female, married and the mother of one child, is admitted for the third time to the hospital. Nine years ago, it was noted that she had a heart murmur. She had a history of rheumatic fever as a child. Some time ago, she experienced symptoms of weakness, fatigue, increasing dyspnea upon exertion, paroxysmal nocturnal dyspnea, hemoptysis, and mild chest pain. These symptoms progressed rapidly, although she had slight relief with digoxin and diuretics for her congestive heart failure. Eight years ago, she had a closed mitral valvuloplasty. Over the next four years, she again developed paroxysmal nocturnal dyspnea with increased dyspnea on exertion, orthopnea and, at the end of that period of time, had another valvuloplasty performed. Her symptoms were relieved after that operation with the exception of dyspnea and palpitations. Since the beginning of this year her symptoms have progressively increased and her weight has gone from 125 to 110 pounds. She is now advised to have a replacement of her mitral valve.

PHYSICAL EXAMINATION

The patient is a rather thin female, lying in bed with the head elevated so that it is easier for her to breathe. She is cachectic and does not want to exert herself.

Significant Findings

1. There is dyspnea upon exertion.
2. The patient tires easily.
3. She is cachectic, thin, and has a wasted looking appearance from the head to the hips and edema from the hips down, including the legs and feet.
4. Her left ventricle heaves in motion with every beat; she has a systolic murmur that radiates to her axilla.
5. Her lung fields are relatively clear.
6. She may or may not have calcium on her valves at fluoroscopy.
7. Chest x-ray will show left ventricular enlargement.

DIAGNOSTIC STUDIES

Although the patient's problems are believed to derive solely from mitral insufficiency, routine tests — barium enema and G.I. series, stool for guaiac, and gallbladder series — involving other systems must be performed. In this patient's case, no evidence points to any conditions that require preoperative correction (though preparation for the surgery must be initiated, of course).

1. Chest x-rays reveal clear lung fields and cardiomegaly, which includes left atrium dilatation, left ventricular enlargement, and a small aorta. The left atrium is much larger in this instance than in the case of a patient with mitral stenosis. Moderate right ventricular and pulmonary artery enlargement may be seen as a result of pulmonary hypertension secondary to left ventricular failure.

2. Fluoroscopy may reveal calcium present on the valve leaflets.

3. Left and right cardiac catheterization may be done; angiography may be employed to determine the degree of regurgitation and to determine how long it takes for the left ventricle to empty under existing conditions.

4. Electrocardiogram will show evidence of left ventricular hypertrophy or combined ventricular hypertrophy. Left bundle-branch block and atrial fibrillation may also be seen in the EKG.

5. Pulmonary function studies may reveal that 80 per cent of the lung tissue is functioning.

6. Blood chemistries are done to get a picture of the basic electrolytes and to compare them during the diuretic phase of the patient's treatment.

7. Analysis of arterial blood gases is done to determine:
a. Ventilatory efficiency
b. The baseline for future comparisons of function
c. The ability of the blood to carry oxygen and carbon dioxide
d. The acid-base situation in the body

The healthy individual might have blood gases on the arterial and venous sides of the circulation with the following values:

	P_{O_2} (partial pressure of oxygen)	P_{CO_2} (partial pressure of carbon dioxide)	O_2	O_2 saturation
ARTERIAL	95–100 mm. Hg.	40 mm. Hg.	20 vol. %	100%
VENOUS	35–40 mm. Hg.	45 mm. Hg.	14 vol. %	70%

PROBABLE HOSPITAL COURSE

The patient will be treated concurrently for her congestive heart failure and will also be put through many studies to evaluate the severity of her valvular disease. Usually it takes from 10 days to three weeks to prepare a patient physiologically and psychologically for replacement of a heart valve.

Evaluation by the medical staff will determine the following:

1. A hemodynamically significant valvular lesion demonstrated visually and mathematically.
2. Calcium either present or not present on the valve.
3. A valve replacement to be the surgical operation of choice.
4. Other valves are or are not involved in the rheumatic process.

As soon as the patient's condition is satisfactory and studies are completed, medical and surgical consultants will agree on the necessity for surgery. The patient is then scheduled for open-heart surgery. Both the patient and the family are notified of the decision, and are apprised of the operative risk involved.

PREPARATION FOR SURGERY

In addition to the preparation already noted (in the previous chapters) for the patient having a mitral valvuloplasty, some additional measures must be included in the care of the patient about to undergo a valve replacement.

Prepare the patient for an extensive skin preparation; this will cover an area of the entire chest, front and back, down to and including the perineal area. Both groins are shaved as well as the ankles for cutdown purposes.

Digitalis is withheld one or two days before surgery.

The patient is placed on the seriously ill or danger list the night before her operation. Being on the seriously ill list is a routine procedure before all major surgery in some hospitals. This allows the family to have more flexible visiting privileges. Be sure to explain the meaning of this order to the patient so that she will not become unduly alarmed. The attending surgeon or the resident in charge will speak to the family or nearest relatives to review again the need for the operation and to answer any further questions. Arrangement should be made to have the family in a hospital waiting room the day of surgery. They will be told the outcome of the operation by the surgeon in charge.

The pulmonary therapist will visit the patient preoperatively to teach her remedial breathing and arm exercises; these will be utilized in the postoperative period.

Psychologically, it is most important to prepare the patient for the event of having an endotracheal tube in place postoperatively. Explain to her that this tube will be in and down her throat and that she will not be able to speak during the time it is in place. Emphasize that this tube will serve as an airway and will help her breathe when it is attached to a respirator. This tube will remain in place anywhere from 6 to 24 hours after surgery, depending upon the pulmonary status, the degree of thoracic bleeding postoperatively, and the stability of the neurological signs. If the endotracheal tube is to be in place more than 3 days, a tracheostomy will be done.

Tell the patient that after her surgery is over, she will awaken periodically but then be put back to sleep again with mild sedatives. Morphine sulphate will be used to relieve pain and restlessness. As soon as the endotracheal tube is removed, the patient will be able to talk, but will have a "sore" throat, caused by the irritation of this tube. Nasal oxygen will be administered and a steam mask will be placed over her nose and mouth in order to help liquefy mucous secretions in the respiratory tract. An ultrasonic nebulizer may also be used and this will provide cool steam, which is definitely more comfortable to the patient. Intermittent positive pressure breathing (IPPB) may be used during this period; some surgeons feel that it is better for the patient to deep breathe and cough on her own without this additional boost. If IPPB is used, it must be specifically adjusted (pressures) to the pulmonary compliance of the patient and should operate in such a way that it does not become an effort for the patient to use it.

It is also well to prepare both the patient and family for a typical period of depression that she may experience 5 to 10 days after surgery. This is a transitory experience but it will be less frightening to the patient if she has been warned. The patient will have a high pulse rate and insomnia during the time that she experiences this depression. She will tell you that nothing is familiar to her. She may hallucinate, have nightmares, and have only a few lucid moments during the day. She will complain during this period that she has "nobody to relate to" or that no one understands what she is going through at this particular stage of her recovery. Patients who have gone through these experiences tell us that they know at the time that they are behaving strangely and realize that the feelings will eventually go away.

It is also safe to tell the patient that when she awakens in the intensive care unit, she may be confused or may experience some visual or auditory hallucinations. The patient's reactions to anesthetics, analgesics, and the stress of surgery as well as having been on cardiopulmonary by-pass are good reasons for these responses. These situations must be cautiously explained to the patient as she is being readied for her open-heart surgery; this information must be streamlined to her individual needs and unique personality.

It will be most beneficial for the patient if the nurse organizes and utilizes a *teaching plan*. This might be:

1. Discuss and explain the heart problem that has led to a need for her surgery.
2. Define and explain the surgical procedure to the extent indicated by the wishes of the patient.
3. Impart information and teach skills that will ease anxiety and prepare her for and after surgery.
4. Discuss what the patient may expect in the intensive care unit.
5. Discuss procedures and the patient's responsibilities when she returns to the ward or her room.
6. Discuss the extent of the patient's permissible activities following discharge from the hospital.

PATHOLOGY

Mitral stenosis increases the workload of the right ventricle only, whereas mitral insufficiency greatly increases the work of the left ventricle as well. To compensate for the damaged valve on the left side of the heart (insufficiency), the left ventricle hypertrophies gradually and eventually dilates. The annulus enlarges and increases the pathological process by further increasing the regurgitation through the valve area. These patients (with mitral insufficiency or regurgitation) have greatly enlarged hearts, involving both atria and ventricles.

GENERAL RATIONALE AND SCHEME

In electing surgery for the patient, the surgeon knows that it is essential for him to operate on the heart before the myocardium deteriorates to the point at which the risk of surgery will be excessive for the patient. A new and efficient valve will permit the myocardium to return to normal, reduce cardiac work, enhance cardiac output, and significantly improve the patient's ability to work and exercise.

Scheme

Two surgical teams operate on the patient: one at the chest incision and the other at the groin incision.

1. The mitral valve area can be reached on either side of the heart; thus a right thoracotomy, left thoracotomy (best approach), or midline incision can be elected. This will depend on the preference of the surgeon.

2. The groin will be opened; the femoral artery and vein are exposed, incised, and cannulated in preparation for the patient to be put on the cardiopulmonary by-pass machine.

3. The right side of the heart will be cannulated to allow venous return to the "pump"; the patient will go on by-pass.

4. The atrium on the left side of the heart is opened; extracorporeal circulation will be maintained. The heart will be kept beating throughout the procedure.

5. The diseased valve will be inspected; the type of insufficiency and degree to which it occurs will be noted.

6. The valve will be extracted, leaving the annulus intact.

7. The prosthetic valve will be sutured in place.

8. The heart will be closed with sutures; air will be evacuated through a suction catheter in the left ventricle.

9. By-pass will be gradually terminated; the heart will resume circulatory responsibility.

10. The incision is closed.

Some Aspects of Placing the Patient on Cardiopulmonary By-pass

Cardiopulmonary by-pass allows diversion of the patient's circulation in order to make the heart and its interior directly visible to the surgeon, thereby enabling him to repair or replace cardiac valves more efficiently.

The patient will be placed on "by-pass" in order to accomplish direct surgery on the mitral valve. The purposes or functions of the by-pass machine are that it will perfuse, oxygenate, and cool the blood and keep the patient "alive" during the intracardiac phase of surgery. Venous blood will be taken from the body via the venae cavae and femoral vein; it will flow into the by-pass machine by siphonage or gentle negative pressure. Blood will be returned to the patient in a nonpulsatile flow via the femoral artery and will flow retrograde to the aortic valve. The blood pressure maintained while the patient is kept on by-pass is usually around 80 mm. of mercury. An adequate arterial pressure must be maintained at all times to adequately perfuse the vital organs and the coronary arteries, which arise at the aortic valve. The blood in the "machine" will be heparinized; whole body anticoagulation is achieved by this maneuver. This anticoagulation effect will be reversed when the patient is taken off "by-pass" by the injection of protamine sulphate. Anesthestic agents will be fed into the "machine" while the patient is on by-pass. The patient will have direct hypothermia effects, since the pump will cool all the blood that is being returned to the patient, down to a level as low as 27° Centigrade. Usually, the patient's temperature will be brought down only to 32° Centigrade for most cardiac surgical procedures employing the cardiopulmonary machine. One safety factor utilized in decompressing the heart is a vent in the form of a polyethylene tube; this is inserted into the left ventricle from below. The purpose of this vent is to keep the pressure in the left ventricle from exceeding the pressure in the aorta and thus keep the aortic valve closed and not permit air to escape from the open left ventricle into the systemic circulation. This escape tube or "vent" also prevents overdistention of the left ventricle and allows removal of any air before the defibrillation procedure is initiated when the heart is being resuscitated.

PROCEDURE

1. The first surgical team will make the thoracotomy or median sternotomy incision.

2. If there has been no previous operation, and there is no aortic or tricuspid disease, a left thoracotomy provides excellent exposure.

3. The second surgical team exposes the femoral artery and vein in preparation for cannulation for the cardiopulmonary by-pass machine. The venae cavae are also cannulated so that additional venous blood can be routed to the pump when the patient is on by-pass.

4. The patient goes on partial by-pass; anticoagulation has been accomplished prior to this with heparinization of the blood in the pump.

5. Total by-pass is instituted at the time when the heart is opened; the left atrium is entered and the mitral valve is exposed.

6. The valve is excised circumferentially; care is taken to preserve the valve annulus.

7. The chordae tendineae are palpated and fractured; this helps with the mobility in placing the new prosthetic valve in its location.

8. The prosthetic valve is sutured into place.

9. The atrium is sutured; the heart is allowed to fill with blood, and air is sucked out.

10. The heart is allowed to resume circulation of the blood. (The patient will be taken off total by-pass and both heart and machine will circulate the blood; a condition of partial by-pass will exist again.)

11. Blood pressure is evaluated; the heart action is monitored and evaluated.

12. The patient is taken off the pump; the heart resumes total responsibility for circulating the blood.

13. Chest tubes (2) are inserted through the intercostal space; they are attached to underwater-seal drainage. (A third chest tube may be utilized in the second anterior chest intercostal space.)

14. The thoracotomy or sternotomy is sutured.

15. The patient returns to the intensive care unit with the endotracheal tube still in place; this tube will be attached to a respirator. Nitrous oxide and oxygen will be given through this tube. Arterial and venous lines will also be in place and attached to the appropriate monitors in the I.C.U.

SURGICAL HAZARDS

Cardiac arrest may occur at any time during the operation or in the I.C.U.

Heart-block may be a result of sutures placed near the septum or in the atrioventricular bundle during fixation of the prosthetic valve, or a consequence of edema in the septum.

Peripheral embolization may be due to (a) air, (b) clots, or (c) particles of calcium broken off during the valve replacement. Air embolus is usually associated with open-heart surgery on the left side of the heart; careful evacuation of all air prior to final closure of the heart is therefore imperative.

Hemorrhage has many causes during this type of surgery. Some of these include:

a. Tears in the great vessels and the heart.

b. Dissecting aneurysm of the cannulated vessel.

c. Operative hemorrhage.

d. Defects in the coagulation mechanism as a result of many transfusions and prolonged cardiopulmonary by-pass, resulting in a bleeding tendency due to abnormal fibrinolytic activity.

e. Protamine rebound — when this drug is utilized to neutralize the effects of heparin it may also cause a defect in the coagulation mechanism.

Decrease in the venous return to the cardiopulmonary by-pass machine. The circulating blood should be checked and the possibilities of mechanical obstruction investigated.

Poor arterial perfusion flow rates will cause low blood pressure readings and poor perfusion of the vital organs as well as that of the coronary arteries.

Renal insufficiency may occur for the following reasons:

a. Inadequate perfusion during cardiopulmonary by-pass.

b. Reduced cardiac output following completion of by-pass.

c. Cardiac tamponade, causing a decreased cardiac output.

d. Diminished circulatory blood volume.

e. Use of large quantities of homologous blood in the pump; in effect being a transfusion reaction accompanied by disintegration of the red blood cells from the activity of the pumping mechanism of the machine.

f. Use of cardiopulmonary by-pass for too long a period of time, resulting in increased destruction of red blood cells followed by a release of hemoglobin, causing kidney damage.

IMMEDIATE POSTOPERATIVE PROBLEMS

1. **Hemorrhage.** Postoperative hemorrhage can result from:

a. Technical difficulties encountered during surgery that have not been adequately overcome.

b. Incisions and dissections through past adhesions from previous surgery.

c. Administration of many transfusions during surgery, producing coagulation problems.

2. **Respirator.** While the patient is on the respirator with the endotracheal tube in place, these problems will be minimal. However, the patient may react to the endotracheal tube with some displeasure and get restless. This may occur when she first awakens and realizes where she is and that she cannot speak with the tube in place. She will require sedation administered intravenously.

3. **Cardiodynamics.** Arrhythmias may be visible on the monitor. These may be controlled with many types of drugs, e.g., Digoxin, Xylocaine, and Pronestyl. Pacing wires in the right atrium and the left ventricle may be connected to a temporary battery pacemaker to treat complete heart-block or other arrhythmias. Staff members should be aware that these wires can break and that such an event can lead to pacemaker failure.

4. **Hypothermia.** Usually the patient's body temperature will be in the range of 96° to 97° F. when she first returns to the intensive care unit. There is severe vasoconstriction during this period. The use of warm bath blankets will help to elevate her body temperature to within normal limits in the next 2 to 3 hours.

5. **Cardiac tamponade** may be the result of persistent, excessive bleeding and malfunction of the chest tubes. Sometimes a clot formation will obstruct the flow of blood from the pericardium, which has been partially sutured, and will bring about this effect. Classic signs of cardiac tamponade include:

a. rising venous pressure

b. paradoxical pulse

c. distant heart sounds

6. **Hypotension** can result from peripheral vasodilation, low cardiac output, or hypovolemia.

PROBLEMS WITHIN THE NEXT FEW HOURS

Acid-base balance. This will be evaluated by (1) blood gas levels, (2) the pH of the blood, (3) the neurological status of the patient, and (4) the skin color.

Hypoxia. This will be evaluated by using the criteria listed for acid-base balance.

Kidney function. Oliguria is a typical problem. If cardiac output can be improved, renal function usually is reversible.

Hypotension. This may be due to inadequate replacement therapy; this will be manifested by a low arterial blood pressure or by cardiac failure.

Bleeding. This is mainly shown by the amount of bloody chest tube drainage and a change in vital signs.

Arrhythmias. These will be observable on the monitor and can be reversed by drugs or cardioversion. The prosthetic valve may be a source of irritation on the septum and thus a cause of an arrhythmia. *Postassium imbalances* may cause the following:

a. An elevated $[K]^+$ can cause a decreased cardiac rate, flat P wave, or a peaked T wave.
b. A decreased $[K]^+$ may cause premature ventricular contractions (PVC's), premature atrial contractions (PAC's), or a flat T wave.

Digitalis excess can cause PVC's or an increased heart rate and heart-block.

Fever. The rectal temperature may rise to over 102 degrees. This rise is due to blood reactions, infection, or pulmonary congestion.

COMPLICATIONS

These include:
1. *Congestive heart failure.*
2. *Embolization* occurring during the first 48 hours. This might produce:
a. A cerebral vascular accident — hemiparesis, aphasia, convulsions, or a comatose state.
b. Myocardial infarct — restlessness, EKG changes.
c. Cardiac arrest.
3. *Renal failure.*
4. *Hypotension.*
5. *Infection.*
6. *Respiratory problems* as a result of chronic obstructive pulmonary disease.

POSTOPERATIVE MANAGEMENT

The care given to this patient can be divided into several priorities:
1. Monitoring vital and neurological signs.
2. Observation of cardiac rhythm patterns.
3. Maintaining optimum function of the respiratory tract.
4. Maintaining optimum renal function.
5. Preserving the psyche of the patient.

Monitoring Vital and Neurological Signs

Rectal temperatures are taken at two-hour intervals. Some hospitals use a telethermometer to electrically assess the rectal temperature almost constantly.

A hypothermia blanket may be put on the bottom of the bed prior to the reception of the patient into the intensive care unit. This device is then utilized whenever the patient's temperature is too high and elevates the heart rate physiologically as a result. The doctor may order that vital signs be taken every 20 minutes. Remember that fever is not unusual postoperatively. Aspirin will usually be administered rectally for an elevation over 101°F. Tylenol is another drug which may be administered. Alcohol sponge baths are routinely employed also.

Arterial blood pressure will be measured with a mercury manometer. Heparinized saline will be used in the arterial line to prevent coagulation of blood in the line. A polyethylene catheter will have been inserted preoperatively into the brachial artery; it is attached to a specific type of gauge designed to measure the pressure in this system.

Central venous pressure is measured through a water manometer set-up (5 per cent dextrose in water is the solution usually used). A polyethylene catheter will have been threaded through the antecubital vein up into the right atrium preoperatively; this pressure is taken intermittently in the postoperative period. This measuring device usually is incorporated with the I.V. fluid line.

Intravenous fluids are closely monitored to make sure that the patient is not over-hydrated. The venous pressure line is watched to insure adequate fluid replacement. Venous pressure will also indicate whether the heart is adequately coping with the return flow of blood, which it is receiving from the body. Fluid restrictions (I.V.) may run from 1500 to 2000 cc. daily. It is important to include in the intake record the amount of I.V. fluids that are going in very slowly in order to leave certain lines "open" for either emergency sake or in order to administer medications intravenously.

Urine output is measured hourly; the amount produced is usually above 30 cc. an hour. Specific gravity of the urine is also tested at the same time.

Chest tube drainage is measured hourly and recorded appropriately. The amount and rate at which it is draining from the chest tubes is observed on a more frequent basis. It is most important to get down to the level of the chest drainage in the bottle to accurately visualize the level of fluid at the time it is to be measured. The blood lost by this drainage route is replaced with transfusion, according to the hematocrit reading which will indicate the degree of blood lost.

The patient's neurological status is evaluated to determine the presence of neurological deficits after surgery. The staff must assess the following:

1. *The Level of Consciousness.* This includes the patient's ability to respond to situation, time, place, and person. The patient should be evaluated for her ability to follow one- or two-step commands and to speak knowledgeably and appropriately when questioned. Any slight change in the patient's affect or a change in the pattern of the patient's usual intellectual responses is significant and should be reported. Seizure precautions must be instituted if there is any possibility of seizure activity.

2. *Pupillary Reactions and Size.* These factors must be evaluated together during any neurological check. The pupils should be equal in size and should accommodate to light. They should not be tightly constricted or widely dilated. Any sudden onset of change, such as unilateral dilation, should be brought to the surgeon's attention *at once.* The quality of the patient's vision should be determined, and note of whether it is clear, blurred, or doubled (diplopia) should be made.

3. *Arterial Blood Pressure and Pulse Rate.* These must be compared to determine if the patient's intracranial pressure has increased. Hypertension and bradycardia are significant changes indicative of lesions causing increasing intracranial pressure.

4. *Respiratory Status.* The rate and quality of respirations should be evaluated.

5. *The Ability of the Patient to Move All of Her Extremities Purposefully and Against Resistance.* The nursing staff must evaluate the appearance of changes in muscle tone, such as a drooping eyelid on one side, or an asymmetrical facial expression, or flaccid body muscles.

Observation of Cardiac Rhythm Patterns

A cardiac monitor with leads attached to the patient is used continually to record and evaluate cardiac rhythm patterns on the oscilloscope.

Arrhythmias are often well tolerated in the postoperative period. However, they are usually controlled with the administration of specific cardiac drugs, in order that the rhythm may be reverted to normal as soon as possible. Signs and symptoms of various deviations in rhythm may be indicated by a sudden drop in the cardiac output, development of congestive heart failure, manifestation of pulmonary edema, and specific monitor rhythm pattern changes.

Common arrhythmias to be watched for are atrial fibrillation or flutter, atrioventricular junctional or nodal rhythms, and ventricular tachycardia.

Some surgeons use pacing electrodes in the atrium or on the ventricle for those patients who undergo open-heart surgery. Cardiac pacing may be used in the event that the patient develops transient heart-block postoperatively.

Cardiac output is evaluated by the clinical impression of the patient, blood pressure, hourly urine output, degree of peripheral perfusion, and assessment of acid-base balance.

Maintaining Optimum Function of the Respiratory Tract

The head of the patient's bed is kept elevated from 30 to 45 degrees during the postoperative period. Her body position is changed from side to side every two hours; back care is administered when each change of position is made.

Blood gases (P_{O_2}, P_{CO_2}, pH) will be ordered for analysis to determine the presence of acidosis, hypoventilation, or hypoxia.

The endotracheal tube will be in place and connected to an appropriate respirator cycled to adequately exchange respiratory gases. The patient will be kept on controlled respirations for the first 6 to 24 hours after surgery. The endotracheal tube can still be kept in place up to 72 hours after surgery. However, after that period of time, if there is still need for controlled respiration, a tracheostomy may be performed. An endotracheal tube may cause laryngeal edema or ulceration of the larynx, and the tube may become occluded through blockage of its lumen with thick mucous plugs after this period of time (72 hours).

Suctioning through the Endotracheal Tube

The patient is hyperventilated with the Ambu bag for 15 deep breaths prior to suctioning, in order to:

1. Ventilate all possible alveoli, thereby preventing atelectasis.

2. Facilitate movement of secretions into the bronchi, thereby making the suctioning procedure more successful.

Certain steps are to be followed in suctioning with a cuffed endotracheal tube:

1. Suction out the endotracheal tube *first,* in order to aspirate out all secretions and to prevent partial obstruction of the airway.

2. Next, suction the patient's oropharynx and nasopharynx so that secretions are not aspirated when the cuff of the tube is deflated.

3. Remove the air from the cuff of the tube by aspirating it with a syringe from the exit route tubing of the endotracheal tube. Be aware of how much air has been in the cuff prior to this time and the lumen size of the tube itself.

4. Let the cuff remain deflated for 15 to 20 seconds to relieve the pressure exerted on the trachea.

5. Reinflate the same cuff of the tube *or* the alternate cuff if the endotracheal tube is double-cuffed.

The nurse's notes should record the type and amount of secretions obtained in the suctioning procedure. The notes should indicate that the endotracheal cuff was deflated for a period of time.

The patient will need frequent mouth care with an endotracheal tube in place. In addition, careful attention must be paid to the condition and position of the mouth block used to prevent the patient from biting down on the endotracheal tube itself.

The nursing staff should always make sure that any intubated patient has an Ambu bag (with face mask attachment) accessible for individual use if the need arises for emergency ventilation.

Complications which may arise from a faulty endotracheal tube cuff or from leakage from the cuff are:

1. Air leaks around the endotracheal tube.
2. Aspiration of secretions or saliva.
3. Untimely extubation.
4. Inability to properly aerate the patient with a ventilator or Ambu bag.

Restlessness, increased pulse rate, and skin color changes indicate respiratory distress and must be reversed immediately.

"Sighing" the patient is a maneuver that is done through the respirator while the patient is having respirations controlled. It is performed every 15 to 30 minutes, one to three times at this interval. The purposes of this *hyperventilation* are:

a. To increase tidal volume and hence alveolar ventilation momentarily, and
b. To prevent atelectasis in the immediate postoperative period.

A chest x-ray and a complete 12 lead electrocardiogram are taken the afternoon of surgery when the patient is stabilized and can afford the movement these procedures entail.

Extubation of the Patient

When the patient's vital capacity, tidal volume, minute volume, and arterial blood gases indicate that adequate ventilation is achieved, the respirator is disconnected from the end of the endotracheal tube and an oxygen adapter is put over the tube. The patient has been told prior to this what she is going to experience during the extubation procedure, what to expect, and her utmost cooperation is enlisted. After the respirator is detached, the patient is coaxed to breathe under her own power. Sometimes, she may require manual assistance, that is, with your hands pressing on the thoracic cage in order to help her expel air. Blood gases are again checked (after this procedure), now that the patient is breathing by herself. If the vital capacity, tidal volume, and blood gases are adequate, the endotracheal tube is removed. Nasal oxygen (running at 7 liters) and a steam mask are put in place. Close observation of adequate chest movements and coaxing of the patient to breathe are in order. Medication for pain is imperative before, during, and after this extubation procedure especially if it lasts over a period of hours. Pain and the fear of now having to breathe on her own can be paralyzing to the patient. She needs optimum encouragement and support during this critical period.

The nasal oxygen catheter must be changed at least every 8 hours to ensure patency. Tape the catheter to the nose, and let it dangle as the tube falls naturally. If the patient swallows too frequently, this is an indication that the nasal catheter is too far down her throat. Beware of gastric dilation if this is the case. Turn off the nasal oxygen flow whenever you give *anything* by mouth to the patient.

Maintaining Optimum Renal Function

Adequate postoperative urine output is a specific indicator of sufficient cardiac function and peripheral perfusion. Urine output is directly related to optimum kidney perfusion, which is dependent upon arterial blood pressure being maintained by efficient cardiac output as well as sufficient blood volume and a permissible degree of vasoconstriction. Hourly measurements of urine output, together with specific gravity analysis, form a standard part of the nursing and medical management of the postoperative cardiac patient. If there is a renal problem in the post-operative period, it is usually manifested by *oliguria.* In general, decreased urinary output is the result of the following factors and situations:

1. Hypovolemia due to hemorrhage.
2. Low cardiac output.
3. Hypotension during surgery, which causes inadequate perfusion of the renal parenchyma and resulting acute tubular necrosis.
4. Severe vasoconstriction due to hypothermia or to the administration of vasopressor drugs such as Levophed.
5. Hemolysis as a result of cardiopulmonary by-pass, causing hemoglobinuria.
6. Renal artery embolism.
7. Pre-existing renal disease.

Treatment for decreased urine output must be carried out along these lines:

1. Maintain adequate blood volume; prevent hypotension from occurring.
2. Enhance and potentiate effective cardiac tone and efficiency.
3. Prevent or treat severe vasoconstriction (which results from the stress of surgery as well as from hypothermia endured throughout the cardiopulmonary by-pass) by promoting a normal body temperature and administering vasodilating drugs.
4. Administer diuretic drugs such as Furosemide and Mannitol when necessary.

When *renal failure* is present after mitral valve replacement, treatment consists of:

1. Fluid restriction.
2. Careful monitoring of blood electrolytes.
3. Control of hyperkalemia with the use of ion exchange resins.
4. Intravenous administration of insulin, glucose, and sodium bicarbonate.
5. Peritoneal dialysis.
6. Hemodialysis.

Psychological Support in the Postoperative Period

It is most important to use analgesic drugs frequently (every 2 to 3 hours) during the postoperative period, to ensure confort, relieve pain, and promote optimum breathing with the least amount of pain and discomfort.

The patient usually remains in the intensive care unit for 48 hours after surgery. The atmosphere in the I.C.U. is usually one of bright light, strange noises, no windows, and no clock. The patient may get little sleep during her stay because of overenthusiastic management, and, as a result, she may be subject to hallucinations both of an auditory and visual nature. She may also experience depression, delusions, agitation, and periods of disorientation.

We know from experience that there is a greater incidence of psychological deviations postoperatively in those patients who have a history of previous emotional difficulties. This state may last from 3 to 5 days, when it occurs.

Amnesia for the postoperative period is typical. However, the patient may remember to some degree that she was emotionally disturbed or upset during this recuperative phase.

Removal of the patient from the intensive care atmosphere will frequently solve many of her psychological difficulties and be quite therapeutic for her emotionally.

It is most important, therefore, to reassure the patient while she is in the intensive care unit. Calmness must prevail so that the patient does not equate hush and rush with impending disaster. The environment of the I.C.U. may be quite overpowering and frightening to the patient. Become adept at communicating with a partially anesthetized and sedated patient. Remember that you will have to repeat certain ideas to her because of her somnolent state. Display a personal concern evidenced by your manner in caring for her during this anxious and stressful postoperative phase of care.

Encourage the patient to be cooperative and to be determined to do well and improve. Inform her of the hour to hour progress wherever possible. Arrange your nursing care so she will have periods of time to *sleep* or *rest*. Talk with her in a conversational way. Use terms and words which she understands. Keep her oriented as to the time of day and the date. Be honest with her and with her family.

STUDY QUESTIONS

1. Review the historical development of open-heart surgery.

2. What mechanical developments made this era possible?

3. What extra equipment is necessary in the operating room during open-heart surgery?

4. Review the duties and responsibilities of the following nurses in the care of the patient:
   a. The O.R. supervisor
   b. The circulating nurse
   c. The scrub nurse
   d. The intensive care nurse
   e. The head nurse in the I.C.U.

5. What extra clinical tests are made preoperatively on the person who is to undergo open-heart surgery? Why are such tests necessary?

6. Does the preoperative nursing care of this patient differ from the patient who is to have a mitral valvuloplasty?

7. In the event of a cardiac arrest in the intensive care unit what are the responsibilities of the:
   a. Doctor
   b. Student nurse
   c. Staff nurse
   d. Supervisor

8. Make a list of the specific drugs that would be used during the preoperative, operative, and postoperative periods; note their actions and nursing precautions.

9. Compose a tentative time schedule and nursing care plan for the management and postoperative care of a patient who has had open-heart surgery.

10. What emergencies (other than a cardiac arrest) would you be prepared for in the intensive care unit while caring for this patient?

11. What are the indications for suctioning of the respiratory tract?

12. How is tracheal suctioning accomplished in the following situations?
   a. During surgery
   b. In the I.C.U. for a patient with an endotracheal tube in place
   c. In a patient with a nasal oxygen catheter in place

13. What patterns of cardiac arrhythmias might you see on the cardioscope in the I.C.U. following open-heart surgery? Differentiate between each and be prepared to draw each rhythm pattern.

14. How can atelectasis be prevented in the postoperative period? How is this condition diagnosed?

15. What signs and symptoms would indicate a neurological problem postoperatively in a patient who has had open-heart surgery?

73   THE PATIENT WITH CORONARY ARTERY DISEASE

Operation: Coronary Artery By-pass Graft

TYPICAL HISTORY

A 52-year-old male has experienced progressive angina pectoris and has had three past myocardial infarctions. He now has severe chest pain almost daily and must take many nitroglycerin tablets for relief. He is disabled to the extent that he can no longer carry on his normal daily activities and is not employable. Because of the progressive angina in this patient's case, coronary artery angiography and saphenous vein by-pass graft are contemplated.

PHYSICAL EXAMINATION

The patient is a well-developed, well-nourished male, somewhat apprehensive and in some degree of discomfort due to angina pectoris.

Significant Findings

1. Mild diastolic hypertension is present.
2. Early hypertensive retinopathy is noted.
3. Heart sounds are normal.
4. There is a bruit over the right femoral artery.
5. Dyspnea on exertion is evident.

DIAGNOSTIC STUDIES

The severity of angina pectoris, coronary artery disease, and symptoms of congestive heart failure must be evaluated in a complete medical program of tests and x-rays.

The medical work-up includes the following:

1. Evaluation of Cardiac Status.
   a. Electrocardiograms.
   b. Submaximal graded exercise test while an EKG is administered.
   c. Cardiac catheterization.
      (1) Ventriculography.
      (2) Coronary angiography.
   d. Chest fluoroscopy and routine chest films.
   e. Serum enzymes, e.g., SGOT, LDH.
2. Evaluation of Respiratory Status.
3. Evaluation of Neurologic Status.
4. Evaluation of Peripheral Vasculature Condition.
   a. Aortogram.
   b. Venogram, to assess the condition of the saphenous vein and to rule out the presence of phlebitis in the leg(s).
5. Evaluation of the Overall Dental Condition (to rule out existing oral infection).
6. Thyroid Function Studies.
7. Renal Function Studies.
8. Liver Function Studies.
9. Other Routine Studies.
   a. Complete blood count.
   b. Platelet count.
   c. Prothrombin time.
   d. Bleeding time.
   e. Creatinine clearance.
   f. Blood urea nitrogen (BUN).
   g. Blood electrolytes.
   h. Blood type and cross-matching.
   i. Urinalysis; urine culture.

Coronary angiography reveals occlusion of the right coronary artery proximally as well as occlusion of the left anterior descending coronary artery. In addition, there is a high grade stenosis of the circumflex marginal artery. Distal visualization of both the left anterior descending coronary artery and the right coronary artery suggests a fair amount of distal arterial disease. Because of the patient's progressive angina, coronary artery reconstructive surgery is recommended, and the patient accepts this course of action.

PROBABLE HOSPITAL COURSE

The patient will have cardiac surgery performed while on cardiopulmonary by-pass. A graft from the saphenous vein will be attached to the aorta and anastomosed to the area distal to vessel obstruction, allowing a more adequate blood supply to nourish the myocardium. At the time of surgery, cardiac pacing wires will be placed in the heart muscle. At the completion of surgery, the patient will be taken to the intensive care unit. If no complications ensue in the initial postoperative phase (i.e., immediately after surgery) or on the following morning, certain routines will be carried out:

1. Assessment of arterial blood gases.
2. Extubation of the patient early in the morning.
3. Removal of the Foley catheter.
4. Removal of all peripheral intravenous and intra-arterial lines.
5. Removal of chest tubes or mediastinal tubes.
6. Removal of left atrial line.

The patient is discharged from the intensive care unit and returned to a clinical unit, where provision for private duty nurses will have been made for his continuous postoperative care and observation.

PREPARATION FOR SURGERY

The student is referred to the preceding chapters on cardiac surgery for information on preparation of the cardiac patient.

PATHOLOGY

The heart is a muscle that pumps blood to and from all parts of the body, bringing nourishment and oxygen to all body cells. The heart is composed of 4 chambers and 2 major vessels. There are two collecting chambers (the right and left atrium) and two pumping chambers (the right and left ventricle). Each pumping chamber is separated from its collecting chamber and the major vessels by a one-way valve which keeps blood going in one direction only. The venous blood returns to the heart from the body tissues into the right atrium, passes through the tricuspid valve, and enters the right ventricle. The blood is then forced through the pulmonic valve into the pulmonary artery and vessels, arriving at the lung, where it is oxygenated. The oxygenated blood passes to the left atrium and through the mitral valve to the left ventricle. From here the blood is pumped through the aortic valve into the aorta and then to the body through the system of arteries. To do its work, the heart muscle must have a continuous supply of blood (to provide nourishment and oxygen) through its own system of arteries, named the coronary arteries (Fig. 73-1). The overall performance of the heart is influenced by a variety of factors: heart size, heart rate, blood pressure, body chemistry, and stimulation by nerves and hormones. Through interaction of these factors, the heart can quickly respond with an increased output of blood when the body demands such during work, exercise or emotional stress.

The heart may be affected by disease processes at many of the structural sites that have been mentioned, with resulting abnormalities in cardiac function. Descriptions of the most commonly encountered heart problems follow.

Atherosclerosis. Commonly known as hardening of the arteries, atherosclerosis is a process in which the inner lining of some of the arteries becomes thickened and roughened by fatty deposits such as cholesterol. This narrows the lumen of the arteries, interfering with blood flow.

Coronary Artery Disease. When atherosclerosis affects the arteries which deliver blood to the heart muscle (Fig. 73-1), the result is coronary artery disease. There may be deficient blood flow to an area of heart muscle at rest or during stress. This diminished blood supply may be associated with arrhythmias and angina pectoris. Total cessation of blood flow to a zone may lead to ischemia of a section of the muscle and a myocardial infarction.

Angina Pectoris. This cardiac problem is marked by a recurring sensation of discomfort or chest pain. It usually occurs at a time when the heart is called on to increase cardiac output, such

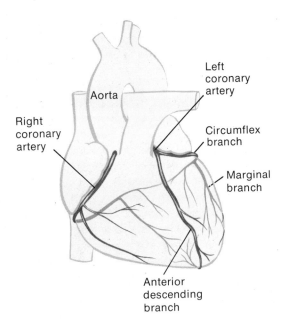

Left
coronary
artery

Aorta

Right
coronary
artery

Circumflex
branch

Marginal
branch

Anterior
descending
branch

FIGURE 73-1 The coronary arteries.

as during physical exercise or in other periods of stress (e.g., emotional tension). Angina occurs when the supply of blood to a part of the myocardium is not enough to meet the body's needs. Anginal episodes are usually brief and are relieved by rest or nitroglycerin.

Coronary Insufficiency. This term refers to episodes of chest discomfort and/or pain that are prolonged and not as responsive to the nitrites or to rest as angina pectoris. There may be an associated prolonged deficit of blood flow to a zone of heart muscle without the gross damage seen in myocardial infarction. Episodes of coronary insufficiency may be the precursor of an imminent "heart attack."

Myocardial Infarction. Irreversible damage to an area of myocardium is the distinguishing characteristic of myocardial infarction (also commonly known as "coronary thrombosis" or "heart attack"). The damage can result from severe ischemia subsequent to cessation of blood flow to the part, such as occurs in coronary artery disease. It can also occur during a hypotensive period in which there is a decreased supply of blood to the coronary arteries, producing ischemia of a section of the myocardium. Another cause of myocardial infarction (MI) is an embolus in a coronary artery that occludes the lumen of the artery, with resulting ischemia of a section of heart muscle. A myocardial infarction is a dangerous medical problem that can have fatal complications.

In the case of a patient with coronary artery disease, the following criteria are used to evaluate whether or not the patient may be a candidate for coronary artery by-pass surgery.

Criteria:

1. Disabling angina pectoris which is not relieved by appropriate medical treatment faithfully followed by the patient.

2. Evidence from coronary angiography of almost complete blockage of the proximal portions of:

    a. the right coronary artery.

    b. the left coronary artery.

    c. the circumflex arteries.

Note: There must be a visibly patent blood vessel distal to the obstructed area.

3. Severe coronary insufficiency, preinfarction angina and evidence of an impending heart attack.

4. Evidence of obvious and severe impairment of left ventricle performance and concomitant cardiogenic shock.

5. A history of chronic cardiac failure from severe coronary artery disease.

GENERAL RATIONALE AND SCHEME

Aortocoronary saphenous vein by-pass surgery for the alleviation of coronary artery disease and the disabling anginal syndrome and pre-infarction angina utilizes reversed segments of an autogenous saphenous vein which is anastomosed directly between the ascending aorta and the patent segments of one or more of the three major coronary arteries (see Fig. 73-2).

The operative field (the heart itself) must be stationary if the delicate anastomoses of the small arteries are to be performed. This is achieved by fibrillating the heart or by anoxic arrest, which is brought about when the ascending aorta is clamped. Fine suture materials and optical magnification permit exact anastomoses between the segments of saphenous vein and each coronary artery chosen to be revascularized.

The by-pass graft establishes myocardial revascularization by providing a ready blood supply to ischemic segments of the myocardium. The patient will have immediate postoperative relief of his angina pectoris. In addition, the great prophylactic advantage of surgery of this nature is that it prevents future myocardial infarcts and allows the patient to maintain his preferred life style (or the style that he has adopted with coronary artery disease).

Scheme

1. A median sternotomy incision is made. When the heart is exposed by opening the pericardium along the midline, it shows considerable evidence of coronary artery disease.

2. A long segment of saphenous vein is harvested from the left thigh.

3. Appropriate cannulae are placed.

4. The first series of anastomoses is performed.

5. The patient is put on by-pass and his body temperature lowered.

6. Ventricular fibrillation is induced.

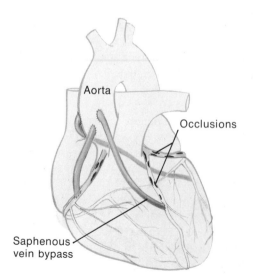

Aorta

Occlusions

Saphenous
vein bypass

FIGURE 73-2 Aortocoronary saphenous by-pass surgery for multiple vessel disease.

7. The second series of anastomoses is performed.

8. The aorta is cross-clamped during repositioning of the heart. The third series of anastomoses is performed.

9. The patient is rewarmed.

10. Cardiopulmonary by-pass is discontinued.

11. Blood flow is assessed. Pacing wires, an atrial line, and chest tubes are inserted.

12. Hemostasis is finalized and the incision is closed in the usual fashion. Chest tubes and pacing wires are brought out through the skin.

PROCEDURE

1. With the patient under general endotracheal anesthesia and in the supine position, a median sternotomy incision is made.

2. Simultaneously, through a series of small incisions the left greater saphenous vein is harvested from the groin to the ankle. Its branches are then ligated in preparation for its use as a by-pass graft.

3. The pericardium is opened along the midline.

4. *Examination of the Heart.* In this patient, the heart is somewhat larger than the heart of a normal, healthy individual. The left ventricle is particularly enlarged, and there is a great deal of fat in the epicardium. There is palpable plaque formation in the proximal left coronary system extending out to the middle third of the left anterior descending system and well down into the branches of the circumflex system. The circumflex marginal branches are very small on the surface of the heart. The right coronary artery is involved to within 2 to 3 cm of the posterior descending artery. There is a small plaque at the bifurcation of the posterior descending artery and the atrioventricular groove branch. While there is no true aneurysm formation present, there is extensive scarring throughout the sclerotic areas.

5. A single venous cannula is placed in the right atrial appendage; an arterial cannula is placed in the ascending aorta.

6. After systemic heparinization, two segments of saphenous vein are reversed and are separately anastomosed to the ascending aorta with running 5-0 Prolene sutures. An excision of a small button of the aorta is used for each anastomosis.

7. When this first series of anastomoses has been completed (vein graft to proximal aorta), the patient is put on cardiopulmonary by-pass. Hypothermia is encouraged, and the patient's temperature is brought down to 28 degrees Centigrade.

8. The left ventricle is drained through the right superior pulmonary vein.

9. The myocardium is protected with a continuous drip of iced Ringer's lactate solution, which (along with hypothermia) induces ventricular fibrillation.

10. The right coronary artery is separated from the atrioventricular groove at the origin of the posterior descending artery. In this patient, the artery is highly sclerotic, with many plaques extending down to the very extremity of the posterior descending artery.

11. The posterior descending artery is opened at a soft spot, in this case at the origin of the artery. There is back bleeding at the point of opening. The distal end of one of the saphenous veins earlier anastomosed to the aorta is anastomosed to the posterior descending artery with running 7-0 Prolene sutures.

12. The left anterior descending coronary artery is separated from the anterior surface of the heart. As in the preceding stage, a soft spot in the artery is sought (in this patient the artery shows a good deal of distal disease).

13. The distal end of the other saphenous vein graft earlier anastomosed to the aorta is anastomosed to the left anterior descending coronary artery with running 7-0 Prolene sutures.

14. The heart is repositioned anteriorly to expose the posterolateral wall of the circumflex marginal artery. The artery is incised directly.

15. During a short period of aortic cross-clamping, the distal end of a third segment of saphenous vein is anastomosed to the circumflex marginal artery with running 7-0 Prolene sutures.

16. The heart is returned to its normal position in the pericardial cavity.

17. The third segment of saphenous vein, the distal end of which has just been anastomosed to the circumflex marginal artery, is anastomosed at its proximal end to the ascending aorta with running 5-0 Prolene sutures. An excision of a small button of the aorta is used to implant the anastomosis of the saphenous vessel.

18. The patient is rewarmed to 37 degrees Centigrade, and spontaneous defibrillation of the heart occurs.

19. Cardiopulmonary by-pass is discontinued (the mean arterial pressure is 80 mm Hg).

20. All cannulae are removed and heparinization neutralized with Protamine.

21. Blood flow through the three vein grafts is measured with a 6 mm electromagnetic flow meter probe.

22. Pacing wires are affixed to the epicardial surface of the right atrium and right ventricle.

23. A left atrial pressure line is placed for purposes of postoperative monitoring.

24. The pericardium is drained with two Tygon chest tubes attached to suction.

25. After hemostasis is established completely, the sternum is approximated with multiple stainless steel wires, the rectus fascia with interrupted Mersilene sutures.

26. The subcutaneous tissue in the chest and legs is closed with running Dexon sutures; the skin is closed with Ethiflex sutures.

27. Sterile dressings are applied and the patient is returned to the intensive care unit with his endotracheal tube in place.

SURGICAL HAZARDS

1. *Arrhythmias.* These are very common before, during, and after surgery. They may be caused by the stress of surgery, the initiation or termination of cardiopulmonary by-pass, myocardial ischemia (caused by inadequate coronary perfusion during by-pass), or sutures in or on the myocardium itself. The most common patterns include:
   a. Atrial fibrillation.
   b. Nodal rhythm patterns.
   c. Ventricular tachycardia.
   d. Extrasystoles (premature ventricular contractions).

2. *Excessive Bleeding.* This can occur as a result of numerous adhesions, excessive anticoagulation, or multiple transfusions.

3. *Cardiac Tamponade.* Tight suturing of the pericardium *must* be avoided intraoperatively in order to guarantee adequate drainage of the sac.

POSTOPERATIVE MANAGEMENT

Problems to be anticipated in the patient who has had coronary artery by-pass surgery involve:
1. Blood gases (going up or down).
2. Blood pressure (hypotension or hypertension).
3. The need for many drugs to be administered intravenously, which requires judicious management of their labeling and individual flow rates.
4. Increased chest drainage (evidenced by rapid filling of the chest drainage collecting bottles).

Nursing care will follow along the lines described in previous chapters. Specifically, the following points must be observed:

1. *Adequate ventilation must be maintained.*
    a. Respiratory care: assisted respirations are provided with a volume respirator.
        (1) The respirator is set at 50 to 60 per cent pure oxygen, delivered at 10 liters per minute.
        (2) Deep endotracheal suctioning should be employed at least once every hour. The patient is hyperventilated by hand for several deep breaths before this procedure is initiated.
        (3) The cuff of the endotracheal tube is deflated after every suctioning (and cleansing of the mouth and pharynx).
2. *Any signs of hypotension must be detected and corrected.*
    a. The essential readings here are of the EKG monitor, the arterial pressure, the left atrial pressure, and the central venous pressure, all checked every 20 minutes.
    b. The pacemaker may be set to work as necessary or at an established rate.
3. *Cardiac arrhythmias must be monitored and controlled.*
    a. Digitalis is given in maintenance dosages or in dosages designed to control the heart rate in atrial fibrillation.
    b. Potassium and lidocaine are used for control of early postoperative arrhythmias.
    c. In some cases, procaine amide is administered for several months after surgery.
4. *Fluid and electrolyte balance must be maintained.*
    a. The patient receives nothing by mouth (mouth care is of course essential).
    b. The intravenous fluid, 5 per cent dextrose in water, is administered at the rate of 50 ml per hour (all I.V. fluids are included in this total).
    c. Packed red cells (pump blood) will be administered in 3 units in the first three hours.
    d. Intake and output are measured every 20 minutes.
    e. The Foley catheter is attached to constant drainage, and the amount of drainage is recorded every hour.
    f. The nasogastric tube is attached to intermittent suction. Patients with coronary artery disease may require larger volumes than would be expected for colloid replacement after surgery, owing to preoperative hypovolemia.
5. *Medications for pain are administered as necessary by intravenous route (morphine is the drug of choice).*
    a. Narcotics should be administered sparingly because of the danger of hypotension or respiratory depression. The intravenous route is the only acceptable route when cardiac output is low, because absorption by other routes may be prolonged, and subsequent doses may then suddenly have a cumulative effect. Morphine administered in doses of 2 to 4 mg at a time is usually satisfactory, although patients on respirators can tolerate much more, provided hypovolemia is not present. Some patients do not require narcotics, but most require small doses to enable them to breathe and cough effectively or to allay restlessness. A patient who becomes restless or apprehensive usually is *hypoxic,* in which case the administration of analgesics or sedatives is absolutely contraindicated.
    b. While the patient is on the respirator, nitrous oxide is administered to control agitation and pain in the immediate postoperative period.
6. *Removal of chest tubes, drains, and lines must be accompanied by appropriate therapy.* Chest tubes are removed on the first day after surgery, and the following procedures are initiated:
    a. Vigorous pulmonary physiotherapy is carried out every four hours.
    b. A heated nebulizer supplies oxygen through a face mask for 8 hours.
    c. Nasotracheal suctioning to prevent atelectasis is used as necessary.

All lines (except I.V. line source) are removed *before* the patient is transferred back to his assigned room on the clinical unit.

SUMMARY

The important areas of concern in the postoperative nursing care of the patient who has had coronary artery by-pass graft surgery include:
1. Extubation of the patient.
2. Monitoring blood pressure.
3. Assessing cardiac stability.
4. Facilitating removal of chest tubes as soon as possible.
5. Administering necessary fluids on the first day after surgery.
6. Providing 2 gm of sodium in the patient's diet when he is able to take fluids and solids.

Complications

Possible complications in the immediate postoperative period include:
1. Myocardial infarction.
a. Clotting of the new saphenous vein graft.
2. Serious ventricular arrhythmias and low cardiac output.
3. Hemorrhage from the incisional path in the chest.
4. Cardiac tamponade.
5. Pulmonary dysfunction.
6. Edema and phlebitis of the leg where the saphenous vein has been removed.

STUDY QUESTIONS

1. Review and discuss the pathology of coronary artery disease and its relationship to angina pectoris.

2. When is surgical therapy necessary in the management of angina pectoris?

3. Describe in detail the medical work-up the patient must have prior to cardiac surgery.

4. List the complications and related nursing care of the cardiac catheterization procedure for the left and right sides of the heart.

5. Is a coronary artery by-pass graft for angina pectoris performed under open-heart technique? Explain.

6. What preoperative teaching measures would you put in a nursing care plan for the patient anticipating a coronary artery by-pass graft?

7. What bearing would congestive heart failure have on whether the patient is chosen for cardiac surgery?

8. Prepare a *checklist* for the preoperative teaching of the patient scheduled for cardiac surgery.

9. Review and be able to define the laboratory tests the cardiac patient would have prior to surgery.

10. What should you tell a patient about his postoperative phase in the intensive care unit?

11. Review and compare the set-ups for chest tube drainage and mediastinal drainage.

12. What types of monitoring devices would be used in the intensive care unit to provide adequate care for the patient in the initial postoperative phase?

13. What arrhythmias would you expect or watch for in the initial postoperative phase? How could they best be treated?

14. What ramifications would the use of the cardiopulmonary by-pass machine during surgery have on the postoperative course of the patient?

15. Design a nursing care plan covering the first 2 days after open-heart surgery.

16. List the general complications which may occur in:
   a. the early postoperative period — up to and including the first day after surgery.
   b. the later postoperative period — from the second day after surgery to the tenth.

17. What psychological responses would you expect from the patient in the first few days after coronary artery by-pass surgery?

18. Make a list of all the drugs which could be used on the patient in the following periods:
   a. preoperative period.
   b. intraoperative phase.
   c. postoperative period.
Indicate why each drug would be used.

19. Review the care of the patient when:
   a. there is an endotracheal tube in place.
   b. he is on controlled breathing via a respirator.
   c. he is receiving anticoagulants postoperatively.
   d. an arterial line is in place.
   e. chest tubes and/or mediastinal tubes are in place.

74

Operation: Transthoracic Vagotomy

TYPICAL HISTORY

A 52-year-old male underwent a subtotal gastrectomy 10 years earlier for a duodenal ulcer. He was well until approximately 8 months prior to admission when he developed recurrent bouts of epigastric pain, heartburn, and belching. A repeat upper G.I. series at that time revealed the presence of a small new ulcer in the gastrojejunostomy stoma. He was placed on a strict ulcer regimen, but the symptoms persisted. At the time of the present admission, he developed anemia and had black, tarry stools. Repeat upper G.I. series revealed a large marginal ulcer in the gastro-jejunostomy stoma. He now enters for evaluation.

PHYSICAL EXAMINATION

The patient is a well-developed, thin male showing signs of recent weight loss.

Significant Findings

1. Pallor and weight loss are obvious.
2. There is tenderness in the epigastrium.
3. Dark stools.

DIAGNOSTIC STUDIES

1. Stool guaiac positive.
2. Liver function studies are normal.
3. Upper G.I. series reveals a marginal ulcer in the gastrojejunostomy stoma.

PROBABLE HOSPITAL COURSE

The patient has been treated conservatively for a recurrent marginal ulcer. The incidence of recurrence of an ulcer in the gastrojejunostomy stoma following subtotal gastrectomy varies from 2 to 10 per cent, depending on the series studied. Should the recurrence be mildly disabling with no evidence of significant bleeding, it can be treated medically, that is, with antispasmodics, antisecretagogues, and alkalis. However, should symptoms become intractable or bleeding recur, surgical intervention must be considered.

A gastric analysis may show a high acid output in spite of the previous subtotal gastrectomy. This indicates that the remnant of stomach left in place is still secreting high levels of acid. In such a case, resection of the vagus nerve may so diminish the acid output as to heal the ulcer and prevent further recurrence. The vagus nerve may be resected transabdominally as well as transthoracically. If no surgery other than vagotomy is contemplated at this time, the preferred approach is transthoracic. This is true for two reasons:

   a. The approach is not marred by any operative adhesions.
   b. Some feel that a more complete vagotomy can be done through the chest.

As soon as the patient's blood volume is brought to reasonably normal levels with transfusion, he may be prepared for transthoracic vagotomy.

PREPARATION FOR SURGERY

1. Levin tube is inserted preoperatively.
2. The patient is typed and cross-matched for three units of whole blood.
3. The skin is prepped down the left side of the chest, including the axilla and the upper abdomen and back. (See Introduction.)
4. A Fleet enema is given preoperatively.
5. *Premedications.* Routine.
6. *Special Medications.* None.
7. *Operating Room Skin Prep.* Includes the left axilla, left back, left chest, and left upper abdomen. (See Introduction.)
8. *Position.* Thoracotomy position with the right side down. (See Introduction.)

PATHOLOGY

There is, of course, no pathological condition found in the chest in association with this operation.

GENERAL RATIONALE AND SCHEME

The vagus nerves are responsible for the *cephalic phase* of gastric hydrochloric acid secretion. Sectioning of both vagus nerves will result in diminution of gastric acidity.

Scheme

1. The chest is opened through the seventh or eighth intercostal interspace.
2. The mediastinal pleura is incised and the vagus nerves are located as they pass in proximity to the esophagus.
3. Both vagus nerves are divided and a section is removed for pathological confirmation.
4. The chest is closed, a thoracic drainage tube being left in place.

PROCEDURE

1. *Skin Incision.* This is a short incision in the seventh or eighth interspace, extending from the anterior to the posterior axillary lines. (See Introduction.)

2. When the chest is opened, a rib retractor is put in place and the rib margins are separated.

3. The inferior pulmonary ligament is divided, allowing the lung to be retracted superiorly.

4. The mediastinal pleura is divided and separated, exposing the esophagus and vagus nerves.

5. Each vagus nerve is grasped with a nerve hook, clamped, divided, and ligated, a small segment of nerve being removed for pathological confirmation.

6. After the main trunks have been divided, the wall of the esophagus is carefully palpated for smaller branches, which should also be divided to complete the vagotomy.

7. A chest tube is placed in the thoracic cavity and brought out through a stab wound below the main incision.

8. A heavy dressing is applied.

SURGICAL HAZARDS

1. Incomplete division of the vagus nerve trunks at the diaphragm.

2. Injury to the spleen and liver.

3. Disruption of the esophageal hiatus, which can produce a hiatus hernia postoperatively.

4. General hazards of any other thoracotomy procedure, such as trauma to the lungs and heart.

POSTOPERATIVE MANAGEMENT

The patient is returned to the recovery room until sufficiently reactive from anesthesia. General postanesthetic measures are carried out. In addition:

1. The chest tube is connected to underwater-seal drainage. (See Introduction for management of chest tube.)

2. The dressing is checked for drainage and the surgeon is notified if bloody drainage soaks through the dressing.

3. The nasogastric tube may be removed the evening after surgery or the following morning.

4. The patient receives nothing by mouth; mouth care should be given at frequent intervals.

STUDY QUESTIONS

1. Define *marginal ulcer.*

2. Discuss the physiology of the vagus nerve with respect to gastric acid secretion.

3. Are there any other physiological mechanisms responsible for gastric acid secretion beside the vagus nerves? Describe these in detail.

4. What are the advantage and disadvantages of a thoracic vagotomy versus an abdominal vagotomy?

5. What is the Hollander test?

6. Describe the make-up and function of a nerve hook.

7. List the essential steps in the performance of transthoracic vagotomy, describing in particular the nurse's role in the operating room.

8. Following transthoracic vagotomy, the nurse notices a good deal of blood in the Levin tube. What are the possible causes of this blood in the Levin tube and what steps should she take?

9. Since the vagus nerves control the rate of cardiac function, are there any cardiac problems that could develop following total transthoracic vagotomy for recurrent ulcer of the stomach? If not, why not?

NEUROLOGICAL SURGERY

75

INTRODUCTION

AREAS OF CONCERN

Because the nervous system is diffused throughout the body, there are, strictly speaking, no boundaries and no limitations to the areas encompassed in the specialty of neurosurgery. Nevertheless, one can consider three separate areas of concern that occupy the neurosurgeon's attention: (1) the brain and cranial nerves, (2) the spinal cord, and (3) the peripheral somatic and sympathetic nerves.

The brain, housed in the thick-walled skull, is accessible only by the lifting of skull flaps, an approach which also serves to make the cranial nerves accessible for various neurosurgical procedures.

Most operative procedures on the back are directly related to the spinal cord or the vertebral column. The vertebral column houses the spinal cord, and all sensory and motor nerves to the neck, trunk, and extremities proceed from the spinal cord through the intervertebral foramina.

The most common symptom of back illness is back pain, either localized to a segment of the back or radiating in the direction of the nerve fibers involved. Frequently, this symptom arises following trauma, such as occurs in a whiplash injury of the neck which is received in an automobile accident. Ruptured intervertebral discs and arthritis of the cervical or dorsal spine, as well as spinal cord tumors, may also cause pain and disability in the back and extremities.

Because of the close relationship of bone to nerve structure in this area, back surgery is relegated to both the neurosurgeon and the orthopedic surgeon. Very frequently, a team of neurosurgeons and orthopedic surgeons performs jointly in the repair of a back injury or an ailment of the spinal cord. For example, it is quite common for a neurosurgeon to remove a ruptured intervertebral disc and then for an orthopedic surgeon to fuse the back in the area of the surgery.

The most common locations for intervertebral disc rupture are in the cervical and lumbar spine. In this section of the book, a typical lumbar disc operation will be described (Chapter 76).

Neurosurgery involves so many distinct procedures marked by so many special features that an introductory overview is impossible. Accordingly, various principles of surgery will be presented with each particular procedure in the chapters ahead.

Operation: Excision of Ruptured Disc

TYPICAL HISTORY

A 48-year-old muscular male has had recurring attacks of acute back pain. Approximately 4 years ago, he noted the sudden onset of acute left low back pain while lifting a heavy object. He fell to the ground and was unable to raise himself. He was brought into the hospital and placed on complete bed rest for 4 weeks. The pain gradually subsided, he was able to ambulate, and he returned to work after an additional 6 weeks of convalescence. On the present admission, he states that the pains now migrate down the left buttock along the left calf and into the foot. He also states that he has had some weakness in the left ankle and knee for approximately 6 months.

PHYSICAL EXAMINATION

A well-developed, heavy, muscular male is admitted complaining of acute back pain and lying quietly in bed.

Significant Findings

1. There is acute tenderness over the lower lumbar spine and some associated spasm of the back musculature.
2. When the patient's legs are raised passively, the right leg can be raised to 50 degrees, with some low back discomfort. The left leg can be raised only to 10 degrees, with extreme low backache and pain radiating down the left thigh and calf.
3. There are diminished knee and ankle reflexes on the left side.
4. The remainder of the physical examination is unremarkable.

DIAGNOSTIC STUDIES

X-ray studies should be deferred until the patient's general condition permits. Submitting him to several x-ray studies at this time would be most uncomfortable for him and would not alter the mode of therapy.

The history and physical examination in this particular case are classic for a ruptured lumbar disc and neurological examination will aid the surgeon in determining exactly which one has been

461

ruptured. Commonly, it is the disc between lumbar vertebrae L4 and L5 or the disc between lumbar vertebrae L5 and L6.

If the surgeon is unable to determine with certainty the location and existence of a ruptured disc, the patient may be submitted to myelographic study.

PROBABLE HOSPITAL COURSE

Because of the long history of recurrent back pain, the patient is suitable for surgical excision of his ruptured disc. If, in the surgeon's judgment, disc surgery is definitely indicated, the patient will be prepared as soon as his general condition permits; on the other hand, if the surgeon feels that a trial of conservative therapy is indicated, the patient may be placed on complete bed rest and on a bedboard, given analgesics and antispasmodics, and observed for 3 to 4 weeks to see if any significant improvement occurs.

PREPARATION FOR SURGERY

1. *Levin Tube.* Not necessary unless the patient has developed significant vomiting due to paralytic ileus.

2. The patient is typed and cross-matched for two units of whole blood.

3. The skin preparation should include the entire lower back from the level of the scapulae down to the buttocks. The skin preparation extends out laterally to the flanks.

4. A Fleet or soapsuds enema is given on the evening prior to surgery.

5. *Premedications.* None.

6. *Special Medications.* None.

7. *Operating Room Skin Prep.* This extends from the level of the scapulae down to the buttocks and out laterally to both flanks.

8. *Positioning.* Surgery is usually done with the patient in the horizontal position, face down.

PATHOLOGY

A disc is a small compressible, fibrous, cartilaginous cushion between the bodies of adjacent vertebrae and provides some elasticity and compressibility to the spinal column. Under normal conditions, this disc is held between the bodies by a strong cartilaginous rim or ridge. Under certain types of stress, the ridge may split, thus permitting the disc to herniate between two vertebral bodies. This protrusion of an intervertebral disc causes compression of the nerves to the back and leg which results in sciatica or root pain.

GENERAL RATIONALE AND SCHEME

Most protruding or herniated discs respond to conservative therapy. The patient is placed on bed rest and given analgesics and antispasmodics. The edema around the disc soon subsides and the disc decreases in size and slides back into the intervertebral area. With care and continued rest, the patient may not have another episode of disc pain. However, when recurrence of acute symptoms is frequent, causing a good deal of work disability, the disc should be surgically excised.

Scheme

1. A vertical incision is made over the appropriate intervertebral body spaces.
2. The lamellae or arches of the vertebrae are removed.
3. The disc material is shelled out.
4. The back is closed with or without fusion.

PROCEDURE

1. *Skin Incision.* This is a vertical incision made over two or three spinous processes in the region of the suspected ruptured disc.

2. The paraspinal muscles and their attachments are dissected free of the spinous processes and retracted laterally with a self-retaining retractor. Bleeding is usually controlled with an electrocoagulating device.

3. The laminae overlying the ruptured disc are excised with rongeur forceps. The offending disc material is next removed with use of spatulas and forceps. The disc material must be removed entirely so that there is no compression of nerve roots.

4. At the conclusion of the disc excision, the surgeon must decide whether fusion is necessary. Usually this is not required.

5. The self-retaining retractors are removed and the paraspinous muscles are allowed to slip back into place. Bleeding is controlled with electrocoagulation and use of Gelfoam. Subcutaneous tissue and skin are closed with interrupted sutures and a heavy dressing is applied.

SURGICAL HAZARDS

1. The most significant surgical hazard is injury to motor roots, which can result in paralysis.
2. Bleeding from epidural veins must be avoided, as this may be difficult to control.

POSTOPERATIVE MANAGEMENT

The patient is returned to the recovery room until he is sufficiently reactive from the anesthetic. General postanesthetic management is carried out. In addition:

1. Motion and circulation in the extremities should be checked each time the vital signs are taken. Check dorsalis pedis and posterior tibial pulses.

2. The patient is turned from side to side and kept off his back. Special care must be taken when moving the patient. Log rolling is essential. Maintenance of good body alignment is necessary in all positions while the patient is in bed.

3. Urinary distention should be anticipated and, if it occurs, a Foley catheter should be inserted and connected to dependent drainage.

4. The patient is allowed liquids as tolerated when he is alert and all his vital signs are stable.

5. Large doses of narcotics may be needed for control of pain.

6. Ace bandages may have been applied to the lower extremities at the time of surgery. Check to see when these may be safely removed.

7. The condition of the body skin should be checked immediately upon the patient's arrival in the recovery room, because the lengthy operating time may have contributed to the formation of pressure areas during surgery.

8. Check patient's ability to void within the 8 to $10°$ limit. The patient may need to be catheterized in the immediate postoperative period and be placed on Foley catheter drainage.

STUDY QUESTIONS

1. Discuss sciatica, listing several medical as well as surgical causes of this condition.

2. What is the anatomy of the intervertebral disc and intervertebral space? Discuss particularly how a disc causes root pain.

3. What is the medical management of a ruptured intervertebral disc?

4. How often and under what conditions do you think surgery for intervertebral disc herniation is necessary?

5. Discuss the essential steps in the excision of a herniated disc.

6. Discuss a nursing plan for the postoperative management and convalescence of a patient who has undergone removal of a herniated disc. How does this plan change if spinal fusion has been carried out?

7. Why is it important to check circulation and motion of the extremities in the postoperative period?

77

THE PATIENT WITH A SUBARACHNOID HEMORRHAGE

Operation: Craniotomy with Clipping of Cerebral Aneurysm (of Circle of Willis)

TYPICAL HISTORY

A 52-year-old female, in good general health, was washing dishes when she experienced the sudden onset of an excruciating bilateral occipital headache which then became generalized and was shortly followed by collapse.

She was hospitalized immediately and was noted to have a stiff neck. A lumbar puncture was performed.

Past history revealed tension headaches.

PHYSICAL EXAMINATION

The patient is a lethargic woman breathing rapidly and complaining of severe headaches.

Significant Findings

1. *Vital Signs.* Early hypertension may occur at the time of rupture of the aneurysm; later the blood pressure may be normal. Pulse and respirations are often increased, and temperature may be mildly elevated.

2. *Mental Status.* The patient is lethargic, poorly oriented to place and time, and is complaining of severe headache.

3. *Ophthalmological Examination.* The pupils are equal and of normal size, and react sluggishly to light. Extraocular movements are full and conjugate. No field cut is demonstrated Funduscopic examination reveals many subhyaloid hemorrhages.

4. *Neurological Examination.* No focal motor or sensory deficits are detectable. Deep tendon reflexes are generally depressed. No pathological reflexes are elicited.

5. *Lumbar Puncture.* Initial pressure usually is high. Cerebrospinal fluid is grossly bloody and when spun down reveals a xanthochromic supernatant.

DIAGNOSTIC STUDIES

1. The patient's history and the physical and neurological examinations should immediately suggest the diagnosis of a subarachnoid hemorrhage. These studies will often give clues as to the location of the ruptured aneurysm.

2. Lumbar puncture, revealing bloody spinal fluid under increased pressure, confirms the clinical suspicion.

3. Angiography, which is highly accurate, is the definitive study. At a minimum bilateral carotid angiography should be performed. The vertebral arteries should be studied if necessary.

4. Additionally, skull x-rays, electroencephalogram, and echoencephalogram may be performed, but these studies are rarely diagnostic and only occasionally of significant value.

PROBABLE HOSPITAL COURSE

The patient is placed at rest in a semi-darkened room. She is kept mildly sedated and is carefully observed for signs of any recurrent hemorrhage. The diet is soft, and tea and coffee are avoided. Bowel softeners may be used. If the patient is deeply stuporous, aspiration and pneumonia are prevented by frequent suctioning and by use of the nasogastric tube.

Lumbar punctures are performed several times until the cerebrospinal fluid pressure is less than 200 to 250 mm.

When the patient becomes alert, surgery should follow. The best results will be achieved by waiting long enough for the patient's condition to improve — i.e., until she is alert and the spinal fluid pressure has returned to normal. The operation should follow, usually about one week after admission, so that it is performed before another hemorrhage occurs.

PREPARATION FOR SURGERY

1. *Psychological Preparation.* A very limited explanation, sufficient to answer the patient's questions about her condition and to allay her anxiety, is offered. However, some responsible member of the family must have a complete understanding of the magnitude and severity of the condition. Specific fears and myths about the shaving of the scalp, cosmetic location of scars, and brain surgery in general are discussed and explained.

2. A general medical evaluation of the cardiopulmonary and renal systems is carried out and any specific problems (e.g., pneumonia or anemia) are corrected, if possible.

3. The patient is typed and cross-matched for 6 to 10 units of whole blood.

4. A Levin tube and enema are rarely necessary.

5. A Foley catheter is inserted.

6. The entire head is shaved.

7. Routine premedication is ordered by the anesthesiologist; no special premedications are necessary.

8. The patient is positioned by the operating surgeon.

9. The standard skin prep for a craniotomy is performed.

PATHOLOGY

So-called "berry" or saccular aneurysms are congenital and usually occur at branches or junctions of vessels when a defect in the media of the vessel wall is present. Ninety-five per cent occur in the anterior part of the Circle of Willis and only five per cent in the posterior portion (Fig. 77–1).

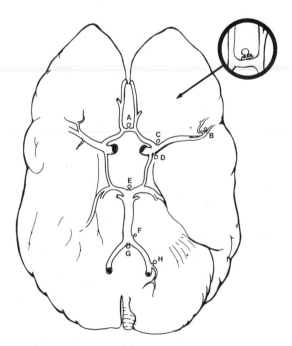

FIGURE 77–1 Multiple sites (A to H) for cerebral aneurysms. The inset shows a clip applied at the neck of an aneurysm to prevent future rupture. *Question:* Can you name the parent vessel for each of the aneurysms shown in this drawing?

Signs and Most Frequent Locations of Specific Cerebral Aneurysms

The findings on neurological examination will vary with the site of the aneurysm and the severity of the hemorrhage (Fig. 77–1).

Internal carotid artery aneurysms (at the branching-off of the posterior communicating artery) often compress nerve III, which passes nearby, resulting in a fixed, dilated pupil on the same side as the aneurysm; in addition, the eye cannot turn toward the nose.

Anterior communicating artery aneurysms may have no localizing signs or may produce profound coma, depending on whether the vessels to the hyopthalamus are affected.

Middle cerebral artery aneurysms cause contralateral hemiparesis in many cases, as they often hemorrhage into adjacent brain tissue.

Together, the three above aneurysms account for 95 per cent of all cerebral aneurysms.

Posterior circulation aneurysms, situated in the vertebral and basilar arteries and their branches, account (approximately) for the remaining 5 per cent. These aneurysms may demonstrate no localizing signs or, in some cases, may produce deep coma.

Multiple aneurysms must always be considered. They probably occur in 20 per cent of all cases of cerebral aneurysms.

GENERAL RATIONALE AND SCHEME

Cerebral aneurysms are the result of defects in the vessel walls of various cerebral arteries. There aneurysms generally grow and produce no symptoms until they suddenly rupture, with the attendant typical history and findings, as depicted here.

If the patient survives the initial subarachnoid hemorrhage, and comes to medical attention, it is imperative that the diagnosis be developed immediately so that proper treatment may be instituted; any suspicions of ruptured aneurysm must be investigated. If left untreated, approximately 65 per cent of patients who survive the initial hemorrhage will succumb to a subsequent one, in most cases within a month. In less than 10 years, the mortality rate for aneurysm surgery has decreased from over 30 per cent to less than 3 per cent.

Scheme

1. The patient is appropriately positioned on the operating table.
2. The craniotomy flap is turned so as to permit exposure of the aneurysm.
3. The aneurysm is prevented from future hemorrhage through suitable procedures (depending on the degree of access to the aneurysm).
4. The craniotomy is closed.
5. A bulky, occlusive dressing is applied.

PROCEDURE

Most aneurysms can be treated through a standard fronto-temporal craniotomy flap, as will be described here.

1. A curvilinear incision is made from above the eyebrow to in front of the ear.
2. The galea and temporalis muscles are similarly incised.
3. Four or five burr holes are made. These holes, arranged in a circular pattern, are then connected with saw cuts. The bone flap then hinges on the base of the temporalis muscle.

4. The dura is opened and the frontal lobe gently elevated. The neck of the aneurysm is identified by following along the parent vessel.

5. If dissecting surgery can free the neck of the aneurysm, a metallic clip is placed across the base of the lesion (see inset in Fig. 77-1). If this is not technically feasible, then the aneurysm may be coated with a fast-setting plastic to prevent further enlargement and future rupture.

6. On some occasions the afferent vessel must be ligated in order to reduce the pressure and the flow in an aneurysm that can be neither clipped nor coated.

7. The frontal lobe retractors are removed; the surgeon must be very meticulous in achieving hemostasis at this stage.

8. The dura is closed.

9. The craniotomy is closed. Use of drains depends on the circumstances and on the surgeon's preference.

10. A standard, bulky dressing is applied to the head.

Adjuncts to Surgery

Modern surgical techniques and instruments, along with improved anesthetics and drug therapy, have combined to effect a tenfold decrease in surgical mortality in less than 10 years.

Corticosteroids. These drugs reduce the preoperative and postoperative increase in intracranial pressure brought on by cerebral edema.

Anticonvulsants. These agents reduce the incidence of pre- and postoperative seizures.

Anesthetic Drugs. Fluothane, Penthrane, Ethrane, and Innovar make the course of surgery smoother, both during the operation and afterward.

Cerebral Dehydrating Agents. The trauma of retraction of the brain is reduced by spinal drainage, which is used to collapse the ventricles, and by Mannitol, Urea, and Glycerol.

Magnification and Improved Illumination. The operating microscope, lamps, and headlamps all markedly improve visualization with less retraction of the brain.

SURGICAL HAZARDS

1. Rupture of aneurysm during dissection and clipping.
2. Spasm of adjacent vessels as a result of manipulation.
3. Cerebral infarction due to occlusion of vessels and/or excessive retraction.

POSTOPERATIVE MANAGEMENT

The patient is transferred to the recovery room, where she is observed until her condition is stable. She is then sent to the intensive care unit for further observation. The anesthesiologist will extubate the patient when the level of consciousness, tidal volume, and return of gag reflexes permit. Extubation may be delayed in the event of persistent coma, in which case the patient may require a tracheostomy.

Maintenance of a good airway with careful attention to suctioning techniques is important, in light of the reaction of the brain to hypoxia: there is an increase in cerebral edema and, secondarily, an increase in intracranial pressure.

1. Skin care, positioning, suctioning, evaluation of vital signs, recording of intake and output, and monitoring of other appropriate laboratory data are as important in this patient as in any other postoperative patient.

2. The neurological evaluation is of critical importance and may be charted on a graph or flow sheet so that trends in the patient's condition may be noted early.

    a. Mental Status.

        (1) Level of Alertness — described in standard, unambiguous terms, such as alert, lethargic, stuporous, comatose — *not* "pretty alert" or "talks ok." Critically ill patients should be examined jointly by incoming and outgoing personnel (as shifts change) so that there is no breakdown in communication.

        (2) Orientation — to person, place, and time.

        (3) Speech — normal, dysphasic, or dysarthric.

    b. Pupils.

        (1) Size — measured in mm.

        (2) Equality.

        (3) Reaction — brisk, sluggish, fixed.

    c. Extraocular movements are evaluated along many lines: are they full? Are they conjugate? Are they abnormal? If so, in what way? For example, does the left or right eye show failure to abduct or adduct?

    d. Paresis or Paralysis

        (1) Area — face, tongue, arm, or leg.

        (2) Side — left or right.

        (3) Degree — slight, moderate, severe, complete.

    e. Dressings and (if present) drains should be checked for any sudden increase in staining or drainage. The surgeon should be notified if such a change occurs, because this may be an early warning sign of recurrent bleeding.

3. The head of the bed may be elevated 30 to 45 degrees, but the surgeon may order a higher or lower range of elevation.

4. The patient must be positioned so that she does not lie on her incision.

5. Large amounts of potent analgesics are both unnecessary and undesirable. Usually, aspirin and codeine will suffice. Narcotics cloud the sensorium, affect pupillary responses, and depress respiration.

6. The Foley catheter may be removed when the level of consciousness warrants a test of spontaneous voiding.

7. Intravenous fluids should be continued until oral intake is adequate and no intravenous medications are being administered. Liquids may be given by mouth when the patient is sufficiently alert, and the diet may be advanced as tolerated. Prolonged stupor or coma may require alimentation via nasogastric tube or gastrostomy.

8. The patient may be allowed to sit up in a chair and then ambulated as soon as her physical and neurological condition permits.

Certain *postoperative complications* must be anticipated, and discovery of these complications should be as rapid as possible. The complications include:

1. *Postoperative Hemorrhage.* The clip may slip from the neck or re-bleeding may occur from a coagulated blood vessel. Any sudden or progressive alteration in level of consciousness or the development of focal neurological deficits should suggest bleeding. Sudden or progressive drainage or staining of dressings may also herald a re-bleed.

2. *Vasospasm.* Progressive focal or diffuse spasm of one or more intracranial vessels may occur as the result of manipulation of vessels or as a response to the release of catecholamines subsequent to the breakdown of blood. Vasospasm leads to diminished cerebral blood flow, and a stroke-like picture develops. The patient usually shows a slow, progressive worsening of the level of consciousness; occasionally, focal neurological deficits are evident.

3. *Communicating Hydrocephalus.* There may be a blockage in the mechanism for absorption of cerebrospinal fluid that is caused by high blood and protein levels in the fluid. The

patient fails to improve or there is a worsening of mental status in the days and weeks following surgery.

4. Electrolyte abnormalities, including diabetes insipidus and the condition associated with inappropriate release of antidiuretic hormone, may be present.

STUDY QUESTIONS

1. Discuss the anatomy of the circle of Willis.

2. What are the dangers of cerebral angiography?

3. Discuss the etiology and the signs and symptoms of diabetes insipidus that develops after surgery for a ruptured aneurysm.

4. Discuss the etiology and the signs and symptoms of inappropriate release of antidiuretic hormone following aneurysm surgery.

78   THE PATIENT WITH HEAD TRAUMA

Operation: Osteoplastic Craniotomy, Repair of Dural Tear, and Reduction of Facial Fracture

TYPICAL HISTORY

A 19-year-old student was driving a car at night. He lost control of the car, and it turned over three times. The police and firefighters extricated him from the car and brought him by stretcher to a rural hospital in a resort area. He is conscious but confused on admission to the emergency room.

PHYSICAL EXAMINATION

The patient is a well-developed, well-nourished male. He is tense, frightened, and seemingly in a confused state in the aftermath of his accident. He holds his hand over a large contused area on his forehead. He is bleeding severely from his nose.

Significant Findings

1. Fresh blood flowing from his nose and mouth.
2. A large contusion on his forehead.
3. A palpable fracture of the left zygoma, with flattening and depression of the left cheek.
4. Superficial abrasions evident on his back and abdomen.
5. Subconjunctival hemorrhage.
6. The patient is alert but frightened and confused.
7. The patient has a fractured mandible which prevents the teeth from meeting properly.

DIAGNOSTIC STUDIES

1. The results of the neurological examination are within normal limits at the time of admission, except for numbness of the left upper lip and the left side of the nose, upper gum, and teeth.
2. Routine laboratory work is normal.
3. Skull films show a fracture curving over the left orbit and extending medially and inferiorly, becoming comminuted as it enters the orbit medially.

PROBABLE HOSPITAL COURSE

The patient was admitted to the hospital and observed for 48 hours. Early efforts were concentrated on maintaining a free airway, which at times was difficult because of extensive bleeding into his mouth and nasopharynx. The patient remained conscious; his temperature ranged between 99 and 100°F. All other vital signs remained stable. Bleeding slowly diminished over the next 8 hours. A large hematoma of the frontal area developed. He was placed on antibiotics. His condition was reevaluated after the initial 48 hours and it was decided to transfer the patient to a large metropolitan hospital where neurosurgery could be carried out. Thus, his initial emergency treatment was geared to preparing him to be transferred to the larger medical facility where definitive surgery could be performed.

When he arrived at the medical center, another history and examination was performed. At this time the examining doctor determined that the patient had been unconscious for the first 7 hours after his accident. His left eye was swollen; his jaw hurt him a great deal and his breathing was difficult. There was decreased sensation on the lateral side of the left nose and left upper lip (hypesthesia).

At present, the patient is in no obvious acute distress. He has pain under his left eye when the zygomatic arch is pressed. There is now slight proptosis of the right eye. Diplopia is present on lateral deviation. His nose is displaced and he breathes poorly. He is unable to open or close his mouth fully without pain. He is oriented to time, place, and person. Motor power is equal and normal in all extremities.

It is recommended that the patient have tomography of the face. This x-ray technique is performed to reveal the condition of structures lying in a predetermined plane of tissue. It eliminates details in images of structures in other planes. It is a particularly helpful diagnostic tool in evaluating the condition of the facial sinuses.

X-rays of the skull, sinus, and facial bones reveal extensive comminuted fractures of the left frontal bone extending across the root of the nose and backwards through the roof and posterior wall of the orbit, which is buckled. There are fractures of the nasal bones with displacement of the right nasal bone toward the midline. There is diastasis of the left zygomatic frontal suture. There are fractures through both maxillary antra with considerable posterior displacement of the left maxillary antrum. There is a fracture of and through the horizontal ramus of the mandible to the left of the midline. The petrous bones of the skull are not involved. There is poor pneumatization of the ethmoid sinuses.

The decision is made by all concerned to perform corrective cranial and facial surgery on the patient.

PREPARATION FOR SURGERY

1. *Physical and Psychological Preparation.* It may be of help to the patient if the various procedures he will undergo and the equipment that is to be used postoperatively are explained to him in the preoperative phase. Tell him that he will have his head shaved (or in the case of the female patient, that hair will be clipped and then the head shaved). This hair will be saved for cosmetic reasons postoperatively. A wig can be used for the female during this postoperative period, since it takes a full year for complete regrowth of hair on the head. The postoperative dressing can be covered by a helmet, usually made of cloth.

The amount of pain the patient will experience after surgery will not be as great as he anticipates. He should be told that he will have a headache, but it will be relieved with analgesic medication. Analgesia will be administered as he requests it.

The chest physical therapist should be notified to see the patient. The patient can then be taught adequate coughing and deep-breathing routines in order to prevent pulmonary complications.

The patient is told that he will remain in the recovery room anywhere from several hours to one day after surgery. Explain how the unit will be set up. Padded side rails, oxygen equipment, and vital signs can be explained in such a way as to impress upon the patient their significance and importance. He may have a Foley catheter in place and be given I.V. fluids after surgery. He can be told that changes in his level of consciousness are to be expected during this time. He may experience or be aware of hallucinations, being confused, or feeling lethargic. If he has muscular twitches, medication (Dilantin) can be administered to control these motions. He may need eye care during this period, since he probably will have one swollen eye on the side of the incision and the trauma. Usually, ice will be applied to the area to help reduce the edema and resulting discomfort. He will be on bed rest for the first 2 days postoperatively. After that time, he will be allowed to ambulate, barring no complications.

Signs such as pupillary constriction and dilatation will be assessed with the use of a flashlight to accurately determine the ability of the eyes to react upon exposure to bright light. Level of consciousness will be determined by asking the patient pertinent questions that relate to the day, time, his name, and where he is. Checking grasp on both hands will be done at frequent intervals.

The surgeon will explain thoroughly why surgery is necessary and what he hopes to accomplish by these procedures. The risk involved and any expected sequelae should be explored at this same time. The dental arch bars and the need for wires and elastics to be attached to the teeth should be discussed with the patient. The patient will be unable to open his mouth to eat solid foods, and his diet will therefore consist solely of enriched liquids for 4 to 6 weeks.

2. *Type and Cross-match.* Four units of blood are to be available for these surgical procedures.

3. *Enema.* Not necessary.

4. *Food and Fluids.* Withheld from the evening before surgery on; if surgery is taking place later in the day, a 6- to 8-hour fast is necessary.

5. *Premedications.* Atropine.

6. *Special Medications.* For patients with head injuries, or those patients with increased intracranial pressure, narcotics are *not* administered. Hypotensive drugs may be given to those

patients with increased intracranial pressure to relieve the condition by decreasing the blood pressure. These drugs also help to decrease the restlessness that is seen when this pressure is increased. Dilantin is administered when a seizure is anticipated. Sedation may be administered to patients who shiver; this mechanism, if allowed to continue, elevates body temperature. This can directly affect the brain by increasing its basal metabolic rate, thus utilizing more oxygen and glucose as nutrients and increasing the work load of an already traumatized and edematous brain. *No* drugs are given to a patient who is already drowsy. Administration of drugs may mask the true level of consciousness in these patients.

7. *Operating Room Skin Prep.* The hair is usually shaved and the skin prepared by the neurosurgeon in the O.R. on the day of surgery. This hair is considered a "valuable" item. It is returned with the patient to his ward and usually kept locked up in the event that it is needed (for the patient who dies postoperatively or for cosmetic reasons later on). Preparation of the site at the time of surgery with the patient anesthetized minimizes psychic trauma and ensures prevention of infection that may occur if the scalp is lacerated during shaving the day or evening prior to surgery.

8. *Position.* The patient is placed on the table in a supine position with his head rotated to the opposite side; he may also be placed in a sitting position with his head supported. Selection of a position depends on the site of incision and the wishes of the surgeon.

PATHOLOGY

For the patient with cerebrocranial head trauma, evaluation and interpretation of presenting signs and symptoms must be repeated at frequent intervals. Diagnostic studies appropriate to the type of injury suspected must be interspersed with frequent observation of vital signs and the level of consciousness. If angiography is to be undertaken, it will be done bilaterally. The incidence of shock in these patients is rare; it may occur if there has been a large scalp laceration or in the person who has received multiple trauma to the viscera or who has fractured bones elsewhere.

It must be remembered that a skull fracture is not a single entity. Rather, it is a complex type of injury which may also involve the scalp, dura, cranial nerves, and cerebral tissues. Fractures may produce deviations in arterial, venous, intracranial, and cerebrospinal fluid circulation.

Ten per cent of all craniocerebral injuries are skull fractures that are amenable to surgical treatment. The optimal time for this type of surgery is generally anywhere from 3 to 6 hours after the trauma has been received. However, surgery may be delayed 24 hours or longer. This should be the case until proper personnel and facilities are available to care for the patient with severe trauma. A patient who has signs and symptoms of shock would also be a candidate for delayed surgery.

A skull fracture usually is accompanied by a dural tear. This tear may extend into the cerebral tissues, or the ventricle, thus establishing a sinus, allowing the passage of air, fluid, and contaminants (such as hair, dirt, and bacteria) to enter. Rhinorrhea may accompany a skull fracture through the frontal sinus. In this instance, pneumocephalus develops. Only 2 to 5 per cent of all skull fractures develop discharge from the nose or middle ear (otorrhea) following head injury. When this happens, the patient complains of severe headache. Infection and meningitis are potential hazards.

Treatment of a depressed and compound or comminuted skull fracture will be surgical as soon as the patient's condition permits. If such is the case, a craniotomy must be performed to remove the bone fragments and repair the dural tear perfectly. The incidence of infection and damage to the brain will be decreased if the surgery is performed as close to the time of injury as possible.

Facial trauma *involving the zygoma* may be the result of injury to the frontal bone, maxilla, or temporal bone. When there is a fracture of the zygoma, facial contour and function as well as the continuity of the orbital floor are jeopardized. Treatment may be a simple reduction of the zygoma articulations with adjacent bones. This can be done under local anesthesia. Most zygomatic fractures compound into the maxillary antrum. A hematoma will collect in this cavity. Any displacement of the zygoma will disrupt the bony orbit. In most instances the orbit will become elongated. The eyeball will fall downward as a result of the inferior displacement of the floor of the cavity. A patient with a zygomatic fracture must be examined closely for eye injury. The possibility of a globe rupture, intraocular hemorrhage, or retinal detachment must be pursued. The eye, then, is the most important structure in the area of zygomatic fracture. Alterations in vision should be recorded and reported.

Signs and symptoms of a zygomatic fracture include:

1. Diplopia or blurring due to eyeball displacement.
2. Paresthesia or anesthesia of the upper lip, ala, upper alveolus, and teeth due to injury to the infraorbital nerve.
3. Inability to open and close the mouth because of impingement of the depressed zygoma upon the coronoid process of the mandible.
4. Contusion, abrasion, or laceration of the cheek.
5. Loss of cheek symmetry due to depression.
6. Emphysema of the cheek owing to air coming from the maxillary antrum into the wound.
7. Eyeball at a lower level on the affected side due to a fracture of the orbital floor and inferior displacement of the orbital fat.
8. Impairment of the eyeball muscle movements as a result of involvement of the nerve supply or pressure on the part from a collection of blood (hematoma) or edema of the involved parts, as well as entrapment of eye muscles in orbital floor fracture.
9. Nasal bleeding on the injured side due to an associated fracture of the maxillary sinus, involving a mucosal tear and bleeding into the nasal cavity.

Management of Penetrating, Craniocerebral Trauma

There are three principles in the over-all plan of care for this type of trauma:

1. *Early, radical debridement with primary closure of the wound.* This will be the usual treatment. If a craniocerebral injury is not recognized initially, and therapy is delayed, complete resection and closure should be undertaken as soon as a diagnosis of this type of injury is made, disregarding the time that has elapsed. The price to be paid for this delay may be a greater chance of infection occurring in the wound.

2. *Prevention of intracranial hemorrhage.* There may be a hematoma formation at or in the site of the injury. This will exert pressure on the surrounding tissues and be the source of undue damage through this direct pressure. It is imperative that definitive neurosurgical therapy be performed within hours after a wound of this type is received.

3. *Prevention of infection.* This complication may be the result of retained bone fragments at the time of injury. The attending neurosurgeon will remove all metallic or other foreign bodies wherever they may be lodged, unless their removal would endanger the patient. If these fragments are allowed to remain, they may be always a potential source of infection.

In the event that there is a combination of penetrating craniocerebral and maxillofacial trauma, a tracheostomy may be performed to insure adequate ventilation and removal of respiratory secretions.

GENERAL RATIONALE AND SCHEME

The diagnosis of a compound, depressed skull fracture with some enophthalmus (recession of the eyeball into the orbit) and prolapse of the left eye will necessitate a craniotomy. This procedure is done to extract the bone fragments that are present and to repair an existing dural tear. A craniectomy can be performed if the incision is put in the temporal region. This type of procedure (where the cranial skull bone is not replaced) can be done here because there is strong, thick muscle covering the skull at this site.

The removal of bony fragments of the fracture is a very important procedure for the patient's well-being. Cerebral abscesses occur in 50 per cent of these patients if these particles are not removed. During the procedure, comminuted portions of the bone will be preserved. Only fragments of particles of bone that have become entirely detached from tissue will be removed. The frontonasal ducts of the sinuses will not be touched; no drains will be used. This decreases the development of infection postoperatively. The typical contour of the frontal sinus will be reestablished. This will be done by gentle manipulation and traction. The less surgery on the frontal sinus, the better. Mucous membrane of the area (cavity) regenerates freely and re-forms its own air pockets during the healing phase. The defects in the other facial bones will be repaired at a later date. Corrective surgery should be postponed for several months after the craniotomy in order to decrease the possibility of sepsis that may occur if the procedure is undertaken too soon after the first operation.

The dural tear must be repaired to stop the possible flow of cerebrospinal fluid and to close off a potential route of infection.

Scheme

1. The original area of injury is incised with a curved incision.
2. The scalp and skull are opened in the usual fashion in this area.
3. Fragments of bone are debrided.
4. Hemostasis will be accomplished perfectly.
5. Possible dural tear will be sutured.
6. The skull and scalp are closed.
7. A compression bandage is applied.

A fractured zygoma will require no special treatment if there is minimal displacement or no associated diplopia. However, usually there are multiple fractures of the maxillary sinus with formation of a hematoma within the antrum. This is often associated with comminuted fractures of the orbit and loss of eyeball support. In severe injuries, the orbital soft tissues are displaced in the maxillary antrum. A fracture of the orbital floor should be treated. Initially, the patient may be asymptomatic. Deformities of the orbit may be the result, if herniation of the fatty tissue of the orbit is not replaced. Alterations in vision must be observed, recorded, and reported to the doctor. A reduction of a zygomatic fracture can be done 7 to 14 days after the injury is received with little or no effects on the patient.

SURGICAL PROCEDURE

Craniotomy

1. Radical excision of all layers of the scalp, inclusive of the periosteum.
2. Craniectomy with resection of all depressed and comminuted bone fragments:
a. Enbloc, excision of the area of the depression and comminution.
b. Open dura to see if there is a subdural or subcortical pathological condition.
3. Excision of dural edges. Point of the dural laceration should not be disturbed until the area has been well exposed. All clots are evacuated. All comminuted bone fragments are removed.

4. Resection of all devitalized and involved brain tissue:

a. Suction and electrocoagulation are used, or

b. Clip and cut method.

5. Removal of all in-driven bone fragments. This is done to prevent infection. It is usually done manually to detect small bone fragments with the sense of touch.

6. A water-tight dural closure is done. A graft of pericranium, temporal fascia, or fascia lata may be needed. This is done to prevent meningeal and intracerebral spread of superficial scalp infection. It is also done to prevent cerebral herniation. Herniation is not likely with small dural tears. Seizures postoperatively may be due to incarceration of a small cortical segment within a very small dural tear.

7. Primary closure of the scalp in individual layers. A scalp rotation flap may be needed.

Reduction of the Zygoma

In most instances, open reduction of a fractured zygoma is accomplished by one or two incisions; the first is made at the lateral end of the brow to provide access to the zygomaticofrontal suture line; the second is made at the inferior margin of the lower lid to permit exposure of the infraorbital rim and inspection of the orbital floor. Direct wiring of the fractures at the frontozygomatic suture and infraorbital rim can be accomplished after the depressed zygoma is made directly visible through both of these incisions. By placing a large, closed, curved hemostat under the zygoma through the brow incision, the bone is elevated until the normal contour of the cheek is restored. Wire sutures are placed at the fracture sites.

The orbital floor can be reconstructed if necessary by placing a silastic implant or a cartilage graft.

SURGICAL HAZARDS

1. Direct brain damage or intracranial bleeding.

2. Severe optic nerve and eyeball injury during zygoma fracture elevation.

3. Infraorbital nerve damage. This nerve runs directly through the maxilla. Damage to this nerve may result in altered sensation or complete anesthesia of the ala (lower extended portions of the wall of the nose).

POSTOPERATIVE MANAGEMENT

1. Check on the operative sheet or the anesthesia record to find out where the incision has been made on the head. Note what type of craniotomy has been performed. If a bone flap has been removed, keep the patient's head off the operative site.

2. Be sure his head is kept elevated for the most part on a plane of 30 to 45 degrees. This maneuver will help venous return of cerebral circulation and facilitate proper respiratory excursions.

3. Suction respiratory secretions as necessary. Rhonchi and dyspnea are indications for this procedure. Beware of increasing the patient's intracranial pressure with aggressive suctioning procedures.

4. One eye may swell postoperatively. Cold may be applied with an ice bag. Methylcellulose may be instilled to keep the sclera and conjuctiva moist. Normal saline (sterile) may be used as an eye irrigant.

5. Check the neurological and vital signs as ordered. This may be on a 15- to 20-minute basis. Blood pressure, pulse, temperature (taken rectally), respirations and their pattern, pupillary reactions and eye movements, hand grasps, the level of consciousness, and response to pain, touch, and verbal commands are included in this assessment.

6. Note if the patient is alert and awake and if he is initiating appropriate responses regarding conversation directed to him. If the patient does not regain consciousness after surgery, the neurosurgeon must evaluate:

a. The nature and location of the lesion that is producing the cerebral depression.

b. The degree to which this process is worsening.

c. The factors or mechanisms that are producing depression of cerebral functions.

7. Orientation to time, place, and person is also determined through purposeful conversation and not that of posing the same questions to the patient over and over again. This may be humiliating and even embarrassing to him during this phase.

8. Ask the patient if he has a headache. Determine its severity, duration, and location.

9. Pain medication must be judiciously administered, but enough given to relieve distressful subjective reactions. (Codeine is usually the analgesic of choice postoperatively.)

10. Note whether the patient is restless, agitated, or uncooperative when stimulated. This may be indicative of cerebral edema or a concurrent respiratory problem during this period. The patient may appear to be in a sleeplike state; this, however, is not comparable to normal sleep and the person may be less responsive to questions, act drowsy, and be lethargic. The *medical management of cerebral edema* involves several steps. It is important to:

a. Prevent further brain damage from hypoxia; promote and provide for an adequate airway. The use of a respirator may be indicated after intubation of the patient.

b. Monitor arterial blood gases to assess the degree of gaseous exchange and the acid/base balance of the body.

c. Correct electrolyte imbalances (on the basis of readings of the levels of blood electrolytes).

d. Administer osmotic diuretics and dehydrating agents (Mannitol and/or Urea); provide a Foley catheter in the urinary bladder so that an accurate record of output can be kept.

e. Use hypothermia to decrease cerebral blood flow and blood needs. (This is optional.)

f. Check for the presence of pulmonary edema whenever cerebral edema is treated aggressively with osmotic diuretics.

g. Remember that dehydrating agents are contraindicated in the patient with severe renal disease.

h. Administer a hygroscopic agent, such as Glycerol (50 per cent dextrose), via nasogastric tube for long-term therapy for cerebral edema. (This is not always necessary.)

i. Use steroids (if indicated) to treat cerebral edema secondary to hypoxia.

j. Sedate the patient with barbiturates.

k. Use the nasogastric tube to feed the patient a high-protein, high-calorie diet.

11. Intake and output measurements and recording should be quite accurate and done on time. The patient will usually be on fluid restriction. It is most important to include all sources of parenteral and oral fluids in this record. Output records should include amounts of drainage from sources other than urinary excretions, such as Levin-tube drainage, dressing drainage, and significant amounts of fluid suctioned from the respiratory tree. Intravenous fluids should be carefully regulated as to their flow rate and time in which certain fluids are to be absorbed by the patient. Marking the I.V. bottle with hours or time levels may be visually helpful to the personnel caring for the patient. Urine volumes may be tested for specific gravity if dehydration or overhydration is suspected.

12. Dressings marked with a special crayon or pen may designate, at the end of each shift or day (as the case may necessitate), the progression of drainage from the wound. Dressings are reinforced with sterile gauze and changed as a rule by the attending doctor.

13. Seizure precautions may be indicated for the patient. The nurse (in this instance) must remain at the bedside during a convulsion. Placing the patient with his head turned to the side and the chin pointed downward has the advantage of keeping the tongue forward, thus eliminating possible blockage of the pharynx during the seizure. Drainage of oral secretions at this time is also facilitated by this position. Use caution with mouth gags! They can serve as an object to block the airway when used in an overaggressive manner. A padded tongue blade or an oral airway is kept at the bedside. Suction apparatus and an Ambu bag should be close at hand to ensure adequate inspiration of air and oxygen when the need arises. When the seizure is occurring, observe the patient's whole body to determine where and what parts are involved in the attack. Note how the attack begins and how long it lasts. Note how it affects the level of consciousness, whether incontinence occurs during the seizure, and the over-all condition of the patient after the attack is over. Padded side rails should be on the bed for the safety of the patient. The medical treatment for seizures encompasses three principles. It is essential to:

    a. Provide adequate oxygenation with and through a patent airway.

    b. Administer tranquilizing drugs (e.g., Dilantin and Valium).

    c. Continue anticonvulsant drug therapy daily.

14. Humidified oxygen will be administered on order. Continuous flows or intermittent administration will depend on the overall condition of the patient.

15. The patient may be intubated with an endotracheal tube before (an elective) tracheostomy is performed. Tracheostomy is used for the patient who has been rendered stuporous by cerebral edema and is therefore not capable of normally exchanging respiratory gases. Establishment of an adequate airway will prevent future hypoxia and hypercapnia. Easy and quick aspiration of respiratory secretions can also be accomplished through this artificial respiratory route.

16. Chest physical therapy in the form of respiratory exercises (deep breathing, coughing, and manual massage of the regions over the lungs) can be a helpful adjunct to reduce the magnitude of possible postoperative pulmonary complications. Suctioning may be employed if the body temperature begins to rise to precarious levels. Generally, deep endotracheal suctioning will be performed by the doctor or by nurses certified to perform this procedure.

17. All extremities should be put through the range of motion periodically if the patient is not capable of these activities himself. This will help reduce the incidence of disuse atrophy and joint contractures that develop so rapidly in some patients.

18. Adequate and frequent oral hygiene at least every 2 hours is a necessity for comfort. Antiseptics may be ordered for the patient who has had an orobuccal reduction of zygoma.

19. A footboard at the bottom of the bed will serve a dual purpose — that of an exercise board and vertical support to keep the feet in the optimum position of function. This simple measure may serve to eliminate footdrop.

20. It is most important to report any significant changes immediately. The most important tasks of the nurse in the immediate postoperative period are

    a. to observe the patient astutely and

    b. to correctly interpret his behavior and all symptoms that she observes.

STUDY QUESTIONS

1. Review the incidence of head injuries incurred in automobile accidents.

2. What measures are indicated in the event that a person is admitted to the emergency room of your hospital with a moderate head injury?

3. What signs and symptoms are particularly dangerous in the case of a person who has suffered a moderate head injury? A severe head injury?

4. What are the signs and symptoms of increased intracranial pressure?

5. Review the facial bones and their relationship to the cranial bones.

6. What types of injuries in general are the bones and related structures of the face subject to in the event of a person receiving a head injury from some external source?

7. What are the various levels of consciousness?

8. How is the level of consciousness determined in an individual?

9. Review the neurological examination that is on a patient's chart.

10. What preoperative preparation must be done for the patient with a fracture of:
    a. The zygoma
    b. The maxillary antrum
    c. The frontal bone

11. What psychological preparation would you give to the person anticipating a craniotomy?

12. How might the doctor determine the extent of the patient's over-all injuries?

13. Review the set-up of the operating room in the event that a craniotomy is to be performed. What additional set-up is needed to enable the surgeon to reduce the patient's facial fractures?

14. Review the types of incisions that could be used in the surgery for:
    a. Orobuccal zygoma elevation.
    b. Frontal craniotomy.

15. What would be the patient's position for each type of procedure? Why?

16. What complications might happen after these procedures?

17. Devise a nursing care plan for:
    a. The preoperative care of a patient with a head injury.
    b. The postoperative care of the patient with a craniotomy and reduction of a fractured zygoma.

MISCELLANEOUS
PROCEDURES

79   INTRODUCTION

No surgical procedure is ever so distinct that it must be grouped apart from all others; however, many surgical procedures belong to areas too highly specialized for an introductory text such as this. In the latter regard, this book has not, for example, discussed reconstructive surgery, transplantation surgery, or surgery of the eye, ear, and nose. Nonetheless, certain procedures, though taken from special areas not otherwise covered in this book, are so commonly performed that it was thought necessary to include them in some section of the book; hence they appear here, with all due apologies to those specialists who perform them and hardly consider them "miscellaneous."

80   THE PATIENT WITH A FRACTURED RIGHT HIP

Operation: Nailing and Plating of Right Hip

TYPICAL HISTORY

A 75-year-old female was unable to rise following a fall suffered in her home on the day of admission. She enters the emergency room of the hospital with acute pain in the right hip and is unable to move her leg.

PHYSICAL EXAMINATION

An elderly female is admitted in acute distress.

Significant Findings

1. The right leg is foreshortened by 3 inches.
2. The right foot is abducted and externally rotated.
3. There is tenderness over the right hip joint.

DIAGNOSTIC STUDIES

Anteroposterior (A-P) and lateral x-rays of the pelvis and hips reveal the presence of an intertrochanteric fracture of the right hip.

PROBABLE HOSPITAL COURSE

It is imperative that the patient undergo surgery as soon as her general condition permits. Failure to appreciate the devastating effects of delayed fixation of a hip with the ensuing lengthy bed rest has often caused the death of elderly patients due to pneumonia, urinary tract infection, and pulmonary embolism.

As soon as the patient's general condition permits, she will be taken to the operating room for repair of her fractured hip. This is usually possible and desirable within 6 to 12 hours of admission.

PREPARATION FOR SURGERY

1. *Levin Tube.* Not necessary unless paralytic ileus has caused nausea, vomiting, or abdominal distention.
2. The patient is typed and cross-matched for four units of whole blood.
3. *Skin Prep.* This includes the entire right hip, the pubis, and the entire thigh.
4. *Enema.* A Fleet or soapsuds enema is given on the evening prior to surgery.
5. *Premedications.* Routine.
6. *Special Medications.* None.
7. A Foley catheter should be inserted in the preoperative period as the patients will either be incontinent or unable to void postoperatively.
8. *Operating Room Skin Prep.* This includes the entire right hip, the pubis, and the thigh down to the knee.
9. *Position.* Horizontal supine.

PATHOLOGY

Fractures of the hip are classified into those which pass just below the head of the femur (subcapital), those which pass through the neck of the femur, and those which pass through the greater and lesser trochanters (intertrochanteric fracture). The operative treatment of these various types of fractured hips differs, depending on the exact location of the fracture and the position of the parts. The indications for nailing and plating versus prosthetic replacement of the femoral head are described in any standard orthopedic textbook.

GENERAL RATIONALE AND SCHEME

The fractured hip in the elderly patient represents a potentially lethal problem. If bed rest is maintained until the patient is able to ambulate, he will almost surely die of pneumonia, urinary tract infection, or phlebitis with pulmonary embolism. Elderly patients do not tolerate prolonged bed rest. Consequently, in spite of their age and usually precarious general condition, they should be operated upon as soon as possible after admission to the hospital. The rationale of the operation is to pin or fix the hip in such a way that early ambulation will be possible.

Scheme

1. Incision is made in the lateral aspect of the thigh down to the fractured bone.
2. A long screw is driven into the fractured segment, pinning it to the neck and head of the femur in its normal socket (acetabulum).
3. A plate is now screwed into the femur and attached to the screw.
4. The skin incision is closed and a dressing applied.

PROCEDURE

1. *Skin Incision.* This is a lateral, vertical incision which extends from the region of the hip joint down the lateral aspect of the thigh.
2. The skin edges should be draped, but towel clips should not be used as these will interfere with the radiography which must be done during the operative procedure.
3. The fascia of the thigh is opened and numerous old blood clots are usually removed.
4. When the fracture sites are located, a long guide wire is driven through the fracture site into the neck and head of the femur. A second wire is also put in place, and A-P and lateral x-rays are taken. (The x-ray machine must be set up and positioned before the patient is draped.)
5. The surgeon awaits development of the x-ray films to determine whether or not the guide wire is properly positioned in the central canal of the neck of the femur and head. It may be that several x-rays must be taken after the guide wire is repositioned and this is done until proper positioning is obtained.
6. The surgeon now obtains the proper nail which passes over the shaft of the guide wire. This nail is driven through the fractured bone into the neck and head of the femur.
7. An appropriate plate is now obtained and screwed into the shaft of the femur. This plate has an adapting neck which fits over the hub of the nail and is screwed into place with a lock nut.
8. At the conclusion of the operative procedure, repeat A-P and lateral films are taken to be certain that positioning is correct.
9. Fascia and muscles are now closed with interrupted or running chromic catgut suture.
10. The skin is closed with interrupted silk or wire suture and a heavy dressing applied.

SURGICAL HAZARD

Rarely, the guide wire may be driven into the pelvis, where it may injure the urinary bladder.

POSTOPERATIVE MANAGEMENT

The patient is taken to the recovery room until sufficiently reactive from the anesthetic. The usual postanesthetic management is carried out. In addition:

1. The Foley catheter is connected to dependent drainage and managed in the usual fashion.

2. The patient frequently develops postoperative pneumonia. Consequently, all efforts must be made to have the patient cough, breathe deeply, and turn from side to side.

3. Sandbags are used to support the extremity so that excessive motion does not occur in the early postoperative period. However, it would be most unusual for a patient to dislodge the nail and plate fixation of the hip.

4. Unless vascular insufficiency of the extremities exists, firm-fitting elastic stockings or Ace bandages should be applied to the lower extremities and leg exercises carried out. There is a high incidence of phlebitis in the elderly patient who has undergone fixation of a fractured hip.

5. Postoperative disorientation, restlessness, and confusion often afflict the elderly patient. While these usually pass in several days, the patient may pull off the dressing or pull out the Foley catheter during periods of restlessness. Consequently, if restlessness does develop, the patient should be given small doses of sedatives such as Sparine and should be restrained if excessively restless. Barbiturates should not be given to the elderly.

6. Intake and output should be charted carefully and intravenous fluids given to supplement any inadequate oral intake.

7. The surgeon may elect anticoagulation for his patient postoperatively; if so, the usual steps are taken.

STUDY QUESTIONS

1. Describe the various types of fractured hips and the appropriate surgical treatment for each.

2. What are the dangers of prolonged bed rest in the management of an elderly patient with a fractured hip?

3. Discuss the essential steps in the nailing and plating of a fractured hip. Can you list some of the orthopedic instruments used in this operative procedure?

4. What are the dangers of using barbiturates in the elderly postoperative patient?

5. It is desirable to operate on patients with fractured hips 6 to 12 hours after admission to the hospital. Is this policy maintained in your hospital? Discuss.

81

Operation: Excision of Pilonidal Cyst and Sinus

TYPICAL HISTORY

A 27-year-old male has noted a painful, tender, draining lump over the coccyx of several months duration. He denies any injury to this area and any previous surgery. He has been in excellent health otherwise.

PHYSICAL EXAMINATION

The patient is a well-developed, slightly obese, muscular male in no particular distress.

Significant Findings

1. There is an indurated tender area over the coccyx and two small fistulae from which can be expressed a small amount of pus.
2. The remainder of the physical examination is unremarkable.

DIAGNOSTIC STUDIES

There are no diagnostic studies used in evaluating this condition; diagnosis is determined by clinical examination.

PROBABLE HOSPITAL COURSE

The patient has a classic history for pilonidal cyst with fistulae; physical examination is confirmatory. Assuming that his general condition permits, he should undergo excision of this cyst and fistula.

PREPARATION FOR SURGERY

1. *Levin Tube.* Not necessary.
2. *Type and Cross-match for Blood.* Not necessary.

3. *Skin Prep.*   The entire lower back and coccygeal area are shaven on the evening prior to surgery. The prep should extend well into the buttock and perianal regions.

4. *Enema.*   A Fleet or soapsuds enema is given on the evening prior to surgery.

5. *Premedications.*   Routine.

6. *Special Medications.*   None.

7. *Operating Room Skin Prep.*   The entire lower back and coccygeal area are prepped in the usual fashion.

8. *Position.*   The Buie position.

PATHOLOGY

There is a good deal of controversy as to the exact etiology of pilonidal cyst and fistula. One school of thought considers this to be a congenital epidermal lining in the region of the coccyx containing small bits of hair which eventually irritate the local tissue and cause infection and formation of a fistula. The second school of thought believes that this is an acquired condition, possibly related to chronic trauma to the area such as occurs in horseback riding, falls on the coccyx, or sitting on the tip of the coccyx too frequently. At any rate, the cyst is usually filled with many hair shafts which cause irritation and finally purulence. The purulent material migrates to the surface where small fistulae eventually develop from which pus escapes.

GENERAL RATIONALE AND SCHEME

The entire cyst wall, which may have many finger-like projections, must be removed along with all the hair shafts to prevent recurrence of this disease.

Scheme

1. A small midline incision is made over the coccygeal area.
2. The entire cyst cavity, the hair shafts, and the purulent material are excised.
3. The skin edges are loosely closed or marsupialized.
4. A heavy dressing is applied.

PROCEDURE

1. *Skin Incision.*   This is a vertical incision extending along the lower back into the coccygeal region. Care is taken to avoid injuring the external musculature of the anus.

2. Skin flaps are dissected down to the presacral fascia.

3. The entire cystic cavity, containing hair shafts and debris, is removed.

4. The edges of the skin are curetted to remove any epidermal cells which may be lining this area.

5. The skin is loosely approximated in the midline with interrupted silk or wire sutures. The skin edges may also be marsupialized, that is, brought down and sutured to the presacral fascia so as to allow a small cleft for the escape of any inflammatory tissue postoperatively.

6. A heavy compression dressing is applied.

SURGICAL HAZARDS

Apart from injury to the external and internal sphincter muscles of the anus, which may result in fecal incontinence, there are no particular surgical hazards associated with the operation.

POSTOPERATIVE MANAGEMENT

The patient is returned to the recovery room until sufficiently reactive from the anesthetic. The usual postanesthetic management is carried out. In addition:

1. The surgeon is notified if the dressing soaks through.
2. The patient may be given a house diet as soon as he is alert.
3. The incision may be quite painful and narcotics in adequate doses should be administered.
4. Watch for acute urinary retention.

STUDY QUESTIONS

1. Discuss the etiology of the development of a pilonidal cyst and sinus.

2. Why is mere drainage of an infected cyst inadequate for the management of this condition?

3. Define the term pilonidal.

4. Define the terms cyst, sinus, fistula.

5. What is the Buie position?

6. Discuss the essential steps in excision of a pilonidal cyst and sinus.

7. Define the term *marsupialization*.

8. Discuss a nursing plan for the postoperative management of a patient who has undergone excision of a pilonidal cyst and sinus.

THE PATIENT WITH HEMORRHOIDS

82

Operation: Hemorrhoidectomy

TYPICAL HISTORY

A 38-year-old male has noted the presence of rectal bleeding and pruritus for 1 year. The bleeding is bright red and occurs after straining at stool. He denies any abdominal cramps, weight loss, or anorexia. Approximately 6 months prior to admission he was given a course of stool softeners and anal suppositories but had no relief. He now enters for surgical excision of his hemorrhoids.

PHYSICAL EXAMINATION

The patient is a well-developed, well-nourished male in no acute distress.

Significant Findings

1. Large, edematous internal and external hemorrhoids are noted with marked excoriation of the surrounding anus.
2. Remainder of physical examination is normal.

DIAGNOSTIC STUDIES

1. Sigmoidoscopy is negative except for the hemorrhoids.
2. Barium enema is unremarkable.

PROBABLE HOSPITAL COURSE

Rectal bleeding must never be assumed to be caused by hemorrhoids only. The surgeon must perform sigmoidoscopy and perform a barium enema to rule out more significant causes of rectal bleeding. If these examinations fail to reveal other conditions, the patient is taken to the operating room for hemorrhoidectomy.

PREPARATION FOR SURGERY

1. *Levin Tube.* Not necessary.
2. Typing of blood is not necessary.

3. *Enema.*   A Fleet or soapsuds enema is given on the evening prior to surgery.

4. *Laxatives.*   Some surgeons prefer to give a mild laxative or stool softener prior to surgery to assure a more comfortable first bowel movement postoperatively.

5. *Skin Prep.*   The anal and perianal areas should be cleanly shaven preoperatively. (See Introduction.)

6. *Premedications.*   Routine.

7. *Special Medications.*   None.

8. *Operating Room Skin Prep.*   Includes the anal, perianal, and perineal regions. (See Introduction.)

9. *Position.*   Lithotomy or reverse lithotomy position. (See Introduction.)

PATHOLOGY

Hemorrhoids consist of dilated and edematous anal veins. The basic cause of this condition is unknown. Precipitating factors include infection, the erect position, pregnancy, and constipation. Two forms of hemorrhoids are distinguished.

External Hemorrhoids.   These are found on the cutaneous side of the anal mucocutaneous junction. They are quite painful and pruritic because the nerve endings in the skin are pain receptors. They usually cause painful bowel movements.

Internal Hemorrhoids.   These are found on the mucosal side of the anal mucocutaneous junction. There are no pain fibers in this area and hence these hemorrhoids cause painless bleeding.

Most cases of hemorrhoids are of the *mixed variety.*

Thrombosis and edema of hemorrhoids often result in a certain degree of surrounding infection (proctitis). In addition, there is often excoriation and thickening of the anal surface due to the marked pruritus often associated with hemorrhoids.

GENERAL RATIONALE AND SCHEME

The majority of patients with hemorrhoids need not undergo surgery. The medical treatment of hemorrhoids includes the following measures:

1. Cortisone suppositories during the acute phase to relieve inflammation and edema.
2. Stool softeners to prevent constipation.
3. Plenty of liquids by mouth to prevent constipation.
4. Anal hygiene, which should include use of Sitz baths daily, as well as gentle soap and water cleansing after each bowel movement.

Indications for hemorrhoidectomy include:

1. Persistent bleeding.
2. Intractable pruritus or anal pain.
3. Associated anal edema and prolapse unrelieved with medical therapy.

Scheme

1. The anus is dilated.
2. Each hemorrhoid is ligated at its base and excised.
3. The mucosal defect is sutured.
4. A compression dressing is applied.

PROCEDURE

1. The patient is placed in the reverse lithotomy position. The anus is dilated to three or four fingers.
2. Any fecal debris remaining is gently cleansed with a Zephiran-soaked sponge.
3. Anal retractors are used to dilate the rectum, exposing the hemorrhoidal groups (often three groups of hemorrhoids are noted).
4. The hemorrhoidal pedicle is grasped and ligated with sutures.
5. The mucosa overlying the hemorrhoid is incised in a V-shaped incision.
6. The hemorrhoid is excised.
7. The mucosal defect is closed with a running suture.
8. The procedure is repeated for the remaining hemorrhoids.
9. A small compression or petrolatum dressing is left in place.

SURGICAL HAZARD

Damage to the internal anal sphincters is a rare hazard but, when it occurs, it may result in a certain degree of fecal incontinence postoperatively.

POSTOPERATIVE MANAGEMENT

The patient is returned to the recovery room until sufficiently reactive from the anesthetic. If spinal anesthesia is used, he may be returned to his room immediately.

1. The dressing should be checked every 2 hours for undue bleeding.
2. If urinary distention occurs, catheterization may be required but only after all conservative means of encouraging voiding have been tried.
3. The patient is given narcotics in sufficient doses for control of pain.

STUDY QUESTIONS

1. Is the medical therapy of hemorrhoids often successful? Discuss in your class.

2. Define fissure in ano and fistula in ano. Is there any relationship between hemorrhoids and these two illnesses?

3. What are the anal crypts and where are they located? Are they in any way associated with hemorrhoids?

4. Describe the essential steps in hemorrhoidectomy.

5. Describe a nursing plan for the postoperative management of a patient who has undergone hemorrhoidectomy.

Operation: Excision of Ganglion

TYPICAL HISTORY

A 23-year-old female noted the onset of tenderness over the wrist in the area of the radial pulse on the right hand. This tenderness developed about 6 months prior to admission and now there is a small tender swelling over the radial pulse which is aggravated at night and when the patient moves the extremity. She denies any previous difficulty with this wrist.

PHYSICAL EXAMINATION

The patient is a well-developed, well-nourished female in no distress.

Significant Findings

1. There is a small, cystic, tender swelling measuring 1 by 1 cm. overlying the right wrist just lateral to the radial pulse. This swelling seems to move on flexion and extension of the thumb.
2. The remainder of the physical examination is unremarkable.

DIAGNOSTIC STUDIES

An x-ray of the wrist may be done but, generally speaking, a ganglion is evident clinically and no other laboratory or x-ray studies are necessary.

PROBABLE HOSPITAL COURSE

As soon as the diagnosis has been established and provided the patient's general condition will tolerate it, she will be taken to the operating room for excision of the ganglion.

PREPARATION FOR SURGERY

1. *Levin Tube.* Not necessary.
2. *Type and Cross-Match of Blood.* Not necessary.
3. *Skin Prep.* The hand, the wrist, and the forearm are prepped in the usual fashion.

4. *Enema.*   Not necessary.

5. *Premedications.*   Routine.

6. *Special Medications.*   None.

7. *Operating Room Skin Prep.*   This should begin in the midforearm and include the entire hand.

8. *Position.*   Horizontal supine with the hand extended.

PATHOLOGY

The ganglion is an extremely common cystic tumor of the hand. It is felt by some surgeons to result from chronic trauma such as occurs in pianists or typists. Others feel there is no evidence to support this theory. Microscopically, the ganglion appears to arise from a tendon sheath or a joint capsule. It consists of a large cystic mass, formed of many separate smaller cysts, each of which contains gelatinous material. Because of its origin deep within the tendon sheath or the joint capsule, the operative procedure is much more extensive than the surface lesion would suggest and consequently it should be done under general or regional block anesthesia.

GENERAL RATIONALE AND SCHEME

Ganglial cysts tend to enlarge with time and to cause progressively greater pain disability to the extremity. Consequently, once diagnosed, the lesion should be excised. Failure to excise the entire lining of the cyst will result in early recurrence. The lesion must be removed completely down to the joint or tendon sheath.

Scheme

1. A small incision is made overlying the cyst which should not be damaged in any way.

2. The cyst is removed down to its attachment to the joint capsule or the tendon.

3. The attachment to the joint capsule or the tendon should be scraped carefully with a periosteal elevator.

4. The skin incision is closed.

PROCEDURE

1. *Skin Incision.*   This is a small incision, often elliptical, sometimes linear, overlying the cystic lesion.

2. Careful subcutaneous dissection is carried out around the entire cyst wall without injuring or perforating the cyst itself. Should the cyst be perforated, gelatinous material would be exuded immediately and the cyst wall would collapse so that it would be extremely difficult to remove the entire cyst.

3. The dissection is carried down to the cystic attachment to the joint capsule or the tendon sheath. This attachment should be carefully excised or scraped with a periosteal elevator to be certain all ganglion cells are removed. Because of this need for meticulous and deep dissection, many surgeons prefer to perform the operation using a pneumatic compression tourniquet.

4. Following excision of the ganglion, the skin is loosely approximated with interrupted Dermalon or Nylon sutures.

5. A small compression dressing is applied.

SURGICAL HAZARDS

1. Injury to the adjacent radial artery sometimes occurs.
2. Injury to nearby extensor tendons to the thumb must be avoided.

IMMEDIATE POSTOPERATIVE MANAGEMENT

The patient is returned to the recovery room until sufficiently reactive from the anesthetic. The usual postanesthesia management is carried out. In addition:
1. The hand is elevated on two pillows.
2. Circulation of the extremity is checked every 2 hours.
3. Liquids to solid diet is allowed as soon as the patient has reacted from his anesthetic.

STUDY QUESTIONS

1. What are some of the common locations for ganglia?

2. What other lesions of the hands may be mistaken for ganglia and what is the treatment of each?

3. Is there any other treatment for ganglia besides surgical excision?

4. Why is there such a high recurrence rate for ganglia?

5. What disabilities may result from failure to excise a ganglion?

Recommended Reading

A good study program begins with the stimulus provided by the individual case under consideration. *The Patient in Surgery* acts as a guide or an outline, and its chapter format suggests many component parts that may be investigated in depth by the student through a proper use of the medical library.

As an illustration, consider the patient with a *perforated ulcer.* The *typical history,* briefly outlined in this book, could lead the student to a full investigation of ulcer symptomatology. The student may wish to obtain an overview of this problem by consulting one of several textbooks on ulcer disease. Perhaps the student finds one aspect of the symptom complex — for example, the relationship of food intake to ulcer pain — intriguing. The various reference indices of the library can be consulted and a fully up-to-date bibliography obtained. The medical librarian can be an invaluable resource to the student who wishes to pursue a certain lead in greater detail. The best set of references is, after all, the one developed by the student. Any catalogue of journal articles and the like that we could provide (at the end of each chapter, as in previous editions) would lose its pertinency all too quickly. Accordingly, we have elected instead to compile a list of references that will lay the groundwork for more intensive investigations. This list includes general texts that have gained wide acceptance for their value as references, journals that have come to be used by many professionals in different aspects of medicine and surgery, and indices that will point the student to other sources of information. Remember: a familiarity with the efficient and intelligent use of the *entire* medical library is the key to further self-education.

GENERAL TEXTBOOKS OF SPECIAL VALUE IN SURGICAL NURSING

Abdominal and Pelvic Surgery

Artz, Curtis P., and Hardy, James D. *Complications in Surgery and Their Management.* Philadelphia: W. B. Saunders Company, 1975.

Bendixon, H. H., et al. *Respiratory Care.* St. Louis: C. V. Mosby Co., 1965.

Committee on Trauma, American College of Surgeons. *Early Care of the Injured Patient.* Philadelphia: W. B. Saunders Company, 1972.

Condon, Robert E., and Nyhus, Lloyd M. *Manual of Surgical Therapeutics.* Boston: Little, Brown and Co., 1969.

Conn, Howard F., ed. *Current Therapy 1974.* Philadelphia: W. B. Saunders Co., 1974.
Flint, Thomas, and Cain, Harvey D. *Emergency Treatment and Management.* 4th edition. Philadelphia: W. B. Saunders Company, 1970.
Hill II, George J., ed. *Outpatient Surgery.* Philadelphia: W. B. Saunders Company, 1973.
Kinney, John M., Egdahl, Richard H., and Zuidema, George D. eds. *Manual of Preoperative and Postoperative Care.* Philadelphia: W. B. Saunders Company, 1971.
Moore, Francis D. *Metabolic Care of the Surgical Patient.* Philadelphia: W. B. Saunders Company, 1959.
Sabiston, David C. ed. *Davis-Christopher Textbook of Surgery: The Biological Basis of Modern Surgical Practice.* 10th edition. Philadelphia: W. B. Saunders Company, 1972.
Thorek, Philip. *An Atlas of Surgical Techniques.* Philadelphia: J. B. Lippincott Co., 1970.

Vascular Surgery

Abrams, Herbert L., ed. *Angiography.* Boston: Little, Brown and Co., 1961
Fairbain II, John F., Juergens, John L., and Spittell, Jr., John A., eds. *Allen-Barker-Hines Peripheral Vascular Diseases.* 4th edition. Philadelphia: W. B. Saunders Company, 1972.
Strandness, D. E. *Collateral Circulation in Clinical Surgery.* Philadelphia: W. B. Saunders Company, 1969.
Wesolowski, S.A., and Dennis, C., eds. *Fundamentals of Vascular Grafting.* New York: McGraw-Hill, 1963.
Winsor, T., and Hyman, C. *A Primer of Peripheral Vascular Diseases.* Philadelphia: Lea and Febiger, 1965.
Wylie, E. J., and Ehrenfeld, W. K. *Extracranial Occlusive Cerebrovascular Disease.* Philadelphia: W. B. Saunders Company, 1970.

Gynecological Surgery

Benson, Ralph C. *Handbook of Obstetrics and Gynecology.* Los Altos, California: Lange Medical Publications, 1971.
Kistner, Robert W. *Gynecology: Principles and Practices.* 2nd edition. Chicago: Year Book Medical Publishers, 1971.
Novak, E., Jones, G. S., and Jones, H. *Novak's Textbook of Gynecology.* 8th edition. Baltimore: The Williams and Wilkins Co., 1970.
Parsons, L., and Ulfelder, H. *An Atlas of Pelvic Operations.* 2nd edition. Philadelphia: W. B. Saunders Company, 1968.

Genitourinary Surgery

Aliapoulios, M. A., and Carroll, Janet. *The Patient in Intensive Care: A Guide for Nurses.* Philadelphia: W. B. Saunders Company, 1975.
Campbell, Meredith F., and Harrison, J. H., eds. *Urology.* 3rd edition. Philadelphia: W. B. Saunders Company, 1970.
Glenn, J. F., and Boyce, W. H., eds. *Urologic Surgery.* New York: Harper and Row, 1969.
Merrill, John P. *The Treatment of Renal Failure.* 2nd edition. New York: Grune & Stratton, 1965
Merrill, John P., and Hampers, Constantine L. *Uremia: Progress in Pathophysiology and Treatment.* New York: Grune & Stratton, 1971.
Winter, Chester C., and Roehm, Marilyn M. *Sawyer's Nursing Care of Patients with Urological Diseases.* St. Louis: C. V. Mosby Co., 1968.

Head and Neck Surgery

Loré, John M. *An Atlas of Head and Neck Surgery.* 2nd edition. Philadelphia: W. B. Saunders Company, 1973.

Breast Surgery

Ackerman, L. V., and del Regato, J. A. *Cancer: Diagnosis, Treatment, and Prognosis.* 4th edition. St. Louis: C. V. Mosby Co., 1970.

Bouchard, R., and Owens, N. F. *Nursing Care of the Cancer Patient.* St. Louis: C. V. Mosby Co., 1972.

Haagensen, C. D. *Diseases of the Breast.* Philadelphia: W. B. Saunders Company, 1971.

Moore, F. D., Woodrow, S. I., Aliapoulios, M. A., and Wilson, R. E. *Carcinoma of the Breast.* New England Journal of Medicine Medicare Progress Series. Boston: Little, Brown and Company, 1967, 1968.

Rubin, Philip, ed. *Carcinoma of the Breast.* New York: American Cancer Society.

Cardiothoracic Surgery

Behrendt, Douglas M., and Austen, Gerald W. *Patient Care in Cardiac Surgery.* Boston: Little, Brown and Company, 1972.

Blades, Brian. *Surgical Diseases of the Chest.* 2nd edition. St. Louis: C. V. Mosby Co., 1966.

Cohn, Lawrence H. *The Surgical Treatment of Acute Myocardial Ischemia.* Mount Kisco, New York: Futura Publishing Co., 1973.

Gibbon, J. H., Sabiston, D. C., and Spencer, F. C., eds. *Surgery of the Chest.* 2nd edition. Philadelphia: W. B. Saunders Company, 1969.

Hurst, J. Willis, and Logue, R. Bruce. *The Heart, Arteries, and Veins.* 3rd edition. New York: McGraw-Hill, 1974.

Norman, John C., ed. *Cardiac Surgery.* New York: Appleton-Century Crofts, 1967.

Peirce, E. C. *Extracorporeal Circulation for Open-heart Surgery.* Springfield, Illinois: Charles C Thomas, 1969.

Phillips, R. E., and Feeney, M. K. *The Cardiac Rhythms.* Philadelphia: W. B. Saunders Company, 1973.

Powers, Maryann, and Storlie, Frances. *The Cardiac Surgical Patient.* New York: The Macmillan Co., 1969.

Sanderson, Richard G., ed. *The Cardiac Patient.* Saunders Monograph In Clinical Nursing #2. Philadelphia: W. B. Saunders Company, 1972.

Neurological Surgery

Carini, Esta, and Owens, Guy. *Neurological and Neurosurgical Nursing.* 5th edition. St. Louis: C. V. Mosby Co., 1970.

Davis, Loyal and Davis, Richard. *Principles of Neurological Surgery.* Philadelphia: W. B. Saunders Co., 1963.

Elliott, Frank A. *Clinical Neurology.* 2nd edition. Philadelphia: W. B. Saunders Co., 1971.

Horwitz, N. H., and Rizzoli, H. V. *Post-operative Complications in Neurosurgical Practice.* Baltimore: The Williams and Wilkins Co., 1967.

Jennet, W. B. *An Introduction to Neurosurgery.* Springfield, Illinois: Charles C. Thomas, 1964.

Kahn, Edgar A., et al. *Correlative Neurosurgery.* 2nd edition. Springfield, Illinois: Charles C Thomas, 1969.

Plum, F., and Posner, J. eds. *Diagnosis of Stupor and Coma.* Philadelphia: F. A. Davis Co., 1972.

Youmans, Julian, ed. *Neurological Surgery.* Philadelphia: W. B. Saunders Company, 1973.

STANDARD SURGICAL JOURNALS

Anesthesiology

Anesthesia (quarterly)

Cardiology

Circulation (monthly)
Progress in Cardiovascular Diseases (bimonthly)

Gastroenterology

American Journal of Digestive Diseases (monthly)
Diseases of the Colon and Rectum (bimonthly)

Gynecology and Obstetrics

American Journal of Obstetrics and Gynecology (semimonthly)

Neurology

Journal of Neurosurgery (monthly)
Journal of Neurosurgical Nursing

Nursing

American Journal of Nursing (monthly)
Nursing Clinics of North America (quarterly)
Nursing Forum (quarterly)
Heart and Lung Journal

Orthopedics

Journal of Bone and Joint Surgery (eight issues per year)

Surgery

American Journal of Surgery (monthly)
Annals of Surgery (monthly)
Annals of Thoracic Surgery (monthly)
Archives of Surgery (monthly)
British Journal of Surgery (monthly)
Journal of Thoracic and Cardiovascular Surgery (monthly)
Journal of Trauma (monthly)
Plastic and Reconstructive Surgery (monthly)
Surgery (monthly)
Surgery, Gynecology, and Obstetrics (monthly)
Surgical Clinics of North America (bimonthly)

Tumors

Cancer (monthly)

Urology

Investigative Urology (bimonthly)
Journal of Urology (monthly)

REFERENCE INDICES

Abridged Index Medicus
Cumulated Index Medicus

Cumulated Index to Nursing Literature
International Nursing Index

SPECIAL NURSING LITERATURE

Ballinger, Walter F., et al. *Alexander's Care of the Patient in Surgery.* 5th edition. St. Louis: C. V. Mosby Co., 1972.

Berry, E. C., and Kohn, M. L. *Introduction to Operating-Room Technique.* 4th edition. New York: McGraw-Hill, 1972.

Burrell, Z. L., and Burrell, L. O. *Intensive Nursing Care.* 2nd edition. St. Louis: C. V. Mosby Co., 1973.

Carini, Esta, and Owens, Guy. *Neurological and Neurosurgical Nursing.* 5th edition. St. Louis: C. V. Mosby Co., 1970.

Given, Barbara A., and Simmons, Sandra J. *Nursing Care of the Patient with Gastrointestinal Disorders.* St. Louis: C. V. Mosby Co., 1971.

Luckman, J., and Sorenson, K. C. *Textbook of Medical-Surgical Nursing.* Philadelphia: W. B. Saunders Company, 1974.

Shafer, K. N., et al. *Medical-Surgical Nursing.* 5th edition. St. Louis: C. V. Mosby Co., 1971.

Watson, J. W. *Medical-Surgical Nursing and Related Physiology.* Philadelphia: W. B. Saunders Company, 1972.

Winter, C. C., and Roehm, M. M. *Nursing Care of Patients with Urologic Diseases.* 3rd edition. St. Louis: C. V. Mosby Co., 1972.

Index